THE MEASUREMENT OF HEARING

McGRAW-HILL SERIES IN PSYCHOLOGY

HARRY F. HARLOW, *Consulting Editor*

John F. Dashiell was Consulting Editor of this series from its inception in 1931 until January 1, 1950. Clifford T. Morgan was Consulting Editor of this series from January 1, 1950 until January 1, 1959.

THE MEASUREMENT
OF HEARING

IRA J. HIRSH, *Central Institute for the Deaf
and Washington University, St. Louis, Missouri; formerly
Research Fellow, Psycho-Acoustic Laboratory, Harvard University*

McGRAW-HILL BOOK COMPANY, INC.

1952   NEW YORK   TORONTO   LONDON

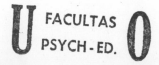

U FACULTAS
PSYCH-ED. O

THE MEASUREMENT OF HEARING

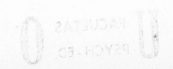

FOREWORD

In 1929 the National Research Council sponsored a conference on "Problems of the Deaf and Hard of Hearing." This conference prepared a series of research recommendations in various areas. One of the areas was "Problems of Sensory Stimulation," and one of the classes of sensory problems was the measurement of the degree and type of impairment of hearing. It is worth quoting from these recommendations of the conference of twenty-two years ago.

Improvement and standardization of methods of acoumetry [audiometry] are necessary. The widely varying results of different surveys made with the same instrument indicate clearly that the psychological factors of the approach to the individual and the method of eliciting his response are of vital importance. The psychological laboratories with their highly developed methods of threshold determination should make a contribution here.

In spite of this appeal there has been little direct contribution from experimental psychology to the art and method of audiometry during the last twenty-two years. A partial approach is seen in the adoption of a series of normal standards for auditory sensitivity, which serve as the base from which we reckon hearing loss and which were accepted by the Consultants on Audiometers and Hearing Aids of the Council on Physical Medicine and Rehabilitation of the American Medical Association. Incidentally, the normal values were based in part on the very surveys mentioned by the National Research Council's conference. Also, a set of rules for the manipulation of the audiometer was adopted, but again these rules were influenced far more by the practical experience of users of audiometers than by the "highly developed methods of threshold determination of the psychological laboratories." There was, and unfortunately still is, a wide cleavage between clinical audiometry and psychophysical experimentation. The rules were a step in advance, but they have been more often honored in the breach than in the observance.

In 1946 a new Committee on Hearing was established under the Division of Medical Sciences of the National Research Council. The membership of that committee was chosen to include otologists, psychologists, and electroacoustic engineers in order to help bridge the gap between them. At the very first meeting of this committee the question of the validity of the standards of normal sensitivity was raised, and the desirability of reformulating and standardizing the methods of presentation of the auditory signals was reaffirmed. It was agreed that this reformulation, taking advantage of advances in instrumentation and in laboratory techniques, was a necessary preliminary to any correction of standards of normality.

It was further agreed that the first practical step toward reformulation should be the preparation, by someone thoroughly trained and experienced in the methods of psychophysics, of a summary of such methods and the fundamental principles on which they are based. The summary should be oriented to the problems of clinical measurements of hearing. It should enable the otologist to understand, talk, and think the language and the ideas of the psychological laboratory.

But who would undertake this task? Fortunately, at this time the idea occurred independently to one of the members of the staff of the Psycho-Acoustic Laboratory of Harvard University that the time was ripe for a book on the measurement of hearing. This book would summarize both the experimental work done in psychological laboratories during and after World War II and the advances in the clinical application of improved technical methods and instruments of audiometry. This man was Dr. Ira J. Hirsh. His objective was rather more ambitious, but it also included the objective sought by the Committee on Hearing.

The Committee on Hearing welcomed the opportunity offered by Dr. Hirsh's interest and encouraged him to proceed with the preparation of his book. Dr. Hirsh consulted with the members of the committee's panel on audiometry and submitted first the general outline of his book and then the manuscript, chapter by chapter, for comment and criticism. Dr. Hirsh's book therefore appears with the blessing of the Committee on Hearing and represents another step in the achievement of an objective laid down by the Conference on Problems of the Deaf and Hard of Hearing twenty-two years ago.

It is written frankly from the point of view of the experimental psychologist, but if it succeeds in bringing this point of view usefully and effectively to the otologist and the audiologist, it will be an important step forward. It may also serve to bring the important problems of clinical measurement of hearing more clearly and forcibly to the attention of other experimental psychologists. These are our hopes, and our hopes are high.

September, 1951

HALLOWELL DAVIS
Chairman, Committee on Hearing
National Research Council
Director of Research, Central Insti-
tute for the Deaf

PREFACE

THIS book is intended to be used as a reference by those who are engaged in measuring and treating disordered hearing and also as a textbook by those who are in training for such clinical work. It is also intended to be used by those students of psychology, physiology, and physics who have an interest in hearing.

Although another textbook on clinical audiometry might be welcomed in the clinical field, the author has felt that at the present time it would be more important and useful for both clinical and experimental workers if the contributions to audiometry of various experimental disciplines were brought together in a single volume. He has attempted to summarize those experimental areas that appear to be basic to both the clinical and experimental measurement of various aspects of hearing.

Anatomy and physiology are not treated in this book, not because they are unimportant for the measurement of hearing, but because they are extensively treated in other contemporary books. Furthermore, psychophysical measurement may be treated more rigorously when we consider that such measurement can be made when only a physical stimulus at the input and a behavioral response at the output are known. There are many instances in the text, however, where references are made to anatomical structures in connection with certain diagnostic problems. It is assumed that the reader comes to this book with at least some knowledge of the anatomy and physiology of the auditory system.

The measurement of hearing cannot be discussed without some mathematical tools. In concrete terms, at least a year of college algebra and some elementary trigonometry are assumed. In addition, some acquaintance with statistical concepts would be extremely helpful.

The treatment of such a large area as the measurement of hearing will depend, of course, upon the knowledge and biases of the author. In the present case, the author's biases lean heavily toward the contribution of experimental psychology to the field of hearing. His treatment of the subject matter has been greatly influenced and aided by his colleagues at the Psycho-Acoustic Laboratory and the Department of Psychology at Harvard University.

The book was written during part of the time that the author was a research fellow at the Psycho-Acoustic Laboratory. He was permitted, for about two years, to devote a large share of his time to the preparation of this book. It is published as report PNR-118, under contract N5ori-76 between Harvard University and the Office of Naval Research, and reproduction by the United States Government for its own use is permitted. It is a pleasure to thank the Office of Naval Research and the Director of the Psycho-Acoustic Laboratory, Prof. S. S. Stevens, for providing the time and substantial facilities for the writing and preparation of the manuscript.

Much help has been received from the panel on audiometry of the National Research Council's Committee on Hearing. The members of this panel, Drs. E. P. Fowler, Jr., J. C. Steinberg, and H. Davis, Chairman, have encouraged and criticized the manuscript as it developed. Professor Davis, in particular, has been extremely generous in offering many suggestions and corrections on the whole manuscript.

This book has developed from a series of lectures in a seminar on the measurement of hearing that was held at the Massachusetts Eye and Ear Infirmary. Drs. D. K. Lewis, M. H. Lurie, P. E. Meltzer, and F. L. Weille of the Infirmary, P. W. Johnston of the Massachusetts Department of Public Health, and other members of the seminar forced much of the difficult material into readable form.

There are some specific debts that are gratefully acknowledged. Professor E. G. Boring, Harvard University, read and criticized Chap. 1. Professor G. A. Miller, then at Harvard University, helped with the rewriting of Chaps. 5 and 7. W. A. Rosenblith, then at Harvard University, contributed greatly to the author's and the reader's knowledge of electroacoustics by almost rewriting Chaps. 2 and 3. Professors B. F. Skinner, Harvard University, and W. G. Hardy, The Johns Hopkins University, read and suggested valuable changes in Chap. 10. Dr. S. R. Silverman, Central Institute for the Deaf, has offered many valuable suggestions, especially in Chap. 11. The wisdom of these helpful colleagues was not always heeded, and undoubtedly faults still remain.

Katherine James Miller typed almost the entire manuscript through several drafts and served as a stubborn editor of the author's use of the English language. This acknowledgment is only a poor recognition of the tremendous work that she has done.

It is a pleasure to thank the authors, editors, and publishers of those journals and books from which figures have been taken with their permission. The details are to be found in the references for each figure, which are given in the bibliography.

Without the encouragement and critical assistance of my wife, Shirley Kyle Hirsh, this book would not have been completed.

St. Louis, Missouri   IRA J. HIRSH
June, 1952

CONTENTS

INTRODUCTION

THE measurement of hearing is of interest to several professional groups. In *otology*, that branch of clinical medicine that has to do with the ear, one is interested in measuring or testing the hearing in so far as this helps in the detection, diagnosis, and correction of diseases of the ear. Indeed, the otologists, or their less specialized ancestors, were probably the first historically to examine hearing in any systematic way. For not so long a time, a second professional group, recently known as *audiologists*, has been concerned with the testing of hearing and the rehabilitation of the deafened. Audiologists have been engaged in developing more and finer tests because their main interest is centered not on the ear, but rather on all the complex facets of the hearing itself. Where surgery or medicine cannot help, the audiologist operates on the hearing directly, first testing and determining various auditory capacities and then training, recommending hearing aids, and helping with the psychological adjustment of his patients. Third, certain groups in *psychology*, *physiology*, and *physics* are interested in measuring hearing as a means of finding out more about how the ear and the whole auditory system works. Furthermore, certain engineers, responsible for designing equipment that is to serve the auditory system (*e.g.*, radios, phonographs, communications equipment, etc.), must be able to measure certain aspects of hearing in order to evaluate the systems they design.

The purposes for which these various groups of people use hearing tests differ according to the specific professional interest. But there is a basic core of information on method and equipment that underlies auditory measurement in all these applications. The otologists and the audiologists are interested in clinical measurement; that is, they wish to know about the difference between the auditory capacities of a patient and those of a normal person. The experimental workers, on the other hand, are interested in describing the auditory capacities of the normal person in order to make generalizations about the normal or average auditory system. Indeed, we find at least two parallel developments in the history of the measurement of hearing: one in the clinical fields of otology and what is now called audiology and the second in the fields of experimental psychology and physiology.

Too often, in recent history, these fields have remained apart, and each has suffered to a certain extent from lack of knowledge of the other. But this divergence is relatively new. Experimental psychologists claim such men as E. H. Weber and Urbantschitsch in the history of their science. But these men were good practicing otologists. Weber not only contributed to psychophysics but also gave otology one of its fundamental tuning-fork tests. Not only did Urbantschitsch carry out important psychophysical experiments; he also was a stout proponent of educational methods for treating his deaf and hard-of-hearing patients.

One of the main purposes of this book is to relate the clinical and experimental fields. This relation is not always possible to establish, because, on the one hand, certain experimental findings have no obvious application in clinical practice, and, on the other hand, certain clinical measurements that have been useful to the experienced clinician may not have been examined in the laboratory. We shall attempt, however, to draw as heavily as possible from the experimental fields in order to write of those principles and facts that are basic to procedures followed in clinical audiometry.

In order to review the various kinds of tests and measurements of hearing that can be made, we must first consider some basic notions, particularly those that have to do with the nature of psychophysical measurement—the measurement of responses and stimuli. Thus in Chap. 1, the development of psychophysics within experimental psychology is related to the present clinical and experimental kinds of audiometry. An attempt is made to show how psychophysical relations are established, what kinds of data are needed, and what kinds of results may be expected.

In Chap. 2, some physical characteristics of the auditory stimulus, sound, and also some basic notions in electricity are considered. This information seems to be necessary because the devices that are used to produce sounds in audiometric tests are rather complicated, and one can use them more intelligently if one knows something of the principles by which they operate. In Chap. 3, some of the principles of sound and electricity which were discussed in Chap. 2 are applied to some of the equipment ordinarily found in clinical practice.

The various types of auditory measurement are considered in Chaps. 4 through 9. Chapters 4 and 5 treat auditory measurements that are most directly related to diagnostic audiometry, namely, the measurement of hearing for pure tones and for speech. Chapters 6 and 7 treat the interrelated subjects of masking, fatigue, and differential sensitivity. Although we cannot say that these three auditory phenomena are now measured in everyday clinical practice, their importance for the theory of hearing and for possible diagnostic and prognostic information justifies their inclusion. Chapter 8 treats the distinction between psychological and physical dimensions and, as an example, considers methods for measuring loudness and its much discussed clinical relative, recruitment. In Chap. 9, the various aspects of hearing that were treated in Chaps. 4 through 8 are reviewed, and the difference, in respect of each of these, between binaural and monaural listening is discussed. As a special case of binaural hearing, the clinically important topic of bone conduction is presented.

A brief Chap. 10 represents an attempt to put the recently developed conditioning techniques of audiometry into the broader frame of reference that is provided by the principles of conditioning in psychology.

Most of the material in the first 10 chapters is drawn from psychophysical experiments. Most of it has been written with an attempt to form a fundamental core of experimental information on which clinical audiometry may be based. It would be difficult, however, for the reader of these first 10 chapters to make clinical audiometric measurements on the basis of this information alone. Rather, we have attempted only to provide him with some principles and criteria that should govern the techniques that he will use for solving various clinical problems.

In Chap. 11, however, an attempt has been made to apply some of the pertinent experimental information in a series of suggested procedures to be used in clinical audiometry. This last chapter is not meant to be a definitive rulebook for standardized audiometric practice. Rather, the procedures are suggested on the basis of implications from experimental results and, in a more limited way, from clinical experience that has been reported in the literature.

In the author's opinion, the first 10 chapters contain the more important information in the book. In these chapters are to be found the problems whose solution might make possible a better Chap. 11 or even a standard audiometric manual. Fortunately, we do not need to wait for all the experimental findings in order to carry out clinical testing programs, but we must not lose sight of the shortcomings of our present technique or of the limitations imposed on our interpretation of the test results.

CHAPTER 1

SENSATION AND MEASUREMENT

THE word *audiometry* has a short but strange history. It is derived from two Latin words, one of which means "to hear" and the other "to measure." *Audiometry* became widely used as a professional term only after the invention of the *audiometer*, an instrument designed to facilitate only one kind of measurement of hearing, namely, the absolute threshold for pure tones. We shall concern ourselves with audiometry in the larger sense that includes all kinds of auditory measurement: absolute thresholds, differential thresholds, hearing for speech, influence of noises, and even a little measurement of psychological dimensions such as loudness and pitch. Not only is this broader conception of audiometry useful for the experimenter interested in hearing, but also it is becoming increasingly clear that the clinician can make better and more complete diagnoses and recommendations for therapy on the basis of tests of hearing that involve measures other than those concerned with the minimum energy required for the detection of a pure tone.

Although the philosophy of psychophysics may have little practical value for the measurement of hearing, its development provides a good basis for understanding some of the foundations of present-day techniques of measurement. Furthermore, most of the specific experimental, metric, and statistical techniques used in audiometry have their origin in the works of the early psychophysicists.

Let us turn now to the development of psychophysics in the history of psychology.

The sense of hearing is one of five (or perhaps more) by which we receive information about the world around us. To get itself most adequately stimulated, each sense department seems to favor a certain kind of physical activity in the environment—sound, light, pressure, etc. The end product of our several sensory systems is the sensation—auditory, visual, tactual, olfactory, or gustatory. Each of us knows what a sensation is, because each of us has sensations. We know what we mean by the "reddishness" of a visual sensation, or the "loudness" of an auditory sensation, or the "sharpness" of a pain. It is difficult, however, for each of us to know about another person's sensations, because we cannot get inside his world of experience very easily. You and I may both say "red" when we see a particular object, but you cannot be sure that my impression of red is exactly the same as yours.

In this book we are going to talk about the measurement of hearing. Hearing is a kind of sensation. But we cannot observe the sensations of others, and we can only measure what we can observe. How then can we measure hearing?

THE MEANING OF MEASUREMENT

What kinds of events or things can we measure? The mathematician's formal definition of measurement tells us that we measure something whenever we assign numerals to things according to any specified rules (Stevens, 1951). These rules are always arbitrary and sometimes may be very simple. In other words, whenever we say that we are going to measure something, we mean merely that we are about to label something with numbers. For example, I may decide to assign numbers to the three chairs in my office. I may call the swivel chair "24," the straight chair "13," and the stool "6." But having done this, I have only named the chairs with numerals. The swivel chair is not *more* than the stool in any sense, because the *rule* for assigning the numerals was only a *naming* one.

If, however, you are told that the swivel chair weighs 24 lb, the straight chair 13 lb, and the stool 6 lb, then the rules by which the numbers have been assigned are specified in terms of formal properties that establish a relation between these measurements and others of weight. Furthermore, there are invoked relations among the numbers themselves that have been agreed upon by the makers of similar measurements. We learned about these rules when we were first exposed to arithmetic and algebra, but there is nothing sacred about them. The rule that 9 represents something greater than 8, or that 20 is twice as great as 10, or that in counting whenever we reach a multiple of 10 we add a number to the second column from the right and then begin over is arbitrary but generally agreed upon. The most precise measurement is made by assigning numerals in accordance with rules that are rigorously defined in arithmetic or algebra. If we use less rigorous rules, like simple naming, our measurements lose various degrees of meaningful information.

Sensations and Responses

Our definition of measurement tells us that we must assign numerals to events. Having determined the rules for assignment, we must now proceed to determine what are the observable events in hearing. Since we cannot observe the sensation that exists in another individual's world of experience, it would seem indeed that we cannot measure sensation. On the other hand, we can twist the meaning slightly and define the sensation in terms of events that we can measure. When a man says, "I see red," we cannot measure the redness of his visual sensation, nor even be sure that he has one, but we can observe his verbal behavior—"I see red." The phenomena of audition may be studied in the same way. We cannot measure auditory sensations that are private, but we can measure sensations that are defined in terms of behavior or observable responses.

The man who studies hearing—be he audiologist, psychologist, physiologist, otologist, physicist, or engineer—must know the capacities of the auditory system. He must know something about the smallest energies that he must present to the ear in order to observe a measurable response. He wants to know what are the highest and lowest frequencies to which the auditory system will respond. Beyond these so-called *absolute thresholds*, he may be interested in the smallest detectable change, whether the change be of frequency, of energy, or of any other physical dimension in which a change can be made. Then there are all the problems about interference, the effect of the presence of one signal on the detectability of another, the judgments of psychological magnitudes like *loudness* and *pitch*, and the intelligibility of spoken language. We define all these in terms of relations between measures of the physical stimulus and responses of the system that we are studying.

One worker may be interested in the over-all auditory system of man or animal, or he may be interested in only a small part of the auditory system, *e.g.*, the *middle ear* or parts of the *central nervous system*. In any case, the worker is faced with the problem of measuring the input-output characteristics of the system in which he is interested. That is to say, he must be able to put in some signal that is physically specifiable and then must provide himself with means for specifying the output of the system in terms of a measurable response.

The general procedures that he will use do not differ very much from those that the engineer uses in the measurement of similar characteristics of a radio or an engine. He does not need to know anything about what is inside the system but rather needs only to specify the input and be able to measure the output. The essential difference between measurements made on the auditory system and those made on a radio lies in the method of measuring the output. In the case of the radio, we measure both input and output with voltmeters and oscilloscopes. The output of the auditory system of a living organism, however, must be measured in terms of other, arbitrarily defined responses—responses that vary in a much more troublesome way than do the voltage responses of a radio or the horsepower responses of an engine. Responses of the over-all auditory system in man may be verbal, or the raising of a finger, or the pressing of a button. Study of a smaller part may involve only a relation between the stimulus and the kinetic response of an *ossicle* or the electrical response of the *cochlea*.

The measurement of hearing or of any sensory process involves the establishment of relations between the responses of individuals and the stimuli that give rise to such responses. It is generally agreed nowadays that we can measure—that is, assign numbers to, according to certain rules—both the dimensions of a physical stimulus that is presented to an observer and the responses of the observer. We can specify relations between two such measurable quantities, but we cannot, scientifically, make these relations extend to private sensations or events in the mind, because we cannot invent operations for getting at such events. The operational definition of the sensation has become the specification of a response.

Psychophysical Measurement

The measurement of observers' responses to measurable stimuli grew up in what is called *psychophysics*, the study of the relations between sensations and the stimuli that produce them. Psychophysics came into being during the middle of the nineteenth century when *experimental psychology* was first becoming experimental. Early investigators in this area were concerned with the study of the average, normal, adult human being. This study was statistical in the sense that investigations sought to describe an average person. Measurements obtained on different people yielded different results, and the main concern was with an average or some other representative measure of central tendency among the results for a particular group of observers.

Differences among people constituted a bother for the early psychophysicists. They would have preferred to throw away this variability or, better yet, to have none in a population where all persons were exactly equal to the average in all respects. Soon after the study of the psychophysics of the average man got under way, however, a group of psychologists broke off from the earlier traditions through an interest in individual differences. Whereas the early psychophysicists were interested in the *average* man and ignored the way in which real persons deviated from this average, the *differential psychologists* ignored the mean (average) almost completely and concentrated on the differences among people.

Today a similar difference exists between the man who seeks experimental results that describe a population of individuals and the clinically oriented worker who, like the differential psychologist, assumes the experimenter's average figure and focuses his interest on the amounts by which different individuals deviate from this average. An experimental average, for example, is incorporated in the audiometer, and the clinician uses the difference between the hearing of an individual and this average to obtain a measure of Hearing Loss. There are certain principles and operations that are basic to *both* the experimental and the clinical approaches to the measurement of hearing. One of the premises of this book is that the essential differences between experimental and clinical audiometry can be understood only after their common factors have become clear.

HISTORY

Philosophy is concerned with human knowledge. In particular, that part of early philosophy that was known as psychology was concerned with how the human mind acquires knowledge. We find explicit in the writings of philosophers from Aristotle[1] through the British empiricists of the nineteenth century the notion that knowledge comes to the mind by way of the senses. This empirical view of the source of human knowledge fostered, in the early philosophical psychologists, a great interest in sensation and the sensory mechanisms.

In the early part of the nineteenth century, things were happening in physiology that were to set the stage for rapid advances in the psychology and physiology of sensation. Early in the nineteenth century Sir Charles Bell and François Magendie discovered that the ventral and dorsal roots of the spinal cord had different functions; the ventral roots served motor functions, while the dorsal roots had to do with sensory functions. This discovery made possible a physiology of sensation that commanded the interest of many important physiologists of the day.

One of them, Johannes Müller, was responsible for the *doctrine of specific nerve energies*, the notion that the kind or nature of a sensation (*e.g.*, visual, auditory, tactual, etc.) is determined by the specific nerve fibers that are stimulated. No matter how the auditory nerve is stimulated, the stimulation gives rise to an auditory sensation. This theory seemed to Helmholtz to be no more valid for the whole system than for parts—*e.g.*, vision and audition. He held not only that auditory nerve fibers were responsible for auditory experience, but also that the quality of a given auditory sensation depended on which of the auditory fibers were stimulated. If we could find the fibers for red in the optic nerve, then no matter how we might stimulate them, a visual sensation of red would be produced.

---

[1] No references will be found in the bibliography for most of the names in this section on History. For original sources, the reader is referred to Boring.

Still another discovery in nineteenth-century physiology was to have a profound effect on the philosophy or psychology of sensation. In 1850, Helmholtz measured the velocity of transmission of the electrical impulse in a nerve. Although the details need not concern us here, we must note that the measured velocity was not that of light but one of a much lower order of magnitude. It was barely conceivable at that time that a measurable amount of time intervened between the occurrence of a stimulus and the experienced sensation. It was humiliating to think that first you willed to move your finger and then, only after the message got to the finger, the finger moved. The worlds of sensation and stimulus were distinctly separate, at least in time.

By the middle of the nineteenth century, then, the way had been opened for experiments on the physiology of sensation. But what about the philosophical psychologists? How far had they come on the problems of sensation and the sensory mechanisms? The thinking of this period was dominated by a dualism that had been made explicit by Descartes in 1650. There were the mind and the body. The brain, that part of the body that had most to do with the mind, interacted with the mind. This notion of interaction was changed by succeeding writers, but the dualism remained. The doctrine that the mind and body are parallel in their respective processes was made explicit by Leibnitz and by Hartley, the British philosopher. It was this parallelism between the experienced world and processes in the body, presumably in the nervous system, that led G. T. Fechner to seek a mathematical expression that would unite the two realms.

Fechner, the physicist, could measure the stimulus. Aware of the difficulty of measuring introspected sensations, he began to measure responses, and, by relating responses to physical changes, he hoped to attach meaningful numbers to sensory qualities. Actually Fechner was concerned with two kinds of relations. First, there was the relation between events in the physical world and the processes of the nervous and sensory systems. Second, there was the relation between these nervous processes and events in the psychological or experienced world. Apparently the physiological processes were assumed to be closely related to those of the physical world, so that the main problem was to establish a relation between experience and the physical world. Specifically, Fechner presented a scheme in his *Elemente der Psychophysik* (1860) whereby the magnitude of a sensation could be computed from objective measurements of physical stimuli and responses. Stimuli and responses could be measured directly, whereas the sensations could not.

The foundation of Fechner's science was what we now know as *Weber's*

Law. E. H. Weber had observed (1834) that in order for a stimulus to appear just noticeably different from a preceding stimulus, the necessary increment had always to be a constant fraction of the original stimulus. Let us consider an example.

Suppose we have a weight resting on an observer's hand. We want to find out how much we must add to that weight in order that the observer will just be able to notice that the weight is different. The *just noticeable difference,* or *jnd,* is a difference that is noticed 50 per cent of the time. According to Weber's Law, the amount of increase divided by the weight that was increased should yield a constant ratio. If we have a weight of 30 oz to begin with and if we find that we must add just 1 oz for our observer to just notice the difference, then to a weight of 30 half-ounces (15 ounces) we should have to add only 1 half-ounce. Also, to a weight of 30 dr we should have to add 1 dr. The constant ratio for weights would be, then, 1:30.

FECHNER'S LAW AND SENSORY MAGNITUDE

Fechner reasoned that if one were to count up just noticeable differences from the absolute threshold on upwards, one would actually be counting up equal sensory units along a psychological scale. Cumulating, for example, successive thirtieths of weight units, beginning with the smallest weight that could just be felt, one would obtain successive sensory units along the psychological scale of "weightiness." One pound does not necessarily seem to be twice as "weighty" as ½ lb, but a weight 20 jnd's above threshold would feel twice as "weighty" as a weight 10 jnd's above threshold.

We probably do not need to mention the tremendous impact made on psychology and physiology by Fechner's Law. The mathematical transposition that is involved in going from Weber's Law to Fechner's Law led to the notion—which subsequently became general—that the responses of human organisms to stimuli vary as the logarithms of those stimuli. Weber's Law stated that a just noticeable difference in any stimulus dimension was obtained from constant increments in the stimulus when those increments were expressed as ratios of the magnitude of change to the absolute magnitude from which the change was made.

$$\frac{\Delta I}{I} = K \text{ (for a jnd)}$$

Fechner now proposed that we cumulate such just noticeable differences to calculate a sensory magnitude. Hence a sensory magnitude could be measured by counting up measurable $\Delta I/I$'s.

The specific relation that Fechner finally proposed, and that we know as Fechner's Law, was

$$S = K \log I$$

where S is the magnitude of sensation, I is a dimension of the stimulus, and K is a constant of proportionality that varies with sense modality.

It is usually held nowadays that Weber's Law is only approximately true and that the Weber fraction is constant over a very small range of the stimulus magnitude. As a matter of fact, with only slight correction Weber's Law is true for hearing over a considerable part of the intensity range, as will be shown in detail when we take up the differential threshold in hearing (Chap. 7).

The more serious objection to Fechner's Law and its application to sensory magnitudes is that the jnd is not necessarily the unit of such magnitude. For example, if one is just able to detect a difference between two intensities that are low and another difference between two intensities that are high, it is not necessarily true that these two differences would constitute equal magnitudes in the judged loudness of a sound. Although an observer may not be able to say directly whether one jnd is greater or less than another, still the difference can become obvious with larger magnitudes when an observer may note that one pair of stimuli 20 jnd's apart seems farther apart than another pair that are also 20 jnd's apart. Neither Fechner nor any of the very early psychophysicists carried out the operations that were necessary to validate the assumption of subjective equality among jnd's. There have been, since Fechner's time, independent operations established for the direct measurement of sensory magnitudes, for example, of loudness. We shall consider them when we come to the measurement of loudness in Chap. 8.

THE CLASSIC PSYCHOPHYSICAL METHODS

Although we may not agree on how successful Fechner was in supplying a mathematical device for measuring psychological dimensions in terms of the physical dimensions of the stimulus, we cannot but agree that the methods that he worked out and formalized for the measurement of the differential threshold, the basic unit of measurement in his argument, represent very valuable tools. It is clear that the methods were first conceived for the purpose of measuring the differential threshold, because this was the important datum to be used in the formula that related sensation to the stimulus. The methods have been extended, however, to the measurement of the absolute threshold and other more complicated psychophysical phenomena. Let us outline very briefly the methods as they would be formulated for the measurement of the difference limen (DL), or differential threshold.

The Method of Adjustment

One of the simplest ways of determining the magnitude of a change in the stimulus that is required for an observer to just detect the change is to give the observer control of the stimulus so that he can adjust the magnitude to satisfy his criterion of detectability. Leaving all auditory examples for later chapters, let us suppose that we have two lengths, one that is fixed and one that can be adjusted by the observer. We ask the observer to adjust the variable length until it appears equal to the fixed length. Since the organism is not a very precise measuring device, a series of such adjustments will show some deviations from physical equality. If we subtract the fixed length from each of the adjusted lengths that the observer has made, we have a series of errors. The difference limen (DL) is defined in this case as the average of these errors calculated arithmetically—*i.e.*, we ignore the sign of direction of the error. Sometimes the standard deviation[1] (σ) is used as the measure of the DL. The reasoning behind such a computational procedure is simply this: if we are to estimate how much of a change is necessary for an observer to detect a difference, we can just as well use a statistic that indicates how poorly he can determine equality. We have computed, therefore, not the just noticeable difference, but rather the just *not* noticeable difference. The computation involved in the method of adjustment for determining the DL has provided another name for this method, namely, the *method of average error*.

The Method of Limits

This method is sometimes called the *method of serial exploration* or the *method of the just noticeable difference*. In this case the observer simply observes, and the experimenter has control of the stimulus. Continuing with our example of the DL for length, we present both the fixed and the variable lengths to the observer. We begin with both lengths physically equal. We gradually increase the variable length until the observer first reports that it looks different from (in this case longer than) the

---

[1] The standard deviation of a set of scores is a measure of the dispersion of the set about the average, or mean, score and is defined as the square root of the sum of the squares of the deviations (*i.e.*, differences between particular scores and the mean score) divided by the number of scores:

$$\sigma = \sqrt{\frac{\Sigma(\bar{X} - X)^2}{N}}$$

where σ is the standard deviation, Σ the symbol for "sum of," $\bar{X}$ the mean, X the individual score, and N the number of scores in the set. The reader who has no background in statistics should consult any good text on elementary statistics.

fixed length. We record the physical difference between the variable and the fixed lengths at the time the observer makes this report. We then set both lengths at equality again and gradually decrease the variable length until the observer again reports that it is different (this time shorter). We repeat this procedure a number of times and get several estimates of the mean difference that is required for the observer to just detect a difference. It may be that the DL for increasing length is systematically different from the DL for decreasing length; such a constant error may be noted in the tabulation of the data. The *method of gradual limits* involves a gradual change from equality that is continued until the observer reports a difference and the subsequent computation of a measure of central tendency (mean or median) within a series of such measurements. We may note at this point that this psychophysical procedure is very close to the traditional technique employed in clinical pure-tone audiometry (see Chap. 4).

The Method of Constant Stimuli

This method was referred to in the earlier years of psychophysics as the *method of right and wrong cases*. What we do is to get a percentage or ratio measure of judgments of "right" and "wrong" or of "equal," "greater," or "less" for several constant stimulus differences, constant in the sense that they do not change in time. We would, for example, present our fixed length of n cm along with the variable-length set at n, $n - 1$, $n + 1$, $n - 2$, $n + 2$ . . . cm and ask the observer each time whether the two lengths were the same, or whether the second was greater or less than the first. Normally we would expect the frequency with which the observer responded "same" to decrease as the difference between the two physical lengths becomes greater.

Guilford has used data from an experiment on lifted weights to obtain the curves shown in Fig. 1.1. Here we see that the frequency with which the variable stimulus is reported to be larger than the standard increases as the variable becomes larger, and the converse is also true. Judgments of "equal" reach a maximum where the judgments of "less" and "greater" appear about equally often. In this case of three categories of judgments, it is usual to define the DL as the interval of uncertainty (or half of it) between the 50-per-cent point on the "less" and the 50-per-cent point on the "greater" curve.

Another variation of this procedure is to force the observer to use only two categories of judgment, *e.g.* "greater" and "less" instead of "greater," "less," and "equal." If there is no constant error in this case, then when the variable and the standard are approximately equal physically, the judgments of "less" and "greater" will be made about equally often. As a matter of fact the cumulative curves would cross each other at 50 per cent. In order to compute a DL in this second case, it is usual to use as an *interval of uncertainty* the range of stimuli between 75 per cent on the "less" curve and 75 per cent on the "greater" (see Fig. 1.2).

The methods of adjustment, limits, and constant stimuli are the three so-called *classic psychophysical methods* that were used in the determination of the theoretically important DL. In the following chapters we shall

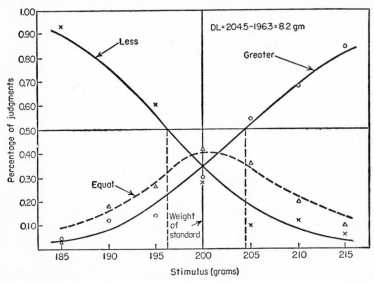

F\scriptsize IG.\normalsize 1.1. Relation between the percentage of judgments and the weight of a stimulus that is compared with a standard weight of 200 gm. The three curves show, for example, that a stimulus weight of 195 gm is judged to be "less" than the standard (200 gm) 60 per cent of the time, "greater" 14 per cent of the time, and "equal" 26 per cent of the time. (*From Guilford, p.* 188.)

be concerned with other data besides the DL. Methods for obtaining these other psychophysical data have been described and formalized by earlier workers. We shall discuss these other methods when we take up the auditory problems to which they are applied.

PSYCHOPHYSICS TODAY

Some psychophysicists of the present day are concerned with methods for computing or measuring psychological dimensions of sensations. Much progress has been made in hearing, vision, space perception, and taste. Many experimenters have denied the necessity for using the jnd as the basic unit for sensory magnitude and have proceeded to use independent operations for the establishment of sensory scales. They may, for example, ask an observer to adjust the physical magnitude of a stimulus until it appears half as loud or half as bright or half as sweet as another, fixed stimulus. Judgments of twice, ten times, etc., have been demanded and recorded reliably. Use of an older technique, the judgment of sense distances, has also figured large in these attempts.

The development of sensory scales represents, however, only a part of contemporary psychophysics. Broadly speaking, psychophysics has

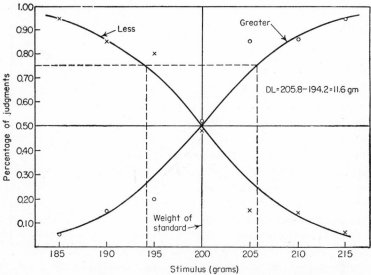

Fig. 1.2. The same relations as those shown in Fig. 1.1, except that in this case the observer is forced to choose between two judgment categories only. Judgments of "less" and "greater" appear equally often when the variable stimulus is equal to the standard. The *interval of uncertainty* is defined as the range of stimulus weights between the two 75-per-cent crossings. The upper or lower DL is defined in terms of the difference between the appropriate 75-per-cent crossing and the point of indifference. (*From Guilford, p.* 196.)

become the study of the relations between the responses of organisms and the stimuli that are presented to such organisms. This sounds almost like a definition of modern experimental psychology, and indeed, it is difficult to separate the two. The influence of behaviorism in American psychology is easily seen in modern psychophysics. We no longer look for relations between stimuli and sensations but rather relations between stimuli and responses. We can observe responses, the elements of behavior, and measure them, whereas the private sensation, which remains as untouchable as it was in Fechner's day, does not concern us. We do not ask whether or not a man hears a tone. We seek only to find whether or not he responds in a specified way to a tone. We can have measurement, then, on both sides of the psychophysical relation. The "psycho" part refers merely to behavior.

We shall have more to say about specific responses when we come to discuss conditioning and its relation to psychophysical measurement (Chap. 10). We should note here, nevertheless, that there are very few observable innate responses to sound. Different components of the startle response may be observed when a very loud sudden sound is presented. Most of the stimuli to hearing that will concern us, however, are of lower intensities than those required to elicit the startle response. We resort, therefore, to training or conditioning techniques in order to elicit the responses that we wish to observe. The audiometrist *tells the patient to raise a finger or press a button* when he hears a tone. Here is an example of a very complicated kind of conditioned or substitute stimulus, and the results of such measurement are valid only in so far as we have faith in the effectiveness of such conditioning.

Responses may be measured in many different ways. Sometimes we use an all-or-none criterion; the response is either made or it is not made. We may, however, go on to record the number of responses that have been made after a given number of stimuli have been presented. The measure of the response then becomes one of frequency of response. Other techniques involve a measure of the amplitude of a single response. We shall meet such a measure when we consider the conditioned galvanic-skin-resistance technique (Chap. 10). Most of the specific types of response measurement that we shall use are discussed in the appropriate chapters.

SUMMARY

To apply numbers to phenomena of experience must have been inconceivable to the early philosophical psychologists. The measurement of sensation has come about only as a result of several gradual transitions, primarily in respect of the way the problem was stated. The dualism that began with Descartes and became the psychophysical parallelism of the nineteenth century made the problem quite clear: there were physical events in the world that gave rise to the sensations of experience; how were the two kinds of events related?

Fechner thought that if he could relate changes in the physical stimulus to changes in the response of an observer, he might be able to write an equation that would relate the physical world with the world of sensation. His basic thesis appears now to have been right, although an apparent mistake was made when he chose the jnd as the crucial response. Perhaps the development of sensory scales as such does not excite us very much, but the fact that they can be and were developed means that we now have a systematic body of method for performing experiments that is based on these apparently dead issues. So far as sensory theory is concerned, the main problems seem to have been distilled into a problem of the appropriate specification of the *real* stimulus and response.

Many of our basic problems have been solved for us. We can approach the measurement of hearing from an operational, behavioristic point of view without worrying about philosophical points on experience and the real world. To measure hearing is to establish a relation between a measure of a stimulus (physical) and a measure of an appropriate response (psychological). Our first job is to examine the nature of the auditory stimulus and to learn something about its production, control, and measurement.

References for Further Study

Boring, E. G. (1942) *Sensation and Perception in the History of Experimental Psychology.* New York: Appleton-Century-Crofts. Chapter 1 traces the beginnings of experimental psychology. There is a section on psychophysics that gives a clear developmental account of the forces that led Fechner to his theory. Chapters 9, 10, and 11 give a detailed account of early experimental work on hearing.

Guilford, J. P. (1936) *Psychometric Methods.* New York: McGraw-Hill. Part I gives a thorough exposition of the classical psychophysical methods as well as an introduction to the concepts of statistics that are needed in psychophysical measurement.

Stevens, S. S. (1948) Sensation and psychological measurement. Chap. 11 in E. G. Boring, H. S. Langfeld, and H. P. Weld (Eds.), *Foundations of Psychology.* New York: Wiley. This chapter in an introductory textbook on psychology presents a broader discussion of the measurement of psychological magnitudes than that attempted in the present chapter.

Stevens, S. S. (1951) Mathematics, measurement and psychophysics. Chap. 1 in S. S. Stevens (Ed.), *Handbook of Experimental Psychology.* New York: Wiley. An even broader coverage of basic points on the relation between concepts of measurement and some of the problems of psychology are provided in this chapter, which is written at a considerably higher level than the previous reference.

CHAPTER 2

THE AUDITORY STIMULUS: SOUND AND ELECTRICITY

PSYCHOPHYSICAL measurement is a two-ended proposition: not only must we know how to observe and measure hearing, or responses to auditory stimuli, but also we must specify the stimulus unambiguously in terms of its physical characteristics. The stimulus for hearing is sound—a vibratory mechanical form of energy. Acoustics, the science of sound, has progressed so rapidly since the invention of the telephone and the vacuum tube that in order to understand how sounds are produced, controlled, and measured these days, one must learn something about electricity. This chapter is an attempt to set down briefly those concepts in acoustics and electricity that are basic to the measurement of the auditory stimulus. Such measurement is an essential part of audiometry in general. In the next chapter we shall put some of these concepts to work in describing how audiometers, hearing aids, and other pieces of everyday electro-acoustic equipment operate.

SOUND

To define *sound* as that stimulating phenomenon that gives rise to an auditory sensation is to give a psychological rather than a physical definition. What is the physical nature of this phenomenon that we call sound? We know that in order to hear, certain parts of the auditory system must be moved. An example of such movement is the inward-outward excursions of the eardrum. If someone sets off an explosion or sticks a pin into a balloon somewhere nearby, we hear something—our eardrums have been moved. How can an eardrum be moved by an explosion that takes place some yards away? There must be some connection between the explosion and the observer's eardrum. In this case, the connecting *medium* is air.

Let us think of the air as consisting of a large number of molecules or small spheres that are distributed fairly evenly throughout the air space and that move about in a random fashion. The air around us exerts an *atmospheric pressure* of about 15 lb/sq in or about 1 million dynes/cm²

(10^6 dynes/cm²). This means that a column of air whose cross section is a 1-in square and whose height is equal to that of the atmosphere exerts a weight (*force*) of about 15 lb. This *pressure* is directly related to the air's *density*, or *mass per unit of volume*. We may think of the density as being proportional to the number of molecules of air in a given volume.

So long as the air in our ear canals (and in the middle ear) remains at atmospheric pressure, we hear nothing. But the explosion changes the state of things. A force is applied to air surrounding the explosion in all radial directions. This force pushes the nearby air molecules away, pressing them against their next outermost neighbors. Such a crowding of molecules results in a *condensation*. If the air were like a mush, with little *elasticity*, the effect of the explosion would stop there: a region of crowded molecules would have been set up around the exploded object, and there they would stay. The air has more elasticity, however, than mush. By that we mean that the air demonstrates a tendency to maintain its normal density in spite of changes that are brought about by external forces. Thus it is that when the air molecules near the explosion become crowded together because of the force acting outward on them, they push other molecules, which in turn push still others.

This is a rough way of describing the process of propagation through an elastic medium. The increase in pressure that was produced near the explosion is transmitted through the air and eventually constitutes the force that moves the eardrum. We have, very superficially, characterized a sound. To be sure, there are simpler examples of sound than an explosion; and we shall now proceed to examine one of them, the *pure tone*. This much we already know: *a sound is a propagated change in the density and therefore in the pressure of an elastic medium*.

Simple Harmonic Motion and Pure Tones

From what we have said so far, we realize that we must deal with motion. When we first studied the motion of bodies in elementary physics, we learned about distance, velocity, acceleration, mass, force, work, and energy in situations where the motion was almost always in a straight line in one direction. We must now review these physical concepts and apply them to motion that changes in both magnitude and direction as time goes on. *Simple harmonic motion*, or *sinusoidal motion*, is sometimes defined as *projected circular motion*, since one simple way to develop this concept is to begin with uniform circular motion and then to project it on a plane. A body is said to be in uniform circular motion when it moves about the circumference of a circle at a constant speed, that is to say, a constant number of degrees of rotation per second.

For a simple example, consider the following not too impossible situation. A ferris wheel at a carnival is rotating at constant speed (see Fig. 2.1). A single passenger in one of the seats holds a flashlight in his hand and points it horizontally at a nearby wall. The flashlight throws a beam on to the wall. We can see that, as the wheel is turned at a constant rate, the spot of light on the wall appears to be moving up and down in a straight vertical line. Now further suppose that the wall is moved past the

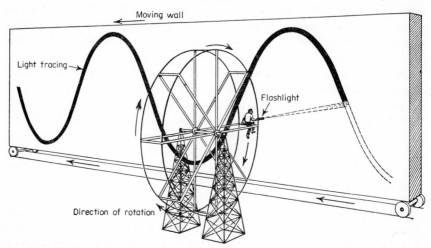

Fig. 2.1. Illustrating the generation of a sinusoid by projecting circular motion. (For explanation see text.)

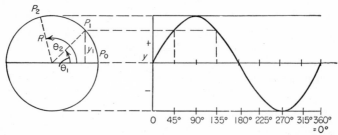

Fig. 2.2. Generation of sine wave, $y = R \sin \Theta$. As P rotates counterclockwise, the horizontal projection of the vertical distance from P to 0 is plotted as a function of degrees of rotation.

wheel at a constant speed. If the wall were coated with a light-sensitive material, we would obtain a negative tracing that would represent the up-and-down path of the light beam as a function of time. This graph of projected circular motion as a function of time is an example of a sinusoid. This particular wave shape is called a sinusoid because its shape is that of a sine wave or cosine wave, depending upon the initial position of the passenger.

Let us carry our example a little further with the aid of the diagram in Fig. 2.2, which is a little more precise but has less scenery. Before we begin rotating our passenger (or point P), we will set him at the position of 0°, the center of the vertical dimension. As we begin rotating counterclockwise, our point P moves from P_0 to P_1 and P_2 and so on around the circle until it returns to 0°, from where the circle is traversed again and again. A single full rotation of 360° is called a cycle. The projection, or sine wave, that is generated on the right of Fig. 2.2 shows the vertical distance of the point P above the horizontal at each position of rotation given in degrees. The abscissa, or horizontal dimension, of the graph is *degrees of rotation*. If the rotation is accomplished at a uniform speed, this dimension will also represent time.

You will remember from trigonometry that the sine of an angle in a right triangle is the ratio of the side of the triangle opposite the angle to the hypotenuse:

$$\sin \theta = \frac{y}{R}$$

Consider the triangle that is formed by the radius of the circle drawn to P_1, the vertical line from P_1 down to the horizontal, and that part of the horizontal between this vertical projection and the center of the circle. The angle θ tells us the number of degrees of rotation that P has moved between P_0 and P_1. The sine of this angle θ would, therefore, be directly proportional to the vertical distance from any P to the horizontal. As a matter of fact, if we set the radius (R) equal to 1, then this vertical distance, the quantity plotted on the vertical scale of the graph on the right of Fig. 2.2, *is* the sine. Its maximum value is 1, when the vertical distance equals the radius; and its minimum value is -1, when the vertical distance is measured in the negative direction. In the graph on the right we have the following relation:

$$y = R \sin \theta$$

This was obvious from the previous equation that gave the definition of the sine of an angle.

Now what does all this have to do with sound in general and with pure tones in particular? We may carry our analogy of projected circular motion into another example that will demonstrate what we mean by a *pure tone*. Consider the large drive wheel of a steam locomotive and its piston rod going into a piston chamber. For the purposes of our example, we will work this mechanism backwards: the turning wheel will drive the piston (see Fig. 2.3). Consider that the point where the piston rod joins the rim of the wheel is moving around the circumference of the circle at a uniform velocity. The circular motion of this point is then 'projected' through the piston rod to the back-and-forth movement of the piston in the chamber. Now suppose we simply couple the piston chamber to an ordinary rubber balloon that is partially inflated. As we turn the wheel at uniform angular velocity, the piston will move back and forth (as did the flashlight beam on the ferris wheel) and the balloon will be subjected to changes in its internal pressure. The outer surface of the balloon will move alternately inward and outward as the piston moves back and forth.

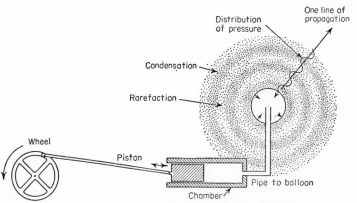

FIG. 2.3. Generation of a pure tone. As the wheel turns, the piston moves back and forth, causing the balloon to contract and expand. The effect of these movements is seen as alternate condensations and rarefactions that are being propagated away from the balloon in all directions. At the instant this 'picture' was taken, the piston was moving to the left, causing the balloon to contract and the layer of air immediately adjacent to rarefy.

In this working condition the balloon is a source of a pure tone (again on the condition that the rod is very long) that can be heard if the balloon is moving in and out fast enough. The strength of the pure tone is related to the distance that the surface of the balloon moves in and out. The frequency of the pure tone is the rate at which the balloon's surface moves in and out and, of course, is also the rate at which the wheel is turning. These two dimensions, *strength* and *frequency*, are the basic variables by which pure tones are differentiated from one another. A third dimension, *phase*, must also be specified in order that a pure tone be defined completely. We must now proceed to consider the way in which these three variables are described and a little about how they are measured.

Magnitude, or Strength, of a Pure Tone. There are several ways of stating the dimension along which a pure tone may be said to be strong or weak, large or small. Consider, for example, the tone that is being produced by the in-and-out movement of the spherical balloon that was discussed above. As the balloon moves outward, the air particles or molecules[1] immediately adjacent to its surface are crowded. This *compression* moves outward. But when the pressure within the balloon falls *below* atmospheric pressure, the air particles just outside the balloon exert a force that produces contraction. In this process they bounce apart, giving rise to a *rarefaction*. The strength of such an in-and-out movement, or increase and decrease in atmospheric pressure, may be specified in terms of the distance that any one (or all) of the particles moves in the course of being pushed, first in one direction and then in the other. The displacement of a particle from its average position, plotted as a function of time, would look like the second curve of Fig. 2.4. The top curve in this figure represents the in-and-out movement of the surface of the balloon, measured relative to the center of the spherical balloon. A given particle will, then, move back and forth according to the movements of the sound source but will not change its general location.

Although *particle displacement* is a rather simple concept to grasp, it is difficult to measure because of the small dimensions involved. A particle that is displaced sinusoidally about an average position (see second curve of Fig. 2.4) must continuously change its velocity, since the displacements in successive time intervals are not all equal or in the same direction. We might therefore specify the strength of a tone in terms of the *particle velocity*, which is simply the amount of displacement (or distance) per unit of time. If the balloon's movements become greater in magnitude, the *particle displacement* increases, and if the displacements are accomplished in the same period of time, the particle velocity also increases. A graph of particle velocity as a function of time is shown in the third curve of Fig. 2.4.

Particle displacement is measured in centimeters, and particle velocity is measured in centimeters per second. In order for a particle to move or change its velocity it must be *accelerated*, and acceleration means applying a *force*. A force of 1 *dyne* is the force required to accelerate a *mass* of 1 *gm* by changing its velocity from V_0cm/sec to $(V_0 + 1)$cm/sec in 1 sec.

$$1 \text{ dyne} = 1 \text{ gm} \times 1 \text{ cm/sec}^2$$

Although it is difficult to measure the small forces required to displace a single molecule, we can make a more gross measure and arrive at the same thing. We can measure the force acting on a large surface, and then, by dividing this force by the area of the surface, we have a measure of *pressure*, which is *force* per unit of *area*. A pressure of 1 dyne/cm² can be measured when a force of 1 dyne acts on an area of 1 sq cm or when a force of 100 dynes acts on an area of 100 sq cm. A constant atmospheric

---

[1] For our purposes we shall ignore the random movements of the air molecules.

pressure of 1 million dynes/cm² exists around the balloon that is moving periodically inward and outward. As it moves outward, the air close by is compressed, whereas an inward movement of the balloon produces a decrease in density. These density changes are equivalent to pressure changes that are transmitted throughout the surrounding medium. In

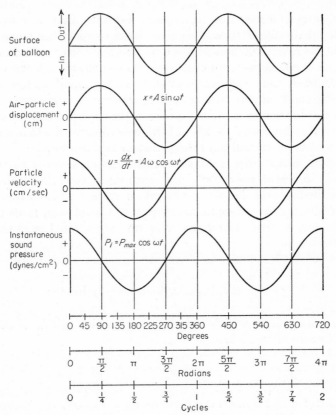

FIG. 2.4. Graphs and equations for particle displacement, particle velocity, and instantaneous sound pressure resulting from sinusoidal movements of a spherical source such as a balloon. Note that the particle velocity and pressure are both 90° out of phase with the displacement. (Particle displacement and pressure are related according to the characteristics of the transmitting medium. See Wave Motion.)

order to measure the strength of a sound, then, one has only to record these small changes in pressure in the medium that surrounds the sound source. The *sound pressure* of the pure tone generated by our balloon is plotted as a function of time in the fourth curve of Fig. 2.4.[1]

[1] The particle velocity and sound pressure are in phase only in plane progressive waves.

Sound pressure is used commonly as a measure of the strength of a sound, since many microphones respond directly to changes in pressure. A more basic measure of strength is given by the *energy* or *power* of *sound waves*. These concepts, as well as the different values that may represent the magnitude of a sinusoid will be discussed when we introduce *wave motion*.

Frequency of a Pure Tone. In many ways the concept of frequency is simpler than any of those that have to do with strength. *Frequency* is simply the rate, in *cycles per second*, at which a sinusoidal motion repeats itself, or at which the circular motion, whose projection is the sinusoid, is accomplished. One cycle of rotation is accomplished when a point has moved from 0° all the way around to 360° or 0° again. The number of times this happens per second is the frequency. Carrying this cycle over to the projection, we note that a full cycle of the sinusoid is represented by a maximum excursion in one direction and in the other. The double movement is explicit in the older frequency notation of tuning, which was in *double vibrations per second*. It is clear that as we speed up the rotation of the wheel in Fig. 2.3, the piston will move back and forth at a correspondingly higher rate and the balloon will be moving in and out at a higher rate, so that the frequency[1] of the pure tone being generated is increased.

If a full cycle occurs in ½ sec, the frequency of the pure tone is 2

---

[1] A cycle in frequency notation is made up of either 360° or 2π radians. Any angle formed by two radii of a circle may also be expressed in *degrees* or in *radians*. An angle is equal to 1 radian when the intersection of the two sides of the angle with the circumference of the circle yields an arc whose length is equal to that of the radius. Since the circumference of a circle is equal to 2π times the radius, there are obviously 2π radians in a full cycle of rotation. Therefore 2π radians is equal to 360°. The sine wave in the upper curve of Fig. 2.5 plots the sine of an angle as a function of the size of the angle measured in either degrees or radians (both these units are shown on the abscissa). Notice that the relation between the sine of an angle and the size of the angle is a relation that applies within each cycle of rotation. Therefore this relation is undisturbed when we change the frequency of rotation of a circle whose projected motion constitutes a sine wave. But now note the lower curve of Fig. 2.5, in which we have plotted the sound pressure of the pure tone that is being generated, through the piston system and the moving balloon, by a particular speed of rotation. Here we find a sinusoidal quantity plotted as a function of time. If one full cycle of the sine wave takes place in ½ sec, the frequency of the pure tone is 2 cps. Note that we can also express frequency in degrees or in radians. A frequency of 2 cps would also be a frequency of 720° per sec and of 4π radians per sec. Multiplying any frequency by 2π would, of course, convert the frequency from cycles per second to radians per second. This particular unit is sometimes called angular velocity. It is essentially the same as the frequency in cycles per second, except that in addition it tells us how many radius lengths are traversed by a moving point on the circumference of the circle per unit time.

cps. The length of time, ½ sec, that is consumed in the occurrence of one cycle of sinusoidal motion is called the *period* of that motion. Since the period is measured in seconds per cycle and the frequency is measured in cycles per second, these two quantities are reciprocally related. A cycle of a pure tone, whose frequency is 1000 cps, has a period of ⅟₁₀₀₀ sec.

You will notice in the lower curve of Fig. 2.5 that we have drawn a complete picture of amplitude as a function of time for a given sine wave,

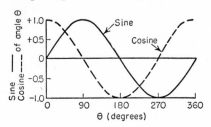

having been given only two pieces of information: the amplitude, or maximum excursion of the sine wave above and below the mid-point, and the frequency. In order to represent this pure tone on a relative time scale (the abscissa), the frequency and the amplitude are the only two quantities needed for a complete description. If, however, our time scale were an absolute one (for example, the actual seconds of a particular day), we should need a third piece of information, namely, the time at which the pure tone began. This kind of consideration leads us to the concept of phase.

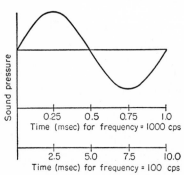

Phase. When we compare one pure tone with another, or mix several pure tones to form a complex tone, we are concerned with the concept of *phase*. Consider, for example, the two pure tones that are represented in the upper graph of Fig. 2.5. They both have the same frequency, but one begins rising from 0° when the other is already at its first maximum. The second tone starts at 0° when the first tone is at 90°. We say that there is a phase lag of 90° between these two tones. This phase relation remains constant, because both these pure tones are of exactly the same frequency, and at any point in time the number of degrees of rotation accomplished by the first sine wave will be 90° more than that accomplished by the second.

FIG. 2.5. A sine wave and a sinusoidal wave. The upper graph shows sine (and cosine) of an angle (θ) as a function of the size of the angle. The second curve shows the sound pressure output of a pure-tone generator as a function of time. (The reciprocal of the time required for one cycle gives the frequency.)

How sensitive is the ear to phase? This question has puzzled workers in this field for about a century. The only thing clearly established is that phase relations do make a difference if the stimulus is sufficiently complex. Phase becomes especially important in auditory measurement when tones of the same frequency and sound pressure are presented to both ears of an observer (see Chap. 9).

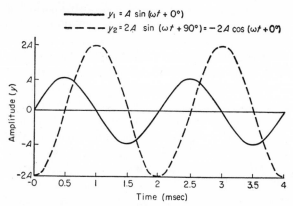

FIG. 2.6. Two sinusoids representing waves of the same frequency but of different amplitude and phase. The dashed curve lags behind the solid curve by 90°. (See text.)

Wave Motion

Having discussed the basic characteristics of pure tones, let us consider how they get themselves propagated through air. Air is, of course, only one of many media through which sound will be propagated. Any medium that has mass, elasticity, and more than a minimum density[1] will transmit sound waves. Normally sounds are conducted through the bones of the head, wood, metal, water, and other materials, but we shall have most to do with sound conducted through air. Returning to our moving balloon, we have said that the first outward movement will push the nearby air molecules against their neighbors, and these in turn will push on others more remote. The mechanical propagation will continue in all directions that are extensions of radii of the sphere.

Speed of Sound. This transmission takes time—the amount of time is determined by the compressibility and density of the medium. The greater the density or the compressibility of a medium, the more slowly sound will travel in it.

$$\text{Speed of sound} = \sqrt{\frac{\text{measure of elasticity}}{\text{density}}} = \sqrt{\frac{1}{\text{density} \times \text{compressibility}}}$$

The speed of sound in air at room temperature at sea level is about 1100

[1] The physicist would say that the "mean free path" (*i.e.*, average distance a molecule travels between collisions) must not be too long.

ft/sec. This means that it will take 1 sec for an increase in pressure produced at the balloon to be detected 1100 feet away.

In considering sound, we have now introduced two quantities that are measured with respect to time: *frequency* is the rate at which sinusoids repeat themselves, and *propagation speed* is the rate at which sound waves are propagated through a medium. We may now proceed to relate these two quantities. The speed of sound is independent of the frequency. A sound wave will travel 1100 ft in 1 sec whether the frequency is 10 cps or 10,000 cps. But the higher the frequency, the greater the number of full cycles that will have been accomplished in a given time or in a given propagated distance. The concept of *wavelength* relates frequency and the speed of sound. The wavelength of a pure tone is the distance that the sound wave travels during one period—the interval of time during which one cycle occurs. A pure tone whose frequency is 1100 cps has a wavelength in air of 1 ft, because one cycle occurs in $\frac{1}{1100}$ sec, and in that time the sound wave has moved 1 ft:

$$\text{Wavelength} = \frac{\text{speed of sound}}{\text{frequency}}$$

In air a tone at 550 cps would have a wavelength of 2 ft, while a tone of 2200 cps would have a wavelength of $\frac{1}{2}$ ft. The speed of sound in water, however, is about 4700 ft/sec. Therefore, whereas in air a 1100-cps tone has a wavelength of 1 ft, in water the same tone has a wavelength of more than 4 ft. Note that the wavelength for a given frequency varies directly with the speed of sound. This means that in less compressible media such as bone and steel, the wavelengths for comparable frequencies will be much longer.

Energy in a Sound Wave. We have already discussed three possible ways of measuring the strength of a sound in air: particle displacement, particle velocity, and sound pressure. As we measure the sound farther and farther away from the sound source, each of these measures will be smaller. What are the rules that govern the strength of a sound as it is propagated away from its source? In order to discuss these rules, we must introduce another measure of strength, namely, *energy.* If a force is applied to a body and the body remains at rest, no work has been done. If, however, the body is moved through a certain distance, then work has been done and the equivalent amount of energy has been expended. *Work* is measured in terms of *force* times the *distance* through which it acts:

$$\text{Work (ergs)} = \text{force (dynes)} \times \text{distance (cm)}$$

Energy is the capacity for doing work; it is numerically and dimensionally identical with work.

Ideally, energy emitted by a sound source, such as our moving balloon, does not change as the sound waves travel through space. Here we have one example of the law of conservation of energy. The earliest sound waves are moving away from the balloon in all radial directions, and the first condensation, for example, is itself the surface of a sphere of compressed air only slightly larger in radius than the balloon. As the sound waves move farther and farther away, the spherical surfaces that are made up of the successive condensations and rarefactions become larger and larger (see Fig. 2.3). If we assume that the energy remains constant, then the energy density, or energy per unit area, must decrease, because the same energy becomes more and more thinly spread over larger and larger spheres.

In solid geometry we learned that the area of a surface of a sphere is related directly to the square of the radius of the sphere. This rule, coupled with the notion of constant energy, gives rise to the *inverse square law*. This law states that the *intensity* of a sound decreases inversely with the square of the distance from the sound source. This intensity is simply the energy that flows through a unit of area per unit of time.

$$\text{Intensity (watts/cm}^2) = \frac{\text{energy (joules)}}{\text{time (secs)} \times \text{area (cm}^2)} = \frac{\text{power (watts)}}{\text{area (cm}^2)}$$

If energy is measured in ergs, then intensity is measured in ergs per square centimeter per second. We have said that the intensity of a sound decreases as the area of the sphere moving away from the sound source increases. If we measure an intensity at a given point and multiply it by the area of the surface of a sphere that intersects that point, we shall have a constant energy or power for all such points. (The *power* is the rate at which work is done—energy per unit of time. We shall have more to say about power when we discuss it in relation to electricity.)

The kinds of sound wave that we have discussed so far are called spherical waves, because the shape of the wave front is that of a sphere. By the time the wave front is a good distance away from the sound source, the sphere has such a large radius that the wave front may be considered a plane. The rules that govern the behavior of *plane progressive waves* or of *spherical waves* apply when the waves are unimpeded by any obstacles or changes in the medium of transmission.

But because we rarely work with sound in such refined environments that these conditions are met, we must always qualify these basic rules. In particular, a room with hard walls upsets the inverse square law, because the measurements of sounds at any particular point in the room are influenced not only by sounds that come directly from the sound source but also by waves that are reflected from the hard walls toward the point of measurement. In the traditional spoken and whispered voice tests that are used by otologists in estimating a man's hearing for speech, for example, the hard walls of the testing room upset the relation between the intensity of the sound at the listener's ear and the distance of the speaker from him. Were these tests given in an anechoic room (a room with soft walls and no echoes), the inverse square law would hold and the reliability of such tests would be improved. Only in such a room can the otologist be sure that when he holds his speech intensity constant, the intensity at the listener's ear is uniquely related to the distance between the two (varies inversely as the square of the distance).

Complex Sounds

Up to now we have discussed pure tones—pure in the sense that they involve only one frequency, only one particular sinusoidal function. By limiting our discussion to pure tones we have been able to describe the individual characteristics of sounds in their simplest forms one at a time. Pure tones, however, are relatively rare acoustic events in our normal environment and are usually produced only by an experimental or clinical investigator who is interested in some very specific relations. The majority of sounds that we ordinarily hear are complex, that is to say, they involve simultaneously more than one frequency. The vibrating structures that act as sources for such sounds—for example, vocal cords, car horns, musical instruments, machines, etc.—do not vibrate in a sinusoidal manner. In other words, the waveforms of these vibrations do not look like sinusoids. The basic question that we must treat here is, can any waveform that is different from a sinusoid be ultimately reduced to a number of sinusoids?

Fourier Analysis. The answer to the preceding question was given early in the nineteenth century by a French mathematician, Fourier, who demonstrated that any waveform that repeats itself periodically, no matter how complex, can be broken down into a finite number of sinusoids of different amplitudes, frequencies, and phases. Each of these frequencies is an integral multiple of the *fundamental frequency*, that frequency whose period is equal to that of the whole complex wave. Examples of some graphic Fourier analyses are shown in Fig. 2.7. By superimposing the sinusoidal waveforms of the individual components of a complex, we can reconstruct the original complex waveform.

Harmonic analysis of complex sounds is usually performed these days by complicated electrical gear, but the basic principles are the same as were incorporated in the mechanical analyzers of fifty years ago. Their basic feature was that they *resonated*—people who like to sing in the bathtub or shower are already familiar with this feature, for bathrooms

and shower rooms resonate too. Most structures, in fact, that have
definite dimensions and normal
modes of vibration (*e.g.*, enclosures
with hard interior surfaces) resonate
well. That is to say, they vibrate
readily at particular frequencies to
which they are 'tuned,' or are resonant, while at other frequencies
their induced vibrations are relatively small.

The old-fashioned way of analyz-
ing complex sounds was to use a
set of Helmholtz resonators. These
are distorted spheres that enclose
different volumes of air depending
on their sizes. A full set of them
covers a wide range of frequencies.
With such a set, one has only to produce the complex sound to be analyzed and then to note which of
these resonators is vibrating and
at what relative amplitudes. The
effect one gets can easily be illustrated with a piano. If you have a
piano at home, try standing close
to the strings and singing a long
"a-a-ah." If the piano's cover is off,
you may note that some strings are
vibrating while most of the others
are not. You have used this rather
complete set of resonators to analyze out those particular frequencies
that were present in your sung
vowel.

The Spectrum. The only graphic
representation of sound that we
have considered so far is the *waveform*, which shows the amplitude,
pressure, intensity, etc., as functions of time. We have said that in

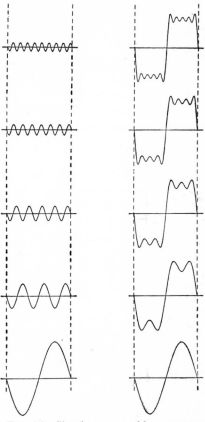

Fig. 2.7. Simple waves add up to complex waves. The first five harmonics of a
single cycle of a 'square wave' are shown
at the left. The series at the right shows
progressive changes from a simple sine
wave as each component is added. If
enough additional odd harmonics were
added, the composite wave would approach a perfectly square shape. (*Reproduction by permission from Newman, E.
B., Chapter 14 in E. G. Boring, H. S.
Langfeld, and H. P. Weld, Eds., Foundations of Psychology, published by John
Wiley and Sons, Inc.*, 1948, *p.* 316.)

some way a sinusoidal waveform is basic and simple and that by harmonic analysis any more complex waveform may be broken down into

a sum of simple sinusoids. It is impossible to perform this harmonic analysis visually by simply looking at a waveform on an oscilloscope or on a piece of graph paper, and we wish therefore to use another kind of graph to indicate what frequencies are present in a given complex sound and at what relative amplitudes.

The waveform for a single frequency is uniquely given in the form of a sinusoid according to the relation

$$y = A \sin (\omega t + \phi)\dagger$$

where y is amplitude at any instant, A is the maximum amplitude of the sinusoid, ωt the angle of rotation in radians, and ϕ the phase. Given a

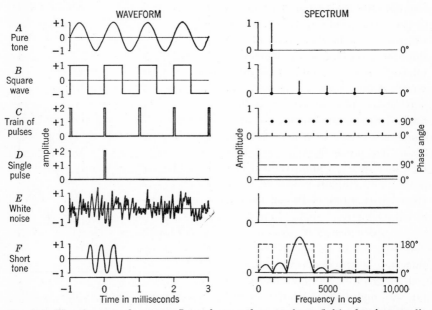

Fig. 2.8. Waveforms and spectra. In each row, the waveform (left), showing amplitude as a function of time, gives the same information as the spectrum (right), which shows amplitude and phase angle as a function of frequency. (*Reproduction by permission from Licklider, J. C. R., Chapter 25 in S. S. Stevens, Ed., Handbook of Experimental Psychology, published by John Wiley and Sons, Inc., 1951, p. 987.*)

single frequency, then, we do not need to plot the waveform but only to specify the frequency, amplitude, and phase.

The *spectrum* is a relation between amplitude and frequency for a given time interval and represents the results of a Fourier analysis. Typical spectra with their associated waveforms are shown in Fig. 2.8.

† $\omega = 2\pi f$. Angular velocity may be given in radians per second (ω) or degrees $\times$ 360/sec (*i.e.*, frequency).

Note that the spectrum for a single frequency or pure tone is a single straight line whose height represents the amplitude and whose position along the abscissa represents the frequency. (The phase may be specified on another ordinate, usually drawn below the base line.)

So long as we deal with complex tones that have regular periods, we will obtain *line spectra* that do not change in time. A line spectrum is one whose vertical lines are separate and represent discrete frequencies. If we 'look' at a complex tone for a time that is longer than one period, we shall obtain line spectra like those of Fig. 2.8. If, however, we look for only a brief time (shorter than one period), we shall have to assume a much more complex spectrum. The simple spectrum of a pure tone is obtained after a relatively long sampling time. The spectra of some sounds change quite rapidly in time, and we should obtain very different spectra from such sounds, depending on the length of time taken to sample the sound for a spectral analysis.

Speech Sounds. The sounds of speech are examples of sounds whose spectra change rapidly in time. These changes occur so rapidly that the analysis of the individual sound components (phonemes) of speech required the development of special equipment that could portray continuously changing spectra as a function of time (Potter, Kopp, and Green). Examples of such spectra from the "visible speech" machines are given in Fig. 5.3. Each part of the "visible speech" pattern represents a spectrum of a speech sound in a small interval of time.

Spectra may also be based on a much longer sampling time, even though the moving spectrum is changing within this longer time interval. An *average spectrum* gives amplitude in each measured frequency band, averaged over a long period of time. The way in which one varies the sampling time varies according to the particular kind of sound being measured. Some electrical meters (see next section) have a very rapid response and can make short-time measurements (microseconds), while others have more highly damped movements, responding very slowly and thus giving long-time measurements. Suppose that we have a sample of conversational English speech. The visible speech patterns tell us how the short-time spectra change in time. We can also make an average spectrum of this over a longer period of time and produce a result like the one shown in Fig. 2.9. Here we see that, on the average over a given period of time, most of the energy in conversational English speech lies below 1000 cps, with special emphasis in frequencies at 400 or 500 cps.

Transients. When the spectrum of a sound is constant over a period of time, the medium through which the sound is propagated is in a *steady state* during that period of time. Transitions in sound from one steady state to another are called *transients*. The pure tone is a steady-state phenomenon while it is on, but in the process of being turned on and off a more complex spectrum is generated, which describes the so-called on- and off-transients. A short transient, produced by most mechanical switches, gives rise to an audible click. Speech, of course, is just a long series of such transient sounds. Some of the vowels in speech may be called steady-state sounds for at least those short periods of time when the vowel is sustained. (The individual components of speech are discussed in Chap. 5.) Suffice it to say now that speech is a complex sound whose spectrum changes in time except for short periods when continuous sounds are sustained.

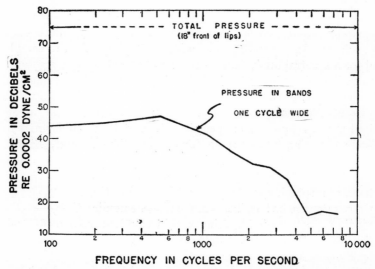

FIG. 2.9. Long-interval acoustic spectrum of male voice saying: "Joe took father's shoebench out; she was waiting at my lawn." Measurement made with microphone 18 in. from speaker's lips. (*After Rudmose et al.; from Miller*, 1951, p. 40.)

A comparison of the steady-state and transient features of speech sounds can be made roughly by examining the waveform of a particular sample of speech (Fig. 2.10). Remember, the waveform shows the amplitude or strength of a sound as a function of time. The relatively large excursions represent vowels sustained for a brief period, while the small wiggles around the base line represent the small energy in the consonants. Note that the rate at which these small wiggles cross the base line is greater than the rate of the larger excursions of the vowels, indicating that the frequencies involved in the consonants are higher. You may have wondered about the measurement of sound pressure in the average spectrum given in Fig. 2.9. To be sure, the sound pressure measured in front of a talker's lips varies, as he talks, from silence between syllables, through the small energies in the consonants, to the higher energies in the vowel sounds. The indicator of the measuring instrument used would therefore bounce between these high and low sound pressures, and detailed measures of the sound pressure in speech must take into account this variability. Average measures, as in Fig. 2.9, ignore it.

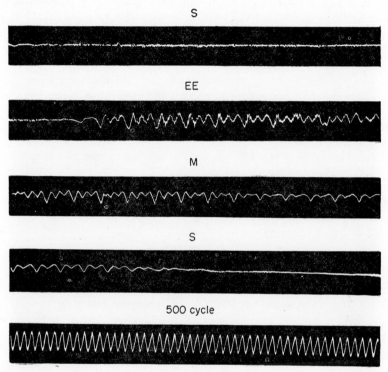

S

EE

M

S

500 cycle

FIG. 2.10. Continuous oscillogram of the spoken word "seems." A time scale is given by the 500-cps wave at the bottom. (*From Fletcher, 1929, p. 30.*)

Noise. A still more complex sound present in our everyday environment is *noise.* We shall not attempt to define noise rigorously, but we may note that a complex sound that has little or no periodicity may be differentiated roughly from the more orderly periodic sounds of musical instruments and speech. To say that a sound is *aperiodic* implies only that the waveform of the sound does not repeat itself at any calculably regular interval of time. An extreme case of aperiodicity is exemplified by a sound that has been called *white noise.* This name comes by analogy from optics, as indeed did the concept of the spectrum.

A monochromatic light beam (sinusoid) gives rise to a pure color or hue such as red, blue, or yellow. If we mix all the pure hues in the visible spectrum together, we obtain white light. In the same way, if we mix all the pure tones in the audible spectrum, we obtain a *white* (also referred to as *random* or *fluctuation*) *noise*. Escaping steam and the hiss of radio receivers are familiar examples of this type of noise. The spectrum of such a noise is characterized by the presence of all the frequencies in the audible range at the same amplitude or pressure. The fluctuations of electrons in resistors and vacuum tubes give rise to random noise. The same holds for the random motions of the air molecules: as a matter of fact, it has been calculated that this latter noise is just barely too faint to be audible.

A summary of the properties of fluctuation noise, which is one of the concomitants of the atomicity of matter and electricity, reads as follows:

1. Waveform: the amplitude varies randomly[1] in time.
2. Spectrum:
   a. The amplitude of the components at different frequencies is uniform.
   b. The phases of the various components are randomly distributed.

There is reason to believe that the future will see an increase in the importance of noise as a tool in scientific research and clinical practice (see Chap. 6).

ELECTRICITY

The mechanical forces that were mentioned in the last section are used to pull or push bodies around. Material bodies are composed of molecules, which in turn are made up of atoms. Each atom has a central nucleus made up of a number of positively charged *protons* and some electrically neutral *neutrons*. Revolving in orbits around the nucleus are negatively charged *electrons*. The number of electrons in each atom is equal to the number of protons in the nucleus. Molecules or larger bodies move primarily under the influence of mechanical forces, whereas the motion of electrons depends essentially upon electrical forces. The negativity of the electron and the positivity of the proton are arbitrarily defined and differentiated in terms of repulsion and attraction: like electrical charges repel, and unlike charges attract. Electrons are attracted to positively charged bodies but are repelled by other electrons. Electrons can be moved through conducting media by the application of an electromotive force (EMF). The general characteristics of such electric conduction are the subject of the first part of this section.

---

[1] The statistically oriented reader might substitute for this statement the more precise one that the distribution of instantaneous amplitudes follows the normal probability curve.

Bell's invention of the telephone in 1876 provided a device that could convert the small mechanical energies of sound into electrical energies and vice versa. When the development of the vacuum tube (*ca.* 1900) provided means for controlling electric currents with much more ease and reliability than had been possible with strictly mechanical methods, the interdependence of acoustics and electronics became apparent. In the modern laboratory or clinic, there is hardly a sound to which an observer or patient listens that has not been produced, modified, or controlled by electrical apparatus.

Dimensions of Electricity

Charge. The negative charge on a single electron is the smallest measurable electrical unit and is not very useful for engineering measurements. The *electrostatic unit* represents the charge on a body that will exert a *force* of one dyne on another body of the same charge when the two bodies are placed 1 cm apart. The *coulomb*, a larger and more practical unit, is equivalent to 3 billion electrostatic units. A *coulomb* also represents the combined charge of 6.3×10^{18} electrons.

Current. The rate at which electrons flow in a *conductor* is the *current*, measured in *amperes* (amps). One ampere of current flows when 1 coulomb of charge moves past a given point in a second.

$$1 \text{ amp (current)} = 1 \text{ coulomb/sec (charge per sec)}$$
$$= 6.3 \times 10^{18} \text{ electrons/sec}$$

When the current flows in only one direction at a constant value, it is called *direct current* (d-c). When it changes direction periodically, it is known as *alternating current* (a-c). Just as the rate at which water flows in a pipe is determined by the size of the pipe as well as the water pressure, so the amount of current flowing in a wire or any conductor is dependent upon the electrical 'pressure' (see next paragraph) and the properties of the conductor.

Voltage. The *electromotive force* (EMF) that is said to move electrons actually does so by imparting energy to them. This EMF, or *voltage*, is measured in *volts*. In so far as a voltage represents a capacity to do electrical work, it is also called *electrical potential*. If the potential difference between two points is 1 volt, then in order to move 1 coulomb from one point to the other we must expend 1 joule of work.

$$1 \text{ volt} = 1 \text{ joule/coulomb}$$

A volt is also defined as that electrical potential that will produce a current flow of 1 amp through 1 *unit of resistance* (ohm).

Resistance.   Not all materials or all sizes of the same material conduct electric current equally well. Those substances (particularly metals) that are good conductors or have high conductivity are characterized by a large number of free electrons. Some materials are very poor conductors; these, we say, have high *resistivity*. Materials with very high resistivity are known as *insulators*. Without laboring the water analogy too long, remember that the greater the cross-sectional area of a pipe, the greater the flow of water per unit of time. The amount of resistivity in a given length of a particular conductor varies inversely with the area of the cross section. *Resistance* is a measure of the opposition to current flow that is offered by an amount of resistivity. The unit of resistance is the *ohm*, 1 ohm being defined as the amount of resistance that will permit 1 amp to flow when 1 volt is applied.

Ohm's Law.   In circuits that involve only direct current, the voltage, current, and resistance are precisely related[1] according to Ohm's Law. In defining voltage and resistance, we have already mentioned these relations. Ohm's Law may be stated in any one of three ways, all of which are algebraically equivalent: if the voltage applied to a circuit remains constant, the current decreases as the resistance is increased; if the resistance of a circuit is held constant, the current increases as the voltage is increased; if the current flowing in a circuit is to remain constant, the voltage applied must be increased as the resistance is increased (see Fig. 2.11). In terms of the symbols that are used to represent current (I), voltage (E) and resistance (R) the relations are as follows:

$$I = \frac{E}{R}$$
$$E = IR$$
$$R = \frac{E}{I}$$

Energy and Power.   Thus far we have discussed only those characteristics of electricity that are peculiarly electrical. But in order to transport charges in a conductor, *energy* has to be expended. If we apply mechanical forces to a wire, such as those that will bend the wire back and forth, we know that the wire will get hot. An electric current passing through the same wire, without any mechanical forces applied, will also produce heat. Heat is produced whenever mechanical forces work against friction or whenever electrical forces work against resistance. The transformation of electrical or mechanical energy into heat provides us with a basic quantity that is important in both electricity and mechanics. *Energy*, like *work*, is measured in joules (1 joule = 10^7 ergs), and, since

[1] We must assume that the resistance in a circuit is unaffected by the current.

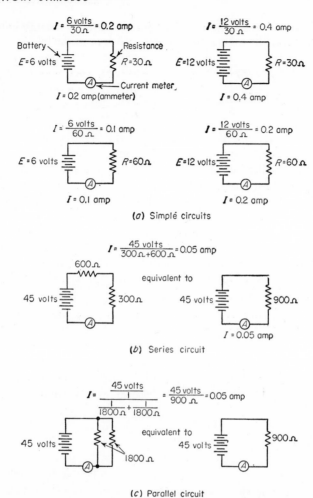

$$I = \frac{6 \text{ volts}}{30\,\Omega} = 0.2 \text{ amp}$$

Battery
E = 6 volts   Resistance
                R = 30 Ω
            (A) ← Current meter
I = 0.2 amp (ammeter)

$$I = \frac{12 \text{ volts}}{30\,\Omega} = 0.4 \text{ amp}$$

E = 12 volts   R = 30 Ω
            (A)
I = 0.4 amp

$$I = \frac{6 \text{ volts}}{60\,\Omega} = 0.1 \text{ amp}$$

E = 6 volts   R = 60 Ω
            (A)
I = 0.1 amp

$$I = \frac{12 \text{ volts}}{60\,\Omega} = 0.2 \text{ amp}$$

E = 12 volts   R = 60 Ω
            (A)
I = 0.2 amp

(a) Simple circuits

$$I = \frac{45 \text{ volts}}{300\,\Omega + 600\,\Omega} = 0.05 \text{ amp}$$

600 Ω
45 volts   equivalent to   45 volts
        300 Ω   900 Ω
    (A)   (A)
                              I = 0.05 amp

(b) Series circuit

$$I = \frac{45 \text{ volts}}{\dfrac{1}{1800\,\Omega} + \dfrac{1}{1800\,\Omega}} = \frac{45 \text{ volts}}{900\,\Omega} = 0.05 \text{ amp}$$

45 volts   equivalent to   45 volts
        1800 Ω   900 Ω
    (A)   (A)

(c) Parallel circuit

FIG. 2.11. Some simple demonstrations of the relations in Ohm's Law. In (a), the four simple circuits show how current (I) is affected by changing the voltage (E), resistance (R), or both. If the voltage is doubled while resistance remains constant, the current is doubled. If the resistance is doubled while the voltage remains constant, the current is halved. If both the voltage and the resistance are doubled, the current remains constant. Simple circuit equivalents are shown for a series circuit [in (b)] and a parallel circuit [in (c)]. The resolution of either of these to a simple circuit is shown in the formulas.

we have already defined the volt as 1 joule/coulomb, energy can also be expressed in terms of *volt-coulombs:*

1 joule (energy) = 1 volt-coulomb (voltage × charge)

Now a coulomb is 1 amp-sec, because an ampere is 1 coulomb/sec. Therefore,

$$\text{Energy} = \text{voltage} \times \text{current} \times \text{time}$$
$$W = E \times I \times t$$

Using other substitutions from Ohm's Law, we obtain the following further equations for energy, or work:

$$W = I^2Rt$$
$$W = \frac{E^2t}{R}$$

It is sometimes convenient to talk in terms of the rate at which energy can be expended or work can be done. This rate is called *power* and is measured in *watts.*

1 watt (power) = 1 joule/sec (energy/time)
$$P = \frac{W}{t}$$

When electrical measurements are made in terms of amperes, volts, and ohms, the energy is measured in joules. By substitution we can define power in terms of any of these basic electrical units.

$$P = EI = I^2R = \frac{E^2}{R}$$

Of course, the electric company does not bill you for power, or the rate at which the work is done, but rather for the actual work done. In other words, you are billed for joules rather than watts. The usual unit that you see is the watt-hour or kilowatt-hour. One watt-hour is the amount of energy expended in 1 hour at the rate of 1 joule/sec. One watt-hour = 3600 joules, both being measures of energy. The concept of power is basic to the measurement of *alternating currents.*

Induction

We have already talked a little about the heating effects of electricity, and we have now to deal with still another effect, namely, the magnetic effect. The relation between electricity and magnetism is reversible: a current produces a magnetic effect, and a magnetic field may give rise to an electric current.

Magnets and Electromagnets. We define a magnet in terms of its behavior relative to the so-called *magnetic north* or *south pole* of the earth. The rules of attraction in magnetism are very much like those of electric charges in that unlike poles of magnets attract each other, whereas like poles repel each other. "North" and "south" have come to be used commonly in talking about the poles of the magnet because of the easy reference to the natural poles of the earth.

As a current flows through a wire, a magnetic field exists about the wire. If you wrap the fingers of your right hand about the wire, holding your thumb in the direction of current flow along the length of the wire, the direction of the magnetic lines of force will be represented by your fingers. This means that the north pole of a magnetic compass, placed anywhere near the wire, will always be pointing in the same direction as

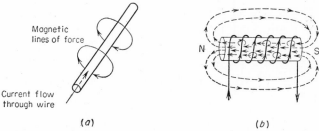

Magnetic lines of force

Current flow through wire

(*a*)   (*b*)

Fig. 2.12. Magnetic fields around wire carrying direct current. The lines of force around a single wire are shown in (*a*). These lines combine when the wire is coiled around a core, giving the magnetic polarity that is shown in (*b*).

your fingers are pointing. Now suppose that we combine many such wires, all connected together, so that these concentric lines of magnetic force are aligned to produce a north pole at one end of this coil and a south pole at the other (see Fig. 2.12). If we insert a soft-iron core in the center of the coil we will have an *electromagnet*. So long as current flows in the wire in a single direction, a north pole exists at one end and a south pole at the other. As soon as the current ceases, the field collapses and the core returns to its neutral status except for some residual effects that may be left.

These simple relations are utilized directly in the construction of meters and motors. Suppose we place such a small electromagnet in a magnetic field that is produced by two permanent magnetic poles, as in Fig. 2.13. With no current flowing through the coil, the core, or armature as it is called in the case of a meter, will remain vertical, being equally attracted by both poles. If, however, a current flows in the wire in one direction, so that the top of the armature becomes a north pole and the bottom a south, the armature will turn in the direction of attraction of unlike poles. The electromagnetic north will go toward the permanent south pole. The number of lines of magnetic force per unit of area (*flux*) that are built up around an electromagnet is directly proportional to the current flowing through the wire. This means, of course, that the amount of turning that will be done as a result of the magnetic attraction will be directly proportional to the current. This little structure, then, is a prototype for a current meter or ampere meter (more briefly, *ammeter*). Almost all meter movements are based on this principle, even though the circuits of some meters may make them suitable for measuring not only current but also, by Ohm's Law, voltage, resistance, and power.

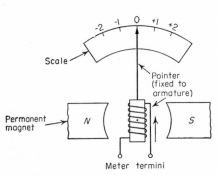

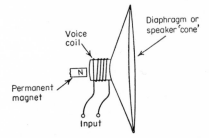

FIG. 2.14. Schematic illustration of an electrodynamic earphone or loud-speaker. If a sinusoidal current flows through the voice coil, the left end of the coil will become alternately *north* and *south*. It will move, therefore, alternately away from and toward the permanent *north pole*. Such movement of the coil moves the diaphragm or 'cone' which, in turn, produces sinusoidal changes in the pressure of the adjacent air.

FIG. 2.13. A basic meter movement. If current flows through the coil in the direction indicated, the top of the coil will become magnetic *north* while the bottom becomes *south*. The combination of this polarity with that of the permanent magnet will produce a movement in the clockwise direction and the needle will register on the positive side of the scale.

The dynamic (moving-coil type) earphone or loud-speaker is another application of electromagnetism. We have seen above that a coil of wire placed in a magnetic field will move when a current is passed through it. Since the particular north or south pole at one end depends upon the direction of the flow of current in the coil, it is clear that if the current is alternating in direction, the poles will alternate in their polarity and the resulting movement will also be alternating. If, for example, we have a small coil fixed to a diaphragm in the vicinity of one pole of a permanent magnet (see Fig. 2.14), a sinusoidal, alternating current through the coil will cause it to move back and forth as the current reverses its polarity. The air in front of the diaphragm will, of course, be propagating a pure tone.

Induced Currents.   We come now to consider an effect that is opposite to the electromagnetic effect discussed in the last paragraph. In this case we begin with a magnetic field and produce an electric effect. This relation has been known at least since the early nineteenth century, when Faraday and Henry demonstrated that when a pole of a permanent magnet is thrust inside of a coil of wire, a current is made to flow in the wire. This is shown in Fig. 2.15a. In order to demonstrate this effect we need three basic things: a magnetic field, a conductor or a coil, and movement of one relative to the other. As a matter of fact, the induced current[1] in any such coil is directly proportional to all these factors, because the current depends upon the number of magnetic lines of force traversed per unit

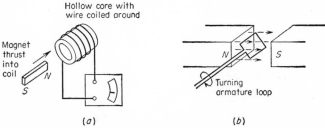

Hollow core with
wire coiled around

Magnet
thrust
into
coil

N

S

N   *S*

Turning
armature loop

(a)   *(b)*

Fig. 2.15. Demonstrations of *induction*. In (a) we see the effect of thrusting a magnet into a coil by observing the deflection of the needle on an ammeter. The needle would move in one direction as the *N* pole enters and in the other direction as the magnet continues and the *S* pole enters. In (b) one loop only from a many-loop armature is seen rotating in a permanent magnetic field; the principle is basic to the operation of a-c generators.

of time. The stronger the magnetic field, or the greater the number of turns of wire in the coil, or the faster the movement, the greater will be the induced current. If you look at Fig. 2.15b, you will see how this principle is involved in the production of electric currents by large commercial generators. In *a*, the magnet moves through the coil; in *b*, the coil moves through a magnetic field.

The direction of the current flow through a wire is determined by the direction of its movement relative to the lines of force in the magnetic field. If a wire moves parallel to the lines of force, no current is induced. If it moves perpendicular to the lines of force, a maximum current is induced. Consider only one piece of wire (on one side of the coil in *b* of Fig. 2.15) that is moving in a circle: as it moves straight up, a maximum current is induced in one direction; as it approaches the top, it is moving parallel to the lines of force and the current drops to zero; as it approaches a straight downward direction, the current again reaches a maximum, but

[1] Voltage is actually induced, but any resistance that is less than infinite will permit a current flow, which is measured.

this time it is in the opposite direction, because the direction relative to the lines of force is reversed. Not only is this principle used by commercial power companies for generating a-c voltage, but also it is clear that this device could be used for producing electric sinusoids analogous to the pure tone. If we were to measure the magnitude and direction of the current flowing in the coil of Fig. 2.15b while it rotates at constant speed, we would obtain a measure as a function of time that would look exactly like the sinusoids that we have considered earlier.

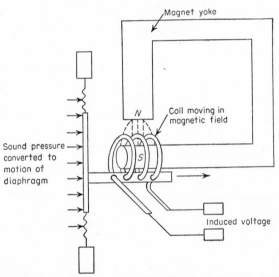

FIG. 2.16. Schematic diagram illustrating the principle of the dynamic (moving-coil-type) microphone. The voltage induced at the output terminals is proportional to the sound pressure that impinges on the diaphragm. Note that dynamic earphones may serve as microphones and vice versa. (*Reproduction by permission from Acoustic Measurement by L. L. Beranek, published by John Wiley and Sons, Inc., 1949, p. 224.*)

Not only uniform circular motion, but also other more complicated forms of movement will induce currents, the variation of which in time will look like the waveform of the original movement. This is the basis on which a magnetic or a dynamic *microphone* operates. The problem is to *transduce* the mechanical energy in the sounds of speech into electrical energy. Such a microphone is shown in Fig. 2.16. There is a small permanent magnet around which there is a coil of wire. The coil is connected to a diaphragm, a large surface against which changing forces in a sound wave work. As pressure in the air near the microphone's diaphragm is changed by the sound waves, the diaphragm will move back and forth. If the magnet is stationary and the coil moves relative to it, a current is induced that is proportional in magnitude and direction to the movements. A faithful microphone is one whose output current, plotted as a function of time, is a replica of the waveform of the sound.

Impedance

Thus far the only kind of impedance, or opposition to the flow of current, that we have discussed is resistance. Electrical energy is dissipated in the form of heat when work is done against resistance. There are, however, other characteristics of electrical components that constitute oppositions to current flow without a loss of energy. In circuits where only direct current is used, the terms *resistance* and *impedance* are equivalent. When, however, the current is changing in magnitude or direction (alternating current) the resistance is responsible for only one component of the total impedance. Let us turn now to two other components of impedance: inductive and capacitative reactance.

Inductance (L). Consider the electromagnet of which we have already spoken: when an alternating current is made to flow through the coil, the magnetic fields are alternately building up and collapsing. From what we have already said about induction, we know that when the fields move relative to the wires, a current is induced. In a device such as an electromagnet, the induced current will flow in a direction that is opposite to that of the current that produced the change in the field; therefore an opposition to the original current would be set up by what is called a "back EMF" or opposing induced voltage. Inductance, measured in *henrys*, is a measure of the opposing voltage, or back EMF, that will be induced by a unit change in the current.

$$1 \text{ henry (inductance)} = \frac{1 \text{ volt (back EMF)}}{1 \text{ amp/sec (current change)}}$$

$$L = \frac{\Delta E}{\Delta I/t}$$

The component of impedance for which such electromagnetic induction is responsible is known as *inductive reactance*. Like resistance, this reactance is measured in ohms. Unlike resistance, it does not cause dissipation of electrical energy into heat but temporarily stores the energy in magnetic form. An electromagnetic device, such as a loud-speaker or an earphone, will have a certain number of ohms of impedance, some of which will be resistance and some of which will be inductive reactance. This opposition or reactance that any coil will offer to a change in current is directly proportional to the inductance in the coil and also to the rate at which the current changes back and forth. That is to say, the inductive reactance of a coil with a given inductance is greater as the frequency of a sinusoidal current is made higher. We know that the opposing voltages that are produced by changes in the magnetic field will be greater as the changes occur more frequently, because we know that induced currents are greater the faster the relative change between a conductor and a magnetic field (see Fig. 2.17).

Inductive reactance (ohms) $= 2\pi$ frequency (cps) $\times$ inductance (henrys)
$$X_L = 2\pi f L$$

Capacitance (C).   We have now to deal with a *condenser* (or *capacitor*), a device that can store energy in electrical form. Suppose we take two metal plates and hold them close together face to face but not touching. We will give them opposite charges by applying a voltage. For example, we can connect the positive terminal of a battery to one plate and the negative terminal to the other. After the battery is disconnected, the voltage (or difference in potential) between the two plates remains, an excess of electrons on one plate and a deficiency of electrons on the other. In order to separate electrical charges, work has to be done. This work is stored as potential electrical energy, much as mechanical potential energy is stored in a body that is lifted to a given altitude above the ground.

We now have a prototype of a charged condenser, two plates separated by a *dielectric medium*. A dielectric, or insulating, medium is one that will not permit free electron flow. The voltage across the condenser imposes a certain stress upon the insulating, or dielectric, medium that separates the plates. If a current meter is connected between the two plates, a brief current will flow during the time when the excess of electrons travels through the conductor to restore electrical equilibrium to the two plates. The measure of the ability of such a device to store electricity is called *capacitance*.[1] Capacitance is dependent upon the area of the conducting plates, the reciprocal of the distance between the plates, and the nature of the dielectric material between them. Capacitance is measured by the amount of charge that can be stored when a voltage of 1 volt is applied to the plates.

$$1 \text{ farad (capacitance)} = \frac{1 \text{ coulomb (stored charge)}}{1 \text{ volt (applied charge)}}$$

$$C = \frac{Q}{E}$$

The *farad* is an impractically large unit, and the condensers that one sees in use are usually marked in *microfarads* or *micromicrofarads*, one

---

[1] A synonym is *capacity*.

millionth (10^{-6}) and one millionth of a millionth (10^{-12}) of a farad, respectively.

So much for the ability to store charges. What about the opposition to current flow of such a device? To direct current (0 cps), the opposition or reactance is infinite. For alternating current, the reactance will be less

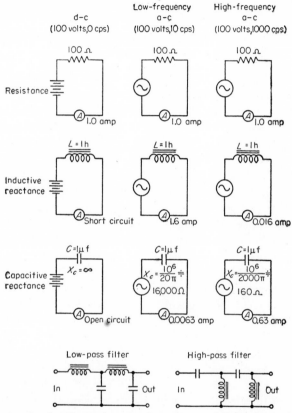

FIG. 2.17. Some circuits illustrating the dependence of inductive and capacitative reactance on frequency. Resistance is independent of frequency. High- and low-pass filters operate on the basis of these dependencies. In the low-pass filter shown, the low frequencies will pass the inductances while high frequencies are stopped by the inductances and shorted out by the condensers. The high-pass filter does the opposite.

as the capacitance is larger, since current is directly related to the ability to store charges. As the frequency of the alternating current is made higher, the reactance of a given capacitance becomes smaller. The component of impedance associated with capacitance is called *capacitative reactance;* it is measured in ohms and is inversely related to the capacitance and the frequency of an alternating current (see Fig. 2.17).

Capacitative reactance (ohms) =

$$\frac{1}{2\pi \text{ frequency (cps)} \times \text{capacitance (farads)}}$$

$$X_C = \frac{1}{2\pi f C}$$

Complex Impedance. When we come to some circuits involving several electrical components in the next chapter, we shall see how different devices have different kinds of impedance. Sometimes the impedance of a single component of a circuit may have resistive, capacitative, and inductive components. The resistance of a given device is independent of the frequency of the alternating current that flows through and remains the same for alternating and direct current. The inductive reactance of a particular coil will increase as the frequency of alternating current increases and is zero for direct current. The capacitative reactance of a condenser will decrease as the frequency of alternating current increases and is infinite for direct current (see Fig. 2.17).

These three kinds of impedance do not add according to simple arithmetic rules. The coil of a loud-speaker, for example, that has a resistance of 3 ohms and an inductive reactance of 4 ohms at a particular frequency will not have a total impedance of 7 ohms, but one of only 5 ohms. If you remember from elementary trigonometry the relations within the so-called 3-4-5 right triangle, you will recognize that we are dealing with a form of geometrical addition. Inductance and capacitance not only impose opposition to current in a circuit but also introduce certain changes in the phase relation between the current and the voltage. The phase changes introduced by an inductance are opposite to those introduced by a capacitance. Therefore, in circuits where the inductive and capacitative reactances are equal, they cancel, leaving only the resistive component responsible for the total impedance. We cannot go into the details of such geometrical or vectorial addition here, but the general principle must be introduced in order that we may proceed to discuss electrical *resonance.*

An understanding of impedance is of extreme practical importance, because most sources of alternating current (*e.g.*, microphones, generators, oscillators, amplifiers) are designed to work into particular impedances. Earphones, loud-speakers, and meters of different kinds constitute the impedances into which such devices work. The improper choice of an impedance for a given device may result in faulty operation.

Impedance Matching and Transformers. Whenever we assemble an apparatus with several components, we must deal with the impedances of the several parts, such as microphones, amplifiers, etc. Again the reader must be referred to the next chapter for specific examples, but we must develop here the concept of *impedance match*. Suppose we have a loud-speaker whose impedance is 5 ohms. It is to receive its electrical energy from an amplifier designed to feed an impedance of 500 ohms. If we connect the loud-speaker directly to the output of the amplifier, the amplifier will be *loaded* with (will work into) 5 ohms only and will not operate properly. We could *match* the impedance of the loud-speaker to that required by the amplifier by inserting a resistance of 495 ohms in series with the loud-speaker, but then $\frac{495}{500}$ of the power would be wasted in the form of heat in the resistance, while only $\frac{5}{500}$ would be delivered to the loud-speaker. The more efficient way to match imped-

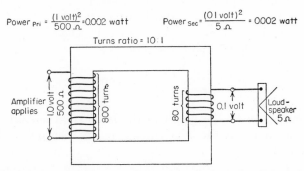

$$\text{Power}_{\text{Pri}} = \frac{(1\ \text{volt})^2}{500\ \Omega} = 0.002\ \text{watt} \qquad \text{Power}_{\text{Sec}} = \frac{(0.1\ \text{volt})^2}{5\ \Omega} = 0.002\ \text{watt}$$

Turns ratio = 10 : 1

Amplifier applies 1.0 volt 500 Ω — 800 turns — 80 turns — 0.1 volt — Loud-speaker 5 Ω

Fig. 2.18. Schematic drawing of an impedance-matching transformer. Both primary and secondary coils are wound on the same core to maximize the inductive coupling between the two. (See text.)

ances involves the use of a transformer, *i.e.*, two coils or inductances that are placed closely enough together so that their magnetic fields overlap.

Figure 2.18 shows two such coils, wound on the same core. The primary coil constitutes the input of the transformer and receives the electrical energy from whatever device is feeding the transformer. The secondary coil constitutes the output and feeds electrical energy to another component. The transformer operates on the principle of induction: fields that are built up in the primary as a result of changing currents will induce currents in the secondary. You remember that the current induced is proportional to the number of turns of wire as well as to other parameters that remain constant here. If both the primary and secondary coils have the same number of turns, then as much voltage will be induced in the secondary as was applied to the primary. If, however, there are fewer turns in the secondary than in the primary, a smaller voltage will be induced in the secondary. As a matter of fact, the ratio of the number of turns in the primary to the number of turns in the secondary will be the same as the ratio of the voltages in the primary and the secondary:

$$\frac{N_p}{N_s} = \frac{E_p}{E_s}$$

Take the specific example in Fig. 2.18. Our amplifier should work into an impedance of 500 ohms, and our loud-speaker has an impedance of 5 ohms. Transformers are very efficient devices, which means that there is little resistance and little consequent heat loss. For the sake of our example, we will assume no resistance in the transformer. The power in this efficient device must, therefore, be the same in the primary and the secondary circuits. Suppose our amplifier applies 1 volt to the primary of a transformer whose turns ratio is 10:1. According to the formula above, the secondary voltage would be 0.1 volt. The secondary power in the loud-speaker coil of 5 ohms would be

$$P_s = \frac{E_s^2}{R_s} = \frac{(0.1)^2}{5} = 0.002 \text{ watt}$$

Since this must also be the power in the primary of our no-loss transformer, we can compute the impedance that has been reflected into the primary circuit:

$$P_p = \frac{E_p^2}{R_p}$$

$$R_p = \frac{E_p^2}{P_p} = \frac{1}{0.002} = 500 \text{ ohms}$$

Such a turns ratio and consequent voltage ratio leads to the conclusion that the 5-ohm impedance of the secondary was made to 'look like' 500 ohms in the primary. Indeed, the impedance-matching transformer does just that by reflecting the impedance of the secondary circuit into the primary circuit according to the square of the turns ratio:

$$\left(\frac{N_p}{N_s}\right)^2 = \frac{Z_p}{Z_s}$$

Had we inserted a 495-ohm resistor in series with the loud-speaker, the total power from the amplifier would have remained 0.002 watt, but the power available to the loud-speaker would have been only $\frac{1}{100}$ of the total, or 0.00002 watt. With the impedance-matching transformer, the total power of 0.002 watt is available to the loud-speaker.

Resonance. After a mechanical force is applied, a body will continue to vibrate, provided that there is not too much friction. Similarly, after a voltage 'kick,' most electrical systems will continue in oscillation for a time, provided that there is not too much resistance. What characterizes such a *resonant circuit*, and what determines the frequency or frequencies to which it will *resonate?* Although we all probably like to sing in bathrooms, we note that some sizes are better than others for booming resonance at our individual natural singing frequencies. The mechanical properties of such hard rooms determine not only how long a given sound will 'ring' after its source has been shut off, but also the frequencies at which this phenomenon will take place with the greatest effect. Similarly, the resistive and reactive properties of electrical circuits determine how fast such an oscillation will die out (the *damping*) and also the frequency at which it will resonate best. An electrical resonant circuit is one in which the inductive and capacitative reactances are equal. Figure 2.19 shows the resistive and reactive components of a resonant circuit as a function of frequency.

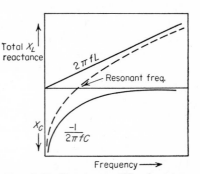

Let us now try to get a picture of how oscillation takes place in such a resonant circuit. Suppose we have a coil and a condenser connected in parallel. If we apply a voltage, the condenser stores energy. As soon as the external voltage source is disconnected, the condenser will discharge through the coil. The increase in current in the coil induces a back EMF, which is in turn applied to the condenser. We have, then, an oscillating current in the circuit because of the fact that the electrical energy is alternately stored in the condenser and in the coil. If there were no

FIG. 2.19. Reactance (X) of a particular inductance (L) and a particular capacitance (C) as a function of frequency. The dashed curve shows the total or combined reactance of the two connected in series (assuming no resistance). The frequency at which the inductive and capacitive reactances are equal (dashed curve intersects abscissa) is the resonant frequency of this particular pair.

resistance in the circuit to dissipate some of the energy in the form of heat, this oscillation would go on forever and we should have an example of perpetual motion. When an instantaneous voltage is applied to a physically realizable circuit, however, the resulting oscillations will be *damped*, *i.e.*, they die out in time. If we wanted to continue the oscillation at a constant amplitude, we should have only to put in the small amount of energy that is dissipated by the resistance in the circuit each time the oscillating cycle occurred.

We can compute the resonant frequency of any combination of inductance and capacitance according to the following formula:

$$f_R = \frac{1}{2\pi \sqrt{LC}}‡$$

Note that a combination of any inductance with any capacitance will yield a frequency of resonance.

Vacuum Tubes

The main reason why we consider electricity at all is that electrical equipment affords easy and precise control of sounds. So far we have considered electron flow through conductors. If our equipment were restricted to components that we have already described, we could not so easily control electric currents as we can with the vacuum tube. Let us consider how this invaluable device operates.

Emission. Molecules of water overcome the cohesive forces in water when the temperature is raised to about 100°C. The result is steam, which is made up of fast-moving molecules that have broken through the barrier of surface tension. In a similar way, we can greatly facilitate the emission of free electrons from certain materials by heating. Having obtained a large number of free electrons, we can then bring a metal plate with positive electrical potential near the emitter; the positive metal plate will attract the electrons and produce an electron flow through the intervening space. This electron flow is usually produced in a vacuum, which prevents molecules of air from impeding the electrons and prevents the emitter from losing its emissive properties.

The simplest kind of vacuum tube is called the *diode* because it has two electrodes: the *cathode,* which is heated by a relatively high current and from which electrons are emitted, and the *plate,* which is made positive with respect to the cathode by means of an external d-c voltage. The voltage used to produce the heating current is called the A voltage and is produced by, for example, the A batteries with which we are familiar. The B battery produces a larger voltage, but the current through the tube (the *plate current*) is not usually nearly so great as that through the heating wires. We shall not take time to discuss the many uses to which diode tubes are put. Suffice it to say that most of these uses depend

‡ For example, to build a circuit that will have a resonant frequency of 1000 cps, a

$$1000 = \frac{1}{2\pi \sqrt{LC}}$$

$$LC = \left(\frac{1}{2000\pi}\right)^2 = 0.000000021$$

coil of 1 henry inductance could be combined with a capacitance of 0.021 microfarads; or 1 millihenry with 21 microfarads.

upon the *rectifying* property of the diode—the fact that electrons flow in only one direction, from cathode to plate, and not the reverse.

Vacuum-tube Amplifiers. If we construct a vacuum tube with three elements, rather than just two, we have a *triode.* Such a vacuum tube provides an extremely important new property, which the British indicate by calling it a *valve:* it amplifies. The problem that the vacuum-tube amplifier solves is that of obtaining relatively large changes in the flow of energy by the application of only small controlling energies. The energy, for example, that is expended when we turn a valve handle in a water system is very small compared with the large amount of energy that becomes available through the opening of the valve.

One important thing to remember is that we are dealing with changing energies, changing currents, and changing voltages. The controller in the vacuum tube is the third element of a triode and is called the *control grid.* It is a spiral of wire interposed between the cathode and the plate. Since like electric charges repel each other, a negative potential on the grid relative to the cathode will tend to repel the electrons that would ordinarily pass by the grid on their way to the plate. The more negative the grid, the fewer electrons will get to the plate, and vice versa. In a valvelike way, then, small energy changes applied to the grid will produce large energy changes in the plate circuit, the circuit through which the electron path is completed from the plate back to the cathode again.

We are not, however, getting something for nothing in the case of the larger energy changes in the output, because, we must remember, there had to be a source of electrical potential (direct current) in the plate circuit in order to have an electron flow at all. The purpose of a vacuum-tube amplifier is to 'magnify' the voltage changes that are applied to the grid so that they appear much larger in the plate circuit. Figure 2.20, for example, shows a single triode amplifier tube that is being used to amplify a small sinusoidal voltage that is applied to its control grid. The voltage gain of the amplifier is given by the ratio of the a-c voltage across the plate resistance (R_p) to the a-c voltage on the grid.

We usually distinguish two general kinds of amplifiers of audiofrequency voltages: the *voltage amplifier* usually comes in the first stages of an amplifying system and is designed primarily to build up large voltages across large impedances without expending much power (*e.g.,* voltage amplifiers ordinarily drive the grid circuits of succeeding vacuum tubes); the *power amplifier* is used to convert relatively large voltage changes in its grid circuit to large changes in power in the output circuit (*e.g.,* power amplifiers are used to drive power-consuming devices such as loud-speakers and earphones).

Besides triodes, many different kinds of vacuum tubes are used as amplifiers. *Tetrodes, pentodes* (see Figs. 2.21 and 2.22), and other elaborate combinations of many kinds of grids are used for special purposes because of their special properties. The fundamental principle of operation of the triode amplifier will suffice, however, to give us a basic understanding of vacuum-tube amplification in general.

The Oscilloscope. An amplifying tube is not the only device that uses electron flow in a vacuum. There are many other applications of the vacuum-tube principle. The one, however, that is most important to us is the *cathode-ray oscilloscope*, for this instrument has become indispensable in acoustics and electronics. It is called an oscilloscope because it gives a visual indication of the waveform of any electrical signal applied to it; it does this because it uses substances (phosphors) that emit light when they are bombarded with electrons. It is described as a cathode-ray

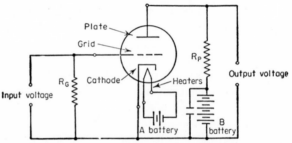

Fig. 2.20. Schematic diagram of a triode vacuum tube used as a voltage amplifier. Voltage input developed across R_G is amplified and a larger voltage is developed across R_P.

oscilloscope because it is a beam of electrons, emitted by the cathode and shaped into a ray by various control anodes, that strikes the phosphorescent screen and thus produces light.

The construction of a simple cathode-ray oscilloscope is shown in Fig. 2.23. The cathode emits the ray of electrons to the screen; the shape of this ray is controlled by the anodes. By adjusting them, one can "focus" a small beam of electrons on the screen and thus produce a spot of light. This spot can be made to move by applying various voltages to the deflecting plates, and these are the most important control elements of the tube. One pair of plates deflects the beam horizontally, and the other deflects it vertically.

To get a picture, say, of a sine wave on the cathode-ray tube, one applies the signal voltage to the vertical plates and a "sweep voltage" to the horizontal plates. The signal voltage makes the spot bob up and down, and with this voltage alone one would see only a line produced by the vertically moving spot. However, by applying a "saw-tooth" wave

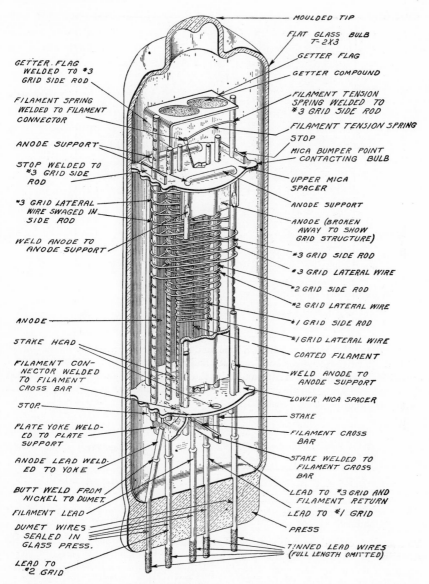

FIG. 2.21. Cutaway drawing of a pentode (three grids) vacuum tube of a type that is used in hearing aids. (*Courtesy of Raytheon Manufacturing Company, Newton, Mass.*)

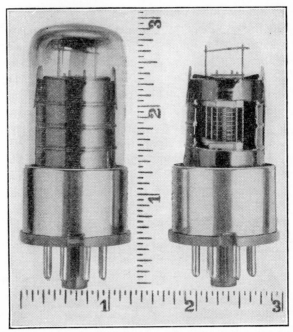

FIG. 2.22. Pentode vacuum tube of a type used in radio receivers. In the picture on the right, the glass envelope has been removed and a window cut in the plate so that the cathode (center) can be seen surrounded by the three grids. The vertical rods on either side of the (thicker) cathode are supports for the grid windings. (*Courtesy of Raytheon Manufacturing Company, Newton, Mass.*)

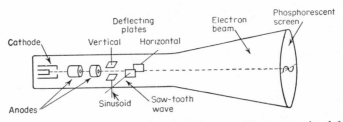

FIG. 2.23. A cathode-ray tube used in an oscilloscope. Electrons emitted from the cathode and accelerated by the anodes bombard the phosphorescent screen. The deflecting plates move the beam of electrons either up and down or from side to side, depending on what deflecting voltages are applied to them.

to the horizontal plates, the spot moves relatively slowly across the face of the screen and then returns quickly back to a "starting position." When this sweeping of the spot across the screen is combined with the movement up and down produced by the signal, one can see, if the signals are properly timed, a perfect picture of the signal. If, for example, we apply a *sinusoidal* voltage to the vertical plates and the saw-tooth wave to the horizontal plates in such synchrony that the spot returns to its original position each time the sinusoid begins from zero, we see on the screen a standing trace of one cycle of the sinusoid.

Obviously an instrument like this is of tremendous value, for its "pictures" can be used to make all sorts of electrical measurements. Indeed it gives us direct information about the frequency, amplitude, phase, and complexity of any given waveform.

Logarithms and the Decibel

Before we proceed to some practical systems that apply the principles of sound and electricity mentioned in this chapter, we must consider certain mathematical transformations that are widely used in these areas. These transformations have to do with the conversion from linear to logarithmic scales, done most often for convenience. The electrical and mechanical energies that are of interest to one studying hearing cover an enormous range of frequencies and intensities. The representation of these large ranges of numbers on linear scales has proved to be extremely clumsy and difficult to handle, and extensive use has therefore been made of the more condensed logarithmic scales.

Linear vs. Logarithmic Scales. The usual kind of *linear scale* consists of successive units that are obtained by *adding* a given unit to each successive number. When we say that we "count by ones," we mean that the unit to be added each time is 1. Thus we count "1, 2, 3, 4," etc. When we count by tens, we still use a linear scale but change the unit of addition to 10: "10, 20, 30, 40," etc. Now suppose that we generate a scale, not by successive addings of a unit, but by successive multiplyings of a unit. If we are to multiply each successive unit in a scale by the number 1, for example, the units of our scale would be "1, 1, 1, 1," etc. If the multiplying unit is 2, we have "1, 2, 4, 8, 16, 32, 64," etc. If it is 10, "1, 10, 100, 1000, 10,000," etc. These scales, whose successive units are multiplied by a particular *base*, are known as logarithmic, or exponential, scales. They are called exponential because any such series may be represented as a certain base number that is raised to successively higher and higher powers (on a linear scale). For example,

$$2^0 = 1 \qquad\qquad 10^0 = 1$$
$$2^1 = 2 \qquad\qquad 10^1 = 10$$
$$2^2 = 4 \qquad\qquad 10^2 = 100$$
$$2^3 = 8 \qquad\qquad 10^3 = 1000$$
$$2^4 = 16 \qquad\qquad 10^4 = 10{,}000$$
$$2^5 = 32 \qquad\qquad 10^5 = 100{,}000$$
$$2^6 = 64 \qquad\qquad 10^6 = 1{,}000{,}000$$
$$2^7 = 128 \qquad\qquad 10^7 = 10{,}000{,}000$$
$$2^8 = 256$$
$$2^9 = 512$$

Such a series should not be strange to anyone who has looked at tuning forks, worked with an audiometer, or had something to do with the piano. We are used to seeing a logarithmic scale of frequency across the top of the audiogram blank. Ordinarily the frequencies are not given in the form of exponents of 2, but rather as 32, 64, 128, 256, etc. It should not disturb us, however, if these same frequencies were to be represented on the audiogram blank as 2^5, 2^6, 2^7, 2^8, etc. Indeed, if it were generally understood that the logarithmic scale of frequency would always be reckoned on the base 2, we would not even have to repeat the 2 but could note our frequencies with the exponent alone. For the same frequencies we should simply have 5, 6, 7, 8, etc.

It is clear from what we have said why such scales are called exponential. But what do they have to do with logarithms? Let us look at the columns of numbers above for the scale of the base 10. Note that the two columns are related to each other in two ways. We can ask the question, What does 10^3 or 10^4 equal? The answer is a number, 1000 or 10,000, respectively. We can also ask the question another way: To what power must 10 be raised in order to yield 1000 or 10,000? This latter question is exactly what one asks when one says, what is the logarithm, to the base 10, of 1000 or 10,000? In other words, the logarithm to a particular base of a number is the power to which the base of the logarithm must be raised for it to equal the number. The $\log_{10}$ (read: "log to the base 10") of 1000 and 10,000 are, respectively, 3 and 4.

The choice of the logarithmic base is a purely arbitrary matter, but there are three bases that are most often used: 10, e, and 2. Logarithms that are based upon $e(e = 2.718.\ldots.)$ are called *natural logarithms* and need not concern us here. Logarithms to the base 2 are used extensively in modern work on the computing machine, and we should recognize that the frequency scale on the old-style audiogram blank is plotted according to such a base. The logarithm to the base 2, for example, of 256 is 8.

The Decibel. The ratio of the power of the loudest sound that we can hear without pain to the power of the weakest sound that we can just detect is about 1,000,000,000,000:1. The inconvenience of writing such a great number of zeros every time we specify a figure of power has been avoided by engineers and physicists by the more convenient notation of writing 10 to some power. We could express the above ratio, for example, as 10^{12}:1. As this notation came to be generally used, it became evident that writing the numeral 10 was waste effort, since it carried no information. It was generally understood that 10 was the base. Thus we find the introduction of the term *bel*, which is simply the exponent alone (with the base 10 understood) that represents a power ratio. The ratio that we have referred to here, for example, is one of 12 bels. It is clear that if we have a power ratio $P_1:P_2$, it may be expressed in bels by the following formula:

$$N \text{ (in bels)} = \log_{10}\frac{P_1}{P_2}$$

The bel was found to be an impractically large unit. For example, a power ratio of 1 bel represents the jump from 100,000 to 1 million or from 1 million to 10 million. Certainly it would be more convenient to use a number that could specify smaller ratios. Therefore the term *decibel* (db) was introduced to represent simply one-tenth the power ratio in bels. Therefore from the previous formula we have

$$N \text{ (in db)} = 10 \log_{10}\frac{P_1}{P_2}$$

If a given power is 100 times as great as another power, the power ratio of 100:1 may be represented as 2 bels or as 20 decibels, because 10 must be raised to the second power in order to yield 100. Dealing with even multiples of 10 we can cite the number of bels immediately, but suppose the power ratio were 6:1. It is difficult to say to what power 10 must be raised in order to yield 6 unless we consult the logarithm tables for the base 10. The $\log_{10}$ of 6 is about 0.78, so a power ratio of 6:1 can be represented as 0.78 bels or 7.8 decibels.

Intensity Level (IL). We have already said that *intensity* (J) is a measure of the energy flow per unit of area per second. But energy per second is power, and so intensity is also a measure of power per unit of area and may be measured in watts per square centimeter. Adding the word "level" to obtain the expression *Intensity Level* (IL) means that we are not talking about an intensity measured in absolute terms of watts per square centimeter, but rather we are talking about a ratio (in decibels) of the intensity in question to a standard intensity. Engineers in telephone work have adopted a particular standard intensity using two criteria: the standard should represent an even power of 10, and it should approximate the weakest sound that can be just heard at a frequency of 1000 cps. The standard reference intensity of 10^{-16} watt/cm²[†] has been adopted. The IL of any sound or of any electrical intensity is the ratio of that intensity (expressed in decibels) to the standard intensity of 10^{-16} watt/cm².

$$\text{IL (db)} = 10 \log_{10}\frac{J_x}{J_0} = 10 \log_{10}\frac{J_x}{10^{-16} \text{ watt/cm}^2}$$

[†] A negative exponent is to be interpreted as the reciprocal of the same number with a positive exponent. Thus, $10^{-16} = 1/10^{16}$.

Sound Pressure Level. During the discussion on measures of the strength of a sound it was pointed out that many measuring and detecting devices in present use operate directly according to the pressure of the sound. We should like to know, therefore, what measure of sound pressure is comparable to the standard intensity, and further, whether or not sound-pressure ratios may be expressed in decibels, as are intensity ratios or power ratios. Intensity and sound pressure are related according to the following formula:

$$\text{Intensity (ergs/sec/cm}^2) = \frac{\text{pressure}^2\ (\text{dynes/cm}^2)^2}{\text{density (gm/cm}^3) \times \text{speed of sound (cm/sec)}}$$

$$J = \frac{p^2}{\rho_0 c} \cos \theta$$

The denominator of this fraction, $\rho_0 c$, is the acoustic impedance of 1 cc of air and is equal, at sea level, at 23°C, to 40 acoustic ohms. You might like to reduce both sides of this equation to grams, centimeters, and seconds in order to show that the relation is valid, at least so far as the units are concerned. If the intensity is measured in watts per square centimeter instead of ergs per second per square centimeter, we shall have to correct by 10^7, since a watt is equal to 10^7 ergs/sec. If we now substitute in the formula to determine what is the sound pressure that corresponds to the sound intensity, in air, of 10^{-16} watt/cm², we have

$$10^{-16}\ \text{watt/cm}^2 = \frac{10^{-7} p^2}{40}$$

If we work out the formula we find that p will be equal to 2 times 10^{-4}, or 0.0002 dyne/cm². This sound pressure is the usual reference[1] for expressing *Sound Pressure Level* (SPL) in decibels.

$$\text{SPL (db)} = 20 \log \frac{p_x}{r_0} = 20 \log \frac{p_x}{0.0002\ \text{dyne/cm}^2}$$

Notice that the coefficient of the logarithm for SPL is 20, whereas for the IL it was 10. Let us see how this comes about. We note from the formula given above that intensity is proportional to the pressure squared. Let us write the formula for SPL taking into account this proportion:

$$\text{SPL (db)} = 10 \log_{10} \frac{p_x^2}{p_0^2}$$

The logarithm of any number squared is equal to 2 times the logarithm of the number. Therefore we have only to remove the 2 from its exponent

---

[1] Another reference that is sometimes used is a sound pressure of 1 dyne/cm², which is also referred to as 1 *microbar*.

TABLE 2.1. SUMMARY OF CIRCUIT ELEMENTS

Component name	Property or function	Symbol	Unit of measure	Unit symbol
Battery	Source of d-c potential		Volt	v
a-c generator	Source of a-c potential		Volt	v
Microphone	Transduce acoustic energy to electric		Volt per dyne/cm²	$\dfrac{v}{dyne/cm^2}$
Earphone	Transduce electric energy to acoustic		Dyne/cm² per volt	$\dfrac{dyne/cm^2}{v}$
Loud-speaker	Transduce electric energy to acoustic		Dyne/cm² per volt	$\dfrac{dyne/cm^2}{v}$
Resistor	Dissipate electric energy by transducing to heat (resistance)		Ohm	Ω
Condenser	Store electric charge, pass a-c, block d-c (capacitance)		Farad; microfarad	f μf
Coil (choke)	Store electric energy in magnetic form, pass d-c, impede a-c (inductance)		Henry	h
Transformer	Change voltage or impedance by transferring electric energy from one coil to another		Secondary voltage: primary voltage	$\dfrac{v_s}{v_p}$
Attenuator	Reduce electric power or voltage		Decibel of attenuation	db
Triode vacuum tube (amplifier)	Amplify electric power or voltage		Decibel of gain	db
Voltmeter	Measure difference in potential (voltage) between two points		Volt	v
Ammeter	Measure current flow through a point		Ampere	a

position after the pressure ratio and multiply the coefficient 10 by the 2. Thus,

$$SPL = 20 \log_{10} \frac{p_x}{p_0}$$

The denominator of these ratios, p_0, will be 0.0002 dyne/cm².

Decibels can, of course, be used to express ratios in electricity as well as those in sound. The ratios having to do with electrical power are treated like those of mechanical power. Since power is related to the voltage squared or the current squared ($P = E^2/R = I^2R$), the coefficient 20 must be used for voltage and current ratios. One can always relate powers by decibels, but voltage or current ratios must always concern voltages and currents acting on or through the same impedance.

References for Further Study

Beranek, L. L. (1949) *Acoustic Measurements*. New York: Wiley. This book treats nearly all the measurements that are made in acoustics and treats as well electrical equipment used in some of these measuring devices. There are excellent basic treatments of microphones, earphones, and loud-speakers.

Kinsler, L. E., and A. R. Frey. (1950) *Fundamentals of Acoustics*. New York: Wiley. This is the most recent introductory work on physical acoustics.

Knudsen, V. O., and C. M. Harris. (1950) *Acoustical Designing in Architecture*. New York: Wiley. This book on sound is very readable and understandable. The acoustic chapters are written for architects who have had no previous background in physics.

Lemon, H. B., and M. Ference, Jr. (1946) *Analytical Experimental Physics* (rev. ed.). Chicago: University of Chicago Press. A clear exposition, together with a good set of illustrations, makes this an excellent source for basic concepts, physics in general, and, of particular interest here, acoustics, wave motion, electricity, and electronics.

Wood, A. (1941) *Acoustics*. New York: Interscience Publishers. This book provides a full treatment of basic concepts in wave motion, propagation velocity, interference, etc. It cannot be read easily by persons without background in general physics and mathematics.

CHAPTER 3

ELECTROACOUSTIC SYSTEMS

IN THE following chapters we shall take up several different kinds of auditory measurement. These measurements are different from one another in the properties of the auditory stimulus that are varied as well as in the responses that are measured. It is the aim of the present chapter to describe some pieces of equipment that are required in the kinds of experimental and clinical measurement that we shall discuss later. The three most important acoustic stimuli that we shall use are pure tones, speech, and noise. We have said something about the distinguishing properties of each of these stimuli in the preceding chapter. We must now consider how we may produce, control, and measure each of these stimuli by means of systems that exemplify some of the principles of acoustics and electricity with which we have been occupied.

TWO BASIC CHARACTERISTICS OF SYSTEMS

We might have discussed certain general properties of electroacoustic systems in the previous chapter, but these particular properties become important only when we deal with actual systems, such as those about to be discussed. No physically realizable system is designed to operate over an infinite range of intensities or of frequencies. Certain limitations are put on both these dimensions by the size and characteristics of the individual components. *Distortion* is introduced when the operation of a given system exceeds the limitations inherent in its design. Two types of distortion are of special interest here.

Frequency Distortion

As we shall see presently, most earphones and microphones do not operate equally well at all frequencies. Mechanical and electrical resonances are responsible for the fact that such devices respond particularly well at one or two frequencies and relatively poorly at all others. When a device produces different amounts of output at different frequencies while the inputs at all frequencies are the same, its response as a function of frequency is said to be nonlinear. The *frequency range* of such a device is that band of frequencies through which the response is essentially linear or flat.

Information on frequency range and frequency distortion is usually given in a graphic representation of the response-vs.-frequency characteristic. Examples will be given in the next section.

Amplitude Distortion

We have spoken above of the situation in which a device performs differently at different frequencies. In an analogous way, certain devices perform differently at different amplitudes. As the electrical signal applied to a loud-speaker, for example, increases, the oscillations of the loud-speaker cannot increase indefinitely. There is a maximum beyond which a loud-speaker cone or diaphragm cannot go. In such a device, then, the response is nonlinear as a function of amplitude, and *amplitude distortion* is introduced. Information about amplitude distortion is usually given in graphic form in a transfer characteristic (see Fig. 5.12).

The range of amplitudes over which a device will perform without introducing amplitude distortion is called the *dynamic range*. In general, microphones, loud-speakers, and earphones operate linearly over rather large dynamic ranges, but electronic equipment such as vacuum-tube amplifiers is usually restricted to smaller ranges.

Unlike usual practice in common law, all components of an electro-acoustic system must be considered guilty of amplitude and frequency distortion until they are proved (by measurement) innocent. Such distortion may be found in the earphones, amplifiers, microphones, and oscillators which we are about to discuss and assemble.

PRODUCTION OF PURE TONES

Some of the most basic psychophysical data in hearing come from experiments in which the pure tone is the stimulus. The fundamental nature of such measurements is related to the simplicity of the pure tone as a physically definable stimulus. The earliest work with pure tones employed the tuning fork. But the tuning fork's output is difficult to control because it does not maintain a constant amplitude: it decreases in time. Other mechanical sources for pure tones were vibrating strings and rods and the siren. Ingenious measurements were made by early workers such as Helmholtz, Rayleigh, Henrici, and Koenig; but not until the application of electroacoustic principles did it become possible to standardize measurement.

The Oscillator-Amplifier-Earphone Combination

We know that an electrical resonant circuit will produce sinusoidally alternating current at a particular frequency. We can measure the amplitude and frequency of this electrical oscillation with an oscilloscope and suitable voltmeters. The problem that then remains is to transduce these electrical oscillations into mechanical oscillations that constitute the pure tone. The two most important devices for accomplishing this transduction are the *loud-speaker* and the *earphone*. We have already mentioned briefly the principle of operation of these two transducers, in particular, the electromagnetic variety. The loud-speaker is less often used in psychoacoustic measurement than is the earphone because the properties of the acoustic environment between the transducer and the listener's ear are more difficult to control when a loud-speaker is several feet away than when an earphone feeds directly into the ear canal.

A fairly complete system for producing pure tones in the ear canal of a listener is represented by the combination of an electronic oscillator to generate sinusoidal voltages, an amplifier to boost these voltages to suitably high levels, an attenuator to control the final voltage on a decibel scale, and an earphone to transduce the electrical voltages into sound pressures. Let us consider each of these components with respect to its role in such a pure-tone-generating circuit.

Earphones.[1] The earphone's job is to transduce into mechanical energy as faithfully as possible the electrical energy that is delivered to it. An earphone is said to be of "high fidelity" if the waveform of the mechanical or acoustic output is a good reproduction of the waveform of the electrical input. Several electroacoustic principles are invoked to produce the three types of earphones most commonly used: crystal, electromagnetic, and electrodynamic.

The *crystal earphone* takes advantage of the fact that certain crystal substances, such as quartz, Rochelle salts, and now some synthetic materials, have what are called *piezoelectric* characteristics. Whenever two faces of a particular cut from one of these crystal substances are moved relative to each other, electrical charges are separated at the two faces, and a voltage is thereby generated across the crystal. Conversely, when a voltage is applied to the crystal there will be inward or outward movement depending on the polarity of the voltage. The cross section of a typical crystal earphone is diagramed in Fig. 3.1A.

Crystal earphones have been used for a great many purposes because of their high efficiency. A relatively large amount of sound pressure can

[1] The term *receiver* is sometimes used to mean an earphone. It will not be used here, in order to avoid confusion with a *radio receiver*.

be generated in the ear canal from the application of a relatively small voltage to such crystals, which ordinarily have high impedance. The main disadvantage of crystal earphones comes from the fact that their resonant frequencies are in the audible range, which means that they perform more efficiently at one or two audible frequencies than at all others. An example is illustrated in the frequency-response curves of Fig. 3.2.

The curves in this figure are the calibration curves of earphones. They tell us how much sound pressure will be generated in the ear canal (or,

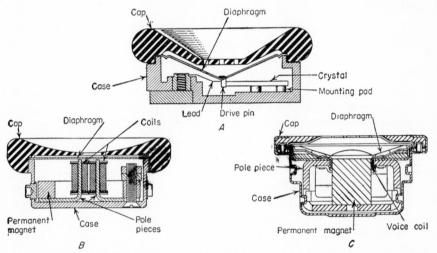

FIG. 3.1. Cross sections of three representative types of earphones: (A) crystal, (B) magnetic, (C) moving-coil, or dynamic. [*Drawings courtesy of Brush Development Company, Cleveland (A); Bell Telephone Laboratories, New York (B); and The Permoflux Corporation, Chicago (C)*.]

more usually, in a standard 6-cc cavity approximating the acoustic impedance of the volume between the eardrum and the diaphragm of the earphone) when a given constant voltage or constant power is applied to the earphone. This quantity is usually given, as it is in Fig. 3.2, as a function of frequency. Curve A of Fig. 3.2 shows the response (as a function of frequency) of one crystal earphone.

The *magnetic earphone*, developed by Bell, is the oldest type of earphone. It is shown diagrammatically in Fig. 3.1B. The moving part is a thin iron diaphragm that is suspended on a circular rim. Underneath the diaphragm, within the shell, there is a small permanent magnet. In addition there is a small electromagnet, the coil of which receives the electrical energy. As the current through this coil varies, the combined strength of the electromagnetic and permanent magnetic fields changes so that the iron diaphragm moves.[1] Magnetic earphones have been found to be very stable; their frequency-response characteristic does not change much over the years, and they are relatively insensitive to rough treatment. A typical frequency-response curve is shown in *B* of Fig. 3.2.

The *electrodynamic earphone*, the standard term for which is now *moving-coil type*, is virtually a little loud-speaker. A sketch is shown in Fig. 3.1*C*. It differs from the magnetic earphone in that its nonmagnetic diaphragm does not move because of attraction or repulsion relative to a magnetic field. Rather, the diaphragm is a thin membrane to which is rigidly connected or cemented a small coil of wire. In the vicinity of this

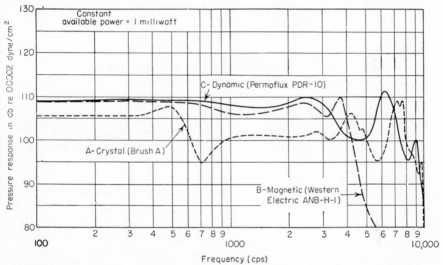

FIG. 3.2. The pressure responses of three types of earphones as a function of frequency. (Crystal, *A*; Magnetic, *B*; Dynamic, *C*.) Constant available power equals 1 milliwatt. (*After Wiener et al.*)

coil is a fixed permanent magnet. As current changes through the coil, fields are built up that cause the coil either to be attracted toward a pole of the permanent magnet or to be repelled away from it. The general principle is, of course, still an electromagnetic one, but the special characteristics of the dynamic earphone provide not only an extensive frequency range but also a relatively flat frequency-response curve (constant as a function of frequency) through that range. The frequency-response curve of a typical high-quality dynamic earphone is given in *C* of Fig. 3.2.

Frequency-response curves are not the only data that reveal the charac-

[1] If there were no permanent magnet, a sinusoidal current through the electromagnet would produce successive 'pulls' on the diaphragm instead of alternating 'pushes' and 'pulls.'

teristics of earphones, but they are the most useful when we are dealing with sinusoidal-voltage inputs and pure-tone outputs. Suppose, however, that we apply a very large sinusoidal voltage to a particular earphone. The diaphragm may be so limited that it cannot satisfactorily complete the excursions that would normally result from this high voltage. In this case, the resulting waveform of the acoustic output would have flattened peaks and troughs. The earphone has thereby introduced amplitude distortion (see previous main section). Amplitude distortion yields additional frequencies, as a Fourier analysis of the distorted sine wave would show.

In order to detect the nonlinearity responsible for such distortion in an earphone, we must first look at the electrical waveform that was applied to the earphone, then look at the acoustic waveform that is produced by the earphone, and finally we must compare the two. Since we are interested in producing the purest tones, we should have some information about the percentage of the output energy that is present in the fundamental frequency and the percentage that is 'wasted' in producing higher harmonics. One other useful datum is the range of intensities between the lowest at which the earphone responds at all and the highest at which it will respond without detectable distortion. This is the *dynamic range*, or the range of linear behavior.

The Oscillator. Now that we have an earphone, we can apply a sinusoidal voltage to it and secure an acoustic pure tone as the output. The next step backward is to generate a sinusoidal voltage. Of course, we might take the 60-cps voltage from a wall plug to begin with, but that limits us in frequency, and the power company is not too particular about the purity of its sinusoid. Instead, let us use the principle of resonance and construct an electric circuit that will oscillate at several frequencies. Suppose, for example, that we wish to generate sinusoidal voltages at the following three frequencies: 500, 1000, and 2000 cps. Using the formula for the resonant frequency of an inductance-capacitance circuit, we obtain the following results:

$$f_R = \frac{1}{2\pi \sqrt{LC}}$$

When $\dfrac{1}{2\pi \sqrt{LC}} = 500$, $\sqrt{LC} = \dfrac{1}{1000\pi}$ and $LC = 0.102 \times 10^{-6}$

When $\dfrac{1}{2\pi \sqrt{LC}} = 1000$, $\sqrt{LC} = \dfrac{1}{2000\pi}$ and $LC = 0.0254 \times 10^{-6}$

When $\dfrac{1}{2\pi \sqrt{LC}} = 2000$, $\sqrt{LC} = \dfrac{1}{4000\pi}$ and $LC = 0.0063 \times 10^{-6}$

The column of three figures on the right tells us the product of inductance and capacitance that will provide resonance at the three corresponding frequencies. If we assume that we have a coil whose inductance is 1 henry, we may use it for all three frequencies in conjunction with three condensers whose capacitances are, respectively, 0.102, 0.0254, and 0.0063 microfarads (farads $\times 10^{-6}$).

In order to keep such a resonant circuit oscillating at its resonant frequency, however, we must replace the energy that is lost in the resistance of the circuit. To do this we connect the resonant circuit to the control grid of a vacuum-tube amplifier. The output of the tube will be greater than the input. Therefore we can take a little of the output and

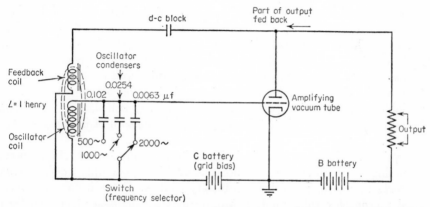

Fig. 3.3. Schematic diagram of a simple oscillator circuit. Three different frequencies of oscillation are available by the combination of any one of three condensers with one fixed coil. Part of the output of the amplifying vacuum tube is returned to the oscillating circuit through the small feed-back coil, which is magnetically coupled to the oscillator coil. (For further explanation see text.)

return it to the grid circuit to keep the resonant circuit oscillating. A simple circuit diagram of such an arrangement is shown in Fig. 3.3. To be sure, this is only one of many possible oscillator circuits. For example, we could have a 'continuous' frequency scale by changing the capacitances in very small steps. A variable condenser, such as the rotating one in your radio, provides very small changes in frequency. Some commercial oscillators take advantage of the special properties of circuits involving the combination of condensers with resistors rather than with coils. But let us continue with what we have and finish the system.

The Amplifier. The vacuum tube in the oscillator circuit is, of course, an amplifier in itself, but we may find that a succeeding power amplifier will give us a larger range of operation. A particular amplifier should provide enough power to the earphone to generate the largest sound pressure that we should ever want to use. For example, if we want SPL's of 130 or 140 db (near the threshold of pain), we have only to consult the calibration curve of our earphone (cf. Fig. 3.2) to determine what the maximum power output of the amplifier should be. In addition, the amplifier must not introduce any distortion (see above) that would cause more frequencies to be put out than were fed in by the oscillator.

Up to this point we have generated some sinusoidal voltages and amplified them to a suitable level. Now we must apply them to our transducer. But what about control? We do not want to present the same frequency and intensity all the time. We have already shown how frequency may be varied, in this case by octaves—and we could have as many different frequencies as we have different condensers. The intensity of the sound, or of the voltage applied to the earphone, must also be changed. This is done most conveniently by means of certain attenuators.

Attenuators. If the radio is playing too loudly, we turn down the *volume control.* Actually, we decrease the amount of voltage that is applied to the grid circuit of an amplifier tube by tapping off only part of a variable resistance. This device is more precisely called a *gain control,* because the end result is obtained by varying the *gain* of the amplifying system.

Equipment, however, that is designed for more precise operations than adjusting the loudness of a radio is more likely to employ *attenuation networks* than gain controls for intensity control. There are at least two good reasons for this. First, not only does a gain control change the signal on a grid, but also a change in gain may produce changes in the characteristics of the amplifier, since these characteristics do not remain constant over wide dynamic ranges (see above, on earphones). Second, an attenuator changes the usable output while maintaining a constant load on the amplifier and permitting the amplifier to operate at constant gain. As the name implies, an attenuator is a weakener. It operates after the amplifier's output. In using an attenuator we set the amplifier at high constant gain for all values of the intensity that we shall use. And we obtain the different values by using different fractions of the energy for our transducer, while the remainder is dissipated in the resistance of the attenuator itself.

One of the most common types of attenuation network, the variable *T pad,* is shown in the output circuit of Fig. 3.4. The arrow on the resistance symbols indicate that they are variable. The design of the network is such that the total resistance into which the amplifier works remains constant, while the percentage of the output that gets to the earphone may be varied. Note that since this is a ratio device, it will give the same results (ratiowise) at high or low levels. Such attenuators are usually calibrated in decibels or some multiple thereof.

The circuit diagram of Fig. 3.4 shows our entire circuit and describes a system that can provide pure tones at any specified SPL and at any of several frequencies. The frequency is determined by the condensers (assuming one coil) and would be marked on a *frequency control*. To specify the SPL of a tone, we have only to measure the voltage that is being applied to the earphone. The frequency-response curve of the

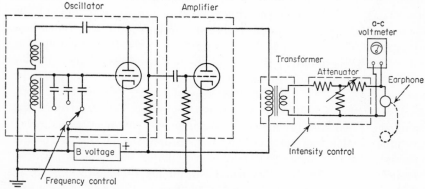

FIG. 3.4. Schematic diagram of apparatus used to produce pure tones. The output of the oscillator is applied to the grid of another amplifying vacuum tube. The output of this tube is fed to an attenuation network so that the variation of the voltage applied to the earphone may be made in decibel steps without changing the impedance to which the power amplifier is coupled. The voltages across the earphone are measured on the voltmeter and may be converted to Sound Pressure Levels by means of a response curve like the ones in Fig. 3.2.

earphone (cf. Fig. 3.2) tells us how much sound pressure corresponds to a particular voltage. In actual operation, we need make the voltage measurement only once, because if the initial level is high enough, we can express an SPL in terms of decibels of attenuation relative to the measured reference pressure.

The Pure-tone Audiometer

What is the difference between the system that we have just described and the clinical audiometer? The answer: very little, especially with regard to basic operation. The essence of pure-tone audiometry is the measurement, at each of several frequencies, of the smallest energy that causes an observer to just hear a tone. The system that is summarized by the diagram in Fig. 3.4 can do just that. How, then, is this system different from commercial audiometers?

Reference Level. The intensity of the tone produced by our home-made system described above is measured on a physical scale with a single physical reference. The manufacturer of audiometers cannot, however, be satisfied with this kind of measure only; he must also build into his system certain properties of a normal auditory system. In other words, our system described above tells us the physical properties of a stimulus that can be just heard, while the clinical audiometer tells us the difference (in decibels) between the SPL of a tone that a listener can just hear and that of a tone of the same frequency that is just heard by a person with normal hearing. On the clinical audiometer, "0 db" is not 0.0002 dyne/cm² but is rather the normal auditory threshold (see Chap. 4). The number of dynes per square centimeter represented by this "0 db" is different at different frequencies because the sensitivity of the ear changes as a function of frequency. A very confusing state of scales!

We must wait until we discuss the concept of the absolute threshold and the attendant problems of measurement before we consider the validity of this 'normal.' At the present time, the "0 db" is specified precisely by the National Bureau of Standards, the American Medical Association's Council on Physical Medicine and Rehabilitation, and the American Standards Association for all manufacturers in this country. It may not represent the hearing of the average man in the United States, but at least it provides a fixed standard against which everybody can make comparable measurements. (See Appendix A.)

Basic Components. The basic parts of the audiometer (see Fig. 3.5A) are essentially those of the system described above. The oscillator circuits may combine either inductance with capacitance (*LC*) or resistance with capacitance (*RC*). The variable frequency control may be continuously variable or adjustable in steps (usually of an octave or half an octave). The amplifying and attenuating systems are different in that the final output with reference to which the attenuators operate must change with frequency as does the normal threshold. In audiometers with fixed frequencies, this compensation that is demanded by the normal sensitivity curve is built in: when the operator switches to a new condenser for a particular frequency, he also switches to an appropriate fixed amount of attenuation for that frequency. In some early audiometers, there was no compensation in the instrument itself; the scale of Hearing Loss in decibels was reckoned from different points on the dial as the frequency was changed. The earphone is ordinarily calibrated as a single unit, and a particular audiometer is designed to work with it. Minute calibrations involve adjustments that can be made only when the over-all system, oscillator-amplifier-earphone, is tested. Thereafter the parts may not be

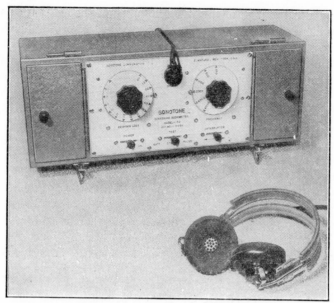

A

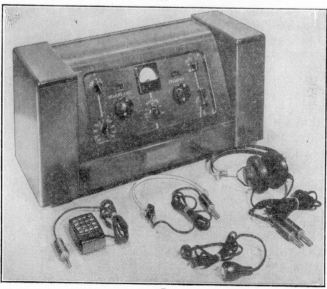

B

FIG. 3.5. Two typical audiometers. In (*A*) is shown a basic (screening) audiometer that is to be used for the measurement of the absolute threshold for tones in the quiet only. In (*B*) is shown a more expensive and elaborate audiometer in which provisions are made for masking, monitored speech, and bone conduction. [*Photographs courtesy of Sonotone Corporation, Elmsford, N. Y. (A); and Audiometer Sales Corporation, Minneapolis (B).*]

interchanged without upsetting the reliability of the calibration relative to the audiometric standard of the National Bureau of Standards.

Additional Features. Clinical audiometers are provided with many extra features (see Fig. 3.5B) that are designed to facilitate clinical measurement. In older audiometers, when the power was turned on, the tone sounded continuously. An interrupter key was provided by means of which the operator could turn off the tone for as long as the key was depressed. It seemed desirable that alternative arrangements should be available in which the tone would normally be off and would be turned on only when the key was depressed. Therefore in newer audiometers both arrangements are provided. Some audiometers have an auxiliary signal light that is turned on by the observer when he hears a tone. The intensity control is marked in decibels of Hearing Loss, so that the operator compares the hearing of his observer directly with that of a normal person. Among other features are devices that are used in bone conduction, masking, loudness matching, and speech audiometry. These will be discussed under these topics in later chapters.

CONTROL OF SPEECH SOUNDS

On many occasions in both the clinic and the laboratory we should like to use, as auditory stimuli, the sounds of speech. Probably the oldest clinical tests of hearing are those that use spoken and whispered speech as test stimuli. Some of the early examinations of hearing that used speech, however, suffered from the shortcoming of using 'live' speech without any monitoring or measuring device to assure the experimenter that successive speech samples were alike.

From what we have already said, it should be clear that at least one way to control the physical characteristics of the speech sounds that are delivered to a listener's ear is to transduce them into electrical voltages and then to apply our controls to the voltages. After we have controlled and measured the electrical phenomena, we may then retransduce to sound. The pure-tone production that was discussed in the last section began with electrical sinusoids, which were then amplified, attenuated, and finally transduced as acoustic tones. Now we must deal with sounds— the sounds of speech—as the beginning product to be amplified, attenuated, measured, etc. Let us first consider the way in which mechanical phenomena, such as the sounds of speech, may be transduced into electrical phenomena.

Mechanoelectric Transducers

Microphones. The device most generally used for changing sound into electricity is the microphone. Operating on the basis of all the principles that were mentioned in our discussion of earphones, the microphone is virtually an earphone in reverse. In describing the physical characteristics of microphones and earphones, the parameter (that which is applied and held constant) of one becomes the dependent variable (that which comes out) of the other. The independent variable may remain frequency. The response of an earphone is sound pressure when a voltage is applied, while the response of a microphone is voltage when a sound pressure is applied.

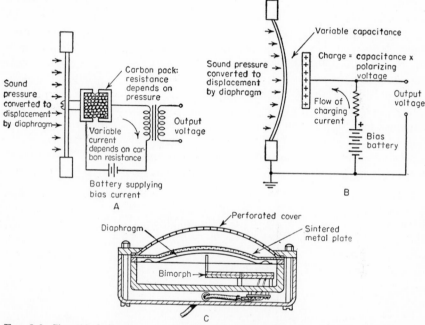

FIG. 3.6. Simplified diagrams of the structure of three basic types of microphones: (A) carbon, (B) condenser, (C) crystal. (*Reproduction by permission from Acoustic Measurements by L. L. Beranek, published by John Wiley and Sons, Inc., 1949, pp. 205, 211, and 240.*)

There are many types of microphones, operating on the basis of more principles than are exploited in the design of earphones. We can do no more than list them and describe them only superficially (see Figs. 2.16 and 3.6). It is impossible to recommend one type over another, because the choice of a microphone for a particular application is always a compromise between the demands of quality, frequency range, sensitivity, and such mundane demands as low cost and small size.

The *carbon microphone* (Fig. 3.6A) is very generally used in military communication systems as well as in telephone systems. The microphone

consists of a small "carbon button" through which flows a direct current
that is supplied by a battery. As sound waves impinge upon the carbon
button, its resistance changes and the magnitude of the current therefore
changes. The changes themselves (a-c component) induce voltages in a
transformer, so that only the current changes corresponding to sound-
pressure changes are found in the output. Two important features that
recommend these microphones are their large output and low cost. Their
mechanical instability is their shortcoming.

The *condenser microphone* (Fig. 3.6*B*) has come to be used as a laboratory standard for making acoustic measurements. This is because of
its extreme reliability and its uniform response through a quite broad
range of frequencies. The microphone is actually a small condenser, made
up of two thin plates, one of which is fixed, the other movable. As sound
waves cause the one plate to move, the capacitance of this condenser
changes because the distance between the plates changes. If a d-c "polarizing" voltage is maintained across the plates, then a change in the
capacitance will produce a small a-c flow, which constitutes the electrical
output of the microphone. The relatively high cost as well as the inconvenient polarizing voltages have prevented the condenser microphone
from coming into very general use, but its appearance in research laboratories is becoming more and more frequent.

The *crystal microphone* (Fig. 3.6*C*) should require little description
because of its similarity to the crystal earphone. We have already said
that the piezoelectric characteristic of most crystal substances is a
reversible process. Not only will movement be produced by the application of voltage (as in the case of the earphone), but also voltages will be
generated across the faces of certain crystals when mechanical stresses
are applied. This characteristic makes certain crystals quite suitable as
microphone elements. Most crystal microphones have a sound-collecting
diaphragm that is mechanically connected to the crystal. As the diaphragm is moved by sound waves, the vibrations are transmitted to the
crystal across which the voltages are produced. Crystals are very unstable
as temperature and humidity change and may be permanently damaged
by high temperatures (*e.g.*, 120°F) and high humidities. Their low cost
and their high efficiency when feeding high impedances contribute to
their very wide use where quality requirements are relaxed.

The *dynamic microphone* (see Fig. 2.16) features high quality and is
probably the most generally used of the types of microphone that we shall
discuss. There are two basic types, both of which depend upon sound
waves that cause a conductor to be moved in the field of a permanent
magnet: the *moving-coil type* has a small coil cemented to a diaphragm
that moves when sound waves strike it; and the *ribbon type* has, instead
of a coil, a small corrugated ribbon of conducting material that is moved

through the magnetic field. Dynamic microphones have low impedance and must, therefore, be matched to amplifier inputs with high-quality step-up transformers. Their stability, combined with relatively good frequency-response characteristics in the audible range, makes them excellent candidates for wide general use in work with speech.

Sound Reproducers. The microphone transduces speech waves into electrical waves. There are other devices, however, that can produce electrical speech waves indirectly (*e.g.*, phonographs and magnetic tape recorders). This is not the time to analyze the different kinds of recording devices and compare them with one another. But we must mention at least one, the phonograph, because of its adaptability to experimental and clinical testing.

You remember that we started off on mechanoelectric transducers because the older tests using speech direct from the speaker's lips were unreliable. To be sure, we can put a voltmeter on the output of a microphone or microphone-amplifier combination in order to monitor or watch our speech output, but these devices can help to cut down on speaker variability only if the speaker is able to correct his speech according to what he sees on the voltmeter or monitoring meter. A better way of ensuring that a speech sample will be the same again and again in repeated tests is to 'can' the speech in some permanent or semipermanent form. This is what we do when we cut a phonograph record. Whereas the movements of an earphone's diaphragm act on a volume of air, the movements of the cutting stylus of a phonograph recorder act on the surface of a blank record in such a way as to engrave the waveform of the speech on the record. If one is interested in how many words of a particular list different individuals can hear, one can record the list and thus be assured that the words will be spoken in the same way each time the list is given to a new listener. Furthermore, the very same test can be given at many places without having to take into account the variability that would result if the speech were to be presented 'live.'

The *phonograph pickup* is the mechanoelectric transducer that changes the recorded wiggles into voltages. The pickup process is, of course, the reverse of the recording process. Generally speaking, then, microphones and phonograph pickups (together with pickups from magnetic tape and wire, etc.) are the transducing gadgets that convert mechanical speech waves into electrical waves. The electrical waves are fed to vacuum-tube equipments that are known as *speech amplifiers*.

Hearing Aids

Perhaps the simplest way to continue our discussion of the processing of speech after transduction is to consider a specific example: a small vacuum-tube hearing aid. First, what is the purpose of a hearing aid?

Sounds that are too weak to be heard by an individual must be made intense enough to become audible to him. The earliest hearing aid was the hand, cupped behind the ear. The ear trumpet performed the same job a little better and was later succeeded by the combination of carbon microphone and crystal earphone. Today the job is done by vacuum-tube amplifiers that are preceded by a transducer such as a microphone and succeeded by an earphone. Let us see, at least superficially, how the modern hearing aid works.

Over-all Characteristics. Most hearing aids provide an acoustic gain of 30 to 50 db. This means that the difference between the SPL that is generated in the ear canal at the output of the hearing aid and the SPL that impinges on the microphone at the input is between 30 and 50 db. Some hearing aids can provide as much as 70 or 80 db of gain, but these are the special ones rather than the run of the mill.

These numbers represent gain averaged over particular ranges of frequencies. The over-all frequency-response characteristics of hearing aids vary greatly from one manufacturer to another and, as a matter of fact, vary quite substantially from instrument to instrument of a given model made by a given manufacturer. The frequency-response characteristic of a hearing aid is a measure of the sound pressure generated by the earphone at each frequency when a constant sound pressure impinges on the microphone.

There has been a great deal of lively discussion over the notion of tailoring the over-all frequency-response characteristic of a hearing aid to particular kinds of hearing loss. Experimental and clinical reports seem not to be reconciled yet, and the battle goes on, but to a lesser degree than in the recent past. The experimental work at the Psycho-Acoustic Laboratory (Davis *et al.*, 1947) has indicated that the closer a manufacturer can come to a smooth, gently rising over-all frequency-response curve, the more successfully will he satisfy the needs of a large majority of the hard-of-hearing consumers. The hearing aids that are presently available still fall short of this requirement, although a good deal of progress toward this goal has been made (see Fig. 3.7).

More noticeable progress has been made by manufacturers in making hearing aids lighter, smaller, and less cumbersome to wear. Batteries and amplifiers now are housed in the same small unit. The conductor leading from the amplifier has been made smaller, sometimes translucent, and generally less noticeable. In addition to their usefulness for bringing amplified sound to hard-of-hearing persons, hearing aids are also useful as examples of a speech-amplifying system.

Hearing-aid Components. A simplified diagram of a typical hearing aid is shown in Fig. 3.8. The sound waves impinge on the face of the microphone, whose output voltage is applied to the grid of the first voltage amplifier. The output of this stage is divided by the gain control, so that only the desired portion of it is applied to the second voltage amplifier. This second stage feeds the final power amplifier, whose output

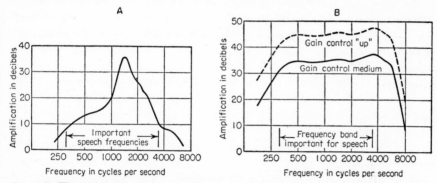

Fig. 3.7. The relation between amplification and frequency in two hearing aids: (A) shows a peaked response; (B) shows a more ideal 'flat' response. (*From Davis*, 1947, *pp.* 173–174.)

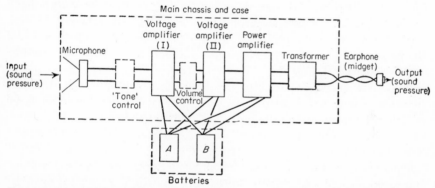

Fig. 3.8. Schematic block diagram of a hearing aid with three stages of amplification. In older aids the batteries were carried in a pack separated from the main case. Newer aids carry the batteries within the main case so that the hearing aid consists of only two main pieces, the earphone and the case with microphone, amplifier, and batteries. Still more recently the microphone has been removed from the main case so that it may be worn outside the clothing while the case itself may be worn underneath. The acoustic gain of a hearing aid (see Fig. 3.7) is the relation between the sound pressure put out by the earphone and the sound pressure put into the microphone.

feeds an impedance-matching transformer. The secondary of the output transformer feeds current through the long connecting cord to the earphone. The earphone is mechanically coupled to a plastic earmold that fits very closely the contours of the wearer's ear canal and part of the outer ear. The filaments of the three vacuum tubes are heated by current produced by a 1.5-volt A battery. The plate voltage for the vacuum tubes is supplied by the larger (22½-, 33-, or 45-volt) B battery.

The *microphone* of the hearing aid is usually a crystal type, although some manufacturers have introduced a magnetic microphone, which is more independent of temperature and humidity than is the crystal. Extremely small crystal microphones can be made inexpensively and are therefore well suited to mass production. It seems fair to say that the greatest bottleneck in the manufacturer's path toward a flat frequency-response characteristic is the small, highly resonant crystal microphone. We must keep in mind that in small components broad frequency range, high fidelity, etc., are constantly pitted against low cost and high output at only certain frequencies.

The *earphone* of a hearing aid is quite different in actual performance from the earphones that we have discussed heretofore, because it is a midget. The relatively good response that is shown in the graphs of Fig. 3.2 is due not only to the characteristics of the transducing elements but also to the design of the cavity of the earphone. With the demand for smaller size and with the advent of the earmold for acoustic coupling to the ear canal, the midget earphones were developed. Inherent in these small devices were the problems of acoustic design in small spaces, and the response of a typical hearing-aid earphone is not nearly so broad or so flat as curves B and C in Fig. 3.2. Most earphones used today are of the magnetic type (see B of Fig. 3.1). Crystals were used more in the past than at present but were found unsatisfactory in operation over large ranges of temperature and humidity. The dynamic hearing-aid earphone has yet to come into general use, although prototype designs have indicated that the dynamic midget earphone should be very satisfactory.

The *amplifier* of a hearing aid usually consists of two stages of voltage amplification and one stage of power amplification. Again we must be reminded that midget versions of vacuum tubes are employed to minimize the required space and battery drain. Probably the greatest limitation on the maximum acoustic power available from a hearing-aid earphone is imposed by the maximum electric-power capacity of the power-amplifier tube. In order to obtain large powers from a vacuum tube, the cathode and plate must be large enough to provide high plate current. Furthermore, electron emission from small cathodes is limited by the available current drain from the A battery.

The *controls* of a hearing aid also operate within the amplifying system. The *volume control* is simply a variable resistance that permits a variable amount of voltage to be applied to the grid of a succeeding amplifier. The *tone control* is a device that switches in different combinations of resistance and capacitance that provide pass bands with different frequency characteristics. Tone controls no longer have the importance that they enjoyed only a few years ago. The experimental work referred to above (Davis *et al.*, 1947) called for no more than two tone positions: the flat frequency-response characteristic and a response rising at the rate of 3 or 6 db per octave.

The hearing aid is not a good example of a system to control sound precisely, because once the hearing aid goes out from the testing laboratory to the user, no measurement is sought or relied on in normal operation. The hearing aid has served us only as an example of an electroacoustic system whose function it is to amplify sounds, particularly sounds that exist in the user's normal environment and that can be picked up by a transducer like a microphone. Now we must turn to another system that amplifies speech but does so with more precise control.

The Speech Audiometer and Group Hearing Aid

The measurement of hearing for speech depends in part upon the availability of speech sounds at known intensities. We have already discussed some of the problems associated with the variability in the instantaneous intensity of speech and will have more to do with such matters in Chap. 5. Let us assume now that we can obtain meaningful averages of the SPL or IL of a given speech sound or series of speech sounds. As in pure-tone audiometry, so in speech audiometry one of the things we wish to know is how little energy we can provide and still have a listener hear some speech, or, more rigorously, correctly repeat speech. The psychophysical problems will be treated later, but now we must concern ourselves with gadgets that can present speech stimuli at known variable intensities so that we can make such measurements.

The progress from crude testing to the most precise technique now available is illustrated in Fig. 3.9. The direct live speech may be made less variable by adding a monitoring meter to the sensory equipment of the talker. Further control is provided by the microphone-amplifier combination that permits adjustment of the level during the speaking. Finally, putting the speech on a record or tape in permanent form and then using the record for testing represents just about the best we can do.

A Typical Speech Audiometer.[1] It is difficult to talk about a typical speech audiometer because there are so few available commercially. Most well-equipped clinics have custom-built equipment, the versatility

---

[1] Specifications for a clinical speech audiometer have been published by the American Medical Association (see Appendix A). Those of the American Standards Association were not available when this book was completed.

of which is equaled by only a few of the commercial products. But again, let us try to build something up from what we know of the parts.

We want to present lists of words at specifiable SPL's. In some situations we shall want the testing procedure to be somewhat elastic and shall therefore use live speech that is monitored and controlled. In other

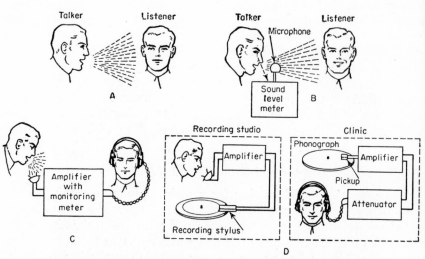

Fig. 3.9. Sketches illustrating the evolution of speech audiometry. (See text.)

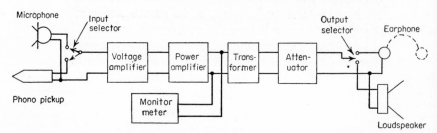

Fig. 3.10. Schematic block diagram of equipment for speech audiometry. The input may be fed from either a microphone or the pickup of a phonograph, and the output may be fed to either an earphone or a loud-speaker. (For further explanation, see text.)

cases, where we can afford to be rigorous, we may use recorded versions of the tests in conjunction with a phonograph pickup. Our speech audiometer should, therefore, have a choice of input: either a microphone which will transduce live speech or a phonograph pickup which will transduce canned speech.

After suitable amplification, as shown in Fig. 3.10, the electrical speech waves are transduced through an earphone for precise testing or through a loud-speaker, which we may wish to use in specific instances, such as the measurement of hearing with and without a hearing aid. (The reliability of testing with a loud-speaker is difficult to interpret, especially in rooms where proper acoustic treatment has been neglected.) If we have a calibration curve of the earphone, we can compute the SPL of the speech from a measure of the speech voltage that is applied to the earphone. When we use recorded speech, this measurement is facilitated by the

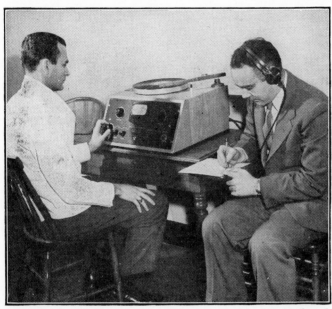

FIG. 3.11. A speech audiometer in use. The source of speech is the phonograph record on top. The monitoring meter, seen on the control panel, permits the operator to adjust the gain of the amplifier so that the level of speech in the earphone can be kept constant. The listener is reporting the words heard by writing them down. (*Photograph courtesy of Grason-Stadler Company, Cambridge, Mass.*)

provision, on the record, of a continuous pure tone whose intensity is known to be the same as the average monitoring level of the speech. With the kind of setup that is summarized in Fig. 3.10 we can find out how much speech sound pressure is needed for a listener to reach a certain criterion of speech hearing, and further, we can present the speech at known fixed levels to measure the amount of intelligibility (see Chap. 5) that a listener can obtain.

The Group Hearing Aid. The important point to be presented here is that we have already, in the last paragraph, described a group hearing aid. Such a speech audiometer can, for example, be used not only as a measuring device but also as a nonportable hearing aid with known amount of gain and output sound pressure. In training situations, where more than one listener is to be accommodated, several earphones may be used in parallel on the output of the amplifying system. The necessary precaution to be taken concerns the new lower impedance of the additional earphones in parallel that must be newly matched to the output of the amplifier or the output attenuator.

Group hearing aids that are available at the present time incorporate the features of a speech audiometer that have been described above. Two

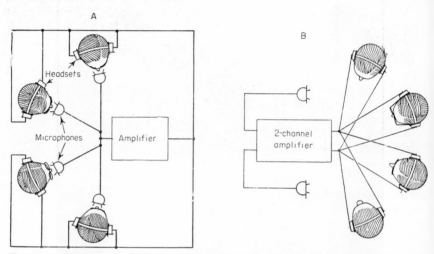

Fig. 3.12. Two types of group hearing aids. (A) Multiple-microphone unit: each student speaks into his own microphone, all microphones feed the same amplifier. and the single amplifier feeds the earphones of all students. (B) Master-microphone unit: in this case, two separate microphones feed separately two amplifiers, one amplifier feeds the right earphone of all headsets, and the other amplifier feeds the left earphone.

general types may be distinguished: the multiple-microphone unit and the master-microphone unit. They are shown in block-diagram form as parts A and B, respectively, of Fig. 3.12. The multiple-microphone unit provides each listener with his own microphone and earphone. The microphones that are used need be no more expensive than the crystal type, and the room in which such apparatus is used need receive no special acoustic treatment.

Recently, improved performance has been reported (Hudgins) with the master-microphone (or two-microphone) group hearing aid, in which a single microphone or pair of microphones suspended from the ceiling pick up the speech of the teacher and all the listeners (see Fig. 3.13). Some

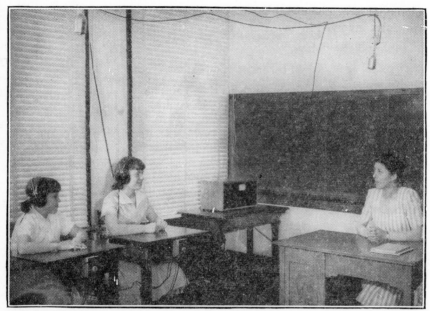

Fɪɢ. 3.13. A master-microphone unit in use. The two microphones, suspended from the ceiling, permit the students and teacher to move their heads freely without having to direct their speech to individual microphones. When such an arrangement is used, certain precautions, such as a rug on the floor, drapes on the windows, and absorbing material on the walls and ceiling, must be used in order to avoid undesirable effects from reverberations. (*Photograph courtesy of Grason-Stadler Company, Cambridge, Mass.*)

increase in the realness of the communicative environment is provided by this arrangement, particularly when each of a pair of microphones feeds separately each of the two earphones in each headset (Hirsh, 1950*b*).

SUMMARY

This chapter was not intended to make the reader a designer of electro-acoustic equipment for the measurement or training of hearing. The basic concepts that have been outlined may, however, serve to make the reader a more intelligent purchaser and user of such equipment. There is not so much difference between the equipment used by the laboratory investigator and that used by the clinical worker as has been implied by some of the misunderstandings in the experimental and clinical literature. Pure tones are produced by amplifying the output of tuned circuits and then transducing the amplified currents. This is true whether a lot of apparatus is spread over a laboratory workbench or is contained in a beautiful wood cabinet. Speech may be produced in measured amounts with the aid of microphones or phonographs and associated amplifying equipment. The principles involved in the design of all such equipment do not change as we move from the laboratory to the clinic or classroom.

References for Further Study

Davis, H. (1947) *Hearing and Deafness.* New York: Murray Hill (now Rinehart). Chapters 6 and 7 discuss some of the equipment that is used in clinical audiometry and auditory training.

Olson, H. F., and F. Massa. (1939) *Applied Acoustics,* 2d ed. Philadelphia: Blakiston. This is an excellent text on the principles of acoustic equipment. It is advanced, however, and requires some background in mathematics.

Watson, L. A., and T. Tolan. (1949) *Hearing Tests and Hearing Instruments.* Baltimore: Williams & Wilkins. Parts I, III, and V discuss audiometers and hearing aids.

CHAPTER 4

ABSOLUTE THRESHOLD FOR PURE TONES:
THE AUDIOGRAM

INTRODUCTION

WE HAVE discussed a class of physical events, called sounds, some of which can be heard by nearly all human beings, others by only some human beings, and still others not at all. This chapter will be concerned with the determination of the physical dimensions of sounds that are *audible*. Sounds that cannot be heard at all are inaudible either because the frequency is too high or because the intensity is too weak. Some persons cannot hear some of the sounds that are audible to most people; these persons constitute the *hard of hearing*. When we determine the physical characteristics of sounds that are audible to *normal* people, we are concerned with the problem of measuring the absolute auditory threshold—with respect to either frequency or intensity. If, on the other hand, we assume that we know the physical requirements for sounds to be heard by the normal man and wish to compare those sounds that are just audible to a particular individual with those sounds that are just audible to the normal individual, we are concerned with the audiogram, a relative kind of threshold.

We shall restrict ourselves in this chapter to those sounds that are known as pure tones. Measurement of pure tones, you will remember, is relatively simple, because a pure tone is characterized by only one intensity and only one frequency. A complete description of a pure tone is given when the frequency, intensity, and phase are specified.

We are now interested in determining the sensitivity of the human auditory system to these sinusoidal pure tones. When we measure the sensitivity of a system, we really do nothing to the system itself but rather do something to the stimulus that we put into it. We do not even measure the system but rather measure the stimulus that is just adequate to evoke some response from the system. This quantitative measure of a stimulus that is just audible *is* the *absolute threshold*. *Threshold* is a quantity of the stimulus that tells us something about *sensitivity*, which is a property of the system. These two measures are reciprocally related. If a person is relatively insensitive to a particular tone, his threshold for that tone is high. When a person is highly sensitive to a particular tone, his threshold for that tone is very low.

The determination of the threshold for a tone of a particular frequency for any one individual is complicated by many problems inherent in psychophysical measurement. For one thing, an adequate description of the stimulus must be given. If we are concerned with the minimum quantity of sound that must be provided for a single frequency, we must decide on the quantitative measure to be used—whether sound pressure or energy (see Chap. 2, Magnitude of a Pure Tone). We must decide further on the locus of the measurement of this quantity—whether at the eardrum, in an equivalent coupler, or in a field.

Not only does the specification of the stimulus present problems, but also the measurement or description of the response is not so simple as it might appear. What do we really mean when we say that a person "hears a tone"? Strictly speaking, we can never mean more than that he responds in a certain way. But what sort of response will we accept as adequate evidence that a person hears? There are many responses in the human repertoire that might be used as evidence of hearing. Some of these responses are easier to observe than others, and some are more easily quantified than others. If he tells us that he hears, we may accept his verbal behavior as an indication of his perception—or, more precisely, we define his perception in terms of his verbal behavior. Sometimes we give verbal instructions with which the observer must comply in order that we may measure his response. Examples are "Extend your index finger" or "Press a signal button" when a tone is heard. Since we have no way of actually observing a sensation taking place in the experience of an observer, we usually take his word that he hears a tone or assume that he has understood our instructions and state that he hears a tone when he raises a finger or presses a button. We measure the *threshold of hearing* by measuring the threshold for responding to sound.

When we say that a person's threshold at 1000 cps is 20 db SPL, what do we mean? Something happens at 20 db that does not happen at 15 db and is qualitatively different from something else that happens at 25 db. We say that this person can "just hear" this 1000-cycle tone at 20 db. Does "just hear" mean that he can hear this tone once, if we present it to him a hundred times, or does it mean that he can hear it a hundred times? Is this tone presented to him continuously, or does the presentation consist of a series of pulses of tone at this particular intensity? When we arrived at the figure 20 were we reducing the intensity or were we increasing the intensity? This group of questions centers around the problem of the psychophysical procedure for making the measurement. Since it is known that the same thresholds will not be obtained under all psychophysical procedures, a rigorous definition of the statement, "He just hears a tone," is required.

It is one thing to measure a single threshold on one individual and quite another to measure *the* absolute threshold for *the* normal human auditory system. *A normal absolute threshold* is a concept that must be inferred statistically from a group of individual thresholds measured on an adequate sample of a particular population. Once we can measure the stimulus and the response, we can specify an individual threshold. But if we wish to compare an individual threshold with that of the *normal listener*, we must previously have obtained some statistical norm from the population with which we wish to make our comparison. For the sake of convenience, we might introduce two terms to distinguish these two kinds of measurement: *experimental audiometry* is concerned with the measurement of thresholds in terms of the physical dimensions of the stimulus, whereas *clinical audiometry* has to do with the measurement of Hearing Loss, *i.e.*, the difference between a particular threshold and a comparable threshold norm.

EXPERIMENTAL AUDIOMETRY

This section will deal with one particular phase of the experimental measurement of hearing, namely, the measurement of the sensitivity[1] of the human auditory system to pure tones of different frequencies. We shall consider first the important factors in the measurement of a set of thresholds for any one individual, namely, description of the stimulus, specification of the response, and the psychophysical procedure. Finally, some statistical considerations will concern certain inferences about a normal threshold.

Measurement of the Stimulus

A determination of the threshold for an auditory stimulus at a particular frequency requires a specification of the quantitative measure of the stimulus that will be used. It will be most convenient for us to restrict ourselves to the concepts of sound pressure and the analogous electrical voltage. All the procedures that we shall discuss concerning the measurement of the absolute threshold will involve the use of devices that produce sound waves by converting electrical energy into mechanical energy. We ignore the tuning-fork tests for the present, not because they are anti-

[1] The word *sensitivity* is used where others have used *acuity*. By analogy to visual acuity, auditory acuity might refer to the ability to separate two auditory stimuli in space, in pitch, or in loudness. To avoid this ambiguity, the use of *auditory sensitivity* with reference to the absolute thresholds seems preferable.

quated and no longer useful, but rather because they are treated fully elsewhere (Fowler, 1947; Bunch) and do not yield the kind of quantitative information that we seek here. Indeed, it is probable that quantification in the field of audition has waited upon the development of electronics and associated areas of electroacoustics: there was marked progress in the measurement of hearing after the advent of the vacuum tube.

Two special applications of the vacuum tube are of interest in this field: (1) its use as an amplifier and (2) a special case of the same, its use as an oscillator or generator of sinusoidal voltages (see Chap. 3).

For the present, we shall concern ourselves with the measurement of the Minimum Audible Pressure (MAP) of pure tones at several different frequencies. Sound pressure is usually measured in *bars* or *dynes per square centimeter* (units of force per unit of area). The range of pressures to which the human auditory system is sensitive covers a great number of dynes per square centimeter. The smallest sound pressure that we can hear may be around 0.0002 dyne/cm², and a very loud sound that is not intense enough to be painful might be 2000 dynes/cm²—a 10-millionfold range! The mere notation of pressure throughout such an extensive range is extremely inconvenient, and the use of a logarithmic scale of decibels is more usual. We should remember from the previous discussion (Chap. 2) that the decibel is a mathematical convenience that allows us to convert a linear scale to a logarithmic scale of base 10. We need not repeat any of the previous discussion on this kind of logarithmic unit, but we should mention here some of the "levels" to which decibel ratios may refer.

In the case of sound pressure, the usual reference is 0.0002 dyne/cm². When we specify a certain sound pressure as being *n decibels SPL*, we mean that 20 times the logarithm of the ratio of the specified sound pressure to 0.0002 dyne/cm² is *n*:

$$n = 20 \log \frac{x(\mathrm{SP})}{0.0002 \ \mathrm{dyne/cm^2}}$$

Most of the measurements discussed in this chapter will be based on a reference of 0.0002 dyne/cm². Some experimenters state sound pressures relative to a reference of 1 dyne/cm². When this is done, this reference is usually stated.

Sensation Level and *Loudness Level* are two other measures of the intensity of a sound relative to a specified reference. The references for both these measures, however, involve the response of a human auditory system (SPL does not). The expression *n decibels Sensation Level* indicates an intensity that is *n* db above the intensity at threshold; *n decibels Loudness Level* (see Chap. 8) indicates a tone that is judged to be equal in loudness to a 1000-cps tone whose SPL is n db. Both Sensation Level and Loudness Level are *physical measures* although their references are determined by a psychological process—*i.e.*, threshold response or judgment of equal loudness (see Chap. 8).

Where and how do we measure the sound pressure? The device that is ordinarily used is a microphone whose output voltage has been measured (by its manufacturer) for given amounts of sound pressure. But since sound pressure varies with distance from the source, we may wonder where to place the microphone.

It is difficult to introduce a microphone and probe tube into the ear canal each time we do an experiment, and furthermore, the equipment needed is beyond the financial capabilities of the many places where psychoacoustic measurements are made. Anyone who buys an earphone, therefore, prefers to compute the sound pressure from a measurement of the voltage that is applied to the earphone. The computation is done by means of the frequency-response curve, such as that in Fig. 3.2. But what is the response, and how did the manufacturer of the earphone measure it?

The response of an earphone is usually measured in terms of the sound pressure developed in a *standard cavity* of 6 cc (see Fig. 1, Appendix A). Such a cavity represents the acoustic impedance that would be presented to the earphone by an average human ear. (The size of the human ear canal varies widely from person to person.) The manufacturer can set up such a cavity in his laboratory and measure the sound pressures in it at any time he wishes. He does not have to depend upon a real ear. The same cavity can be reproduced and used in many different laboratories, so that any measurements made on the cavity can be applied generally and are not limited to the characteristics of a particular individual's ear. The pressure that is developed in a cavity is not the same as the actual pressure generated in a listener's ear canal by the same earphone, but the pressure in the cavity can be measured more easily and more reliably and then can be related to measurements of pressure at the entrance to the ear canal, at several points along the ear canal, and finally at the eardrum.

A typical arrangement of apparatus needed for measuring the response of an earphone that feeds a standard cavity is shown in Fig. 4.1. A particular voltage is applied to the earphone and is measured at the input terminals of the earphone. The earphone is coupled directly to the cavity, and the microphone's face is placed at the opposite end of the cavity. The microphone has been calibrated[1] previously by its manufacturer, and from its calibration curve we know that a pressure of, for example, 1 dyne/cm² impinging on its face will cause a certain voltage to be generated at its output terminals. If, now, we measure the voltage that the micro-

[1] Details of this calibration procedure are given in Beranek, pp. 735–750.

phone puts out when the earphone is producing an unknown pressure on the microphone's face, we can, by referring to the microphone's calibration, compute what the pressure must have been in the cavity.

One way of specifying the sound pressure at threshold for a particular frequency is, then, to specify the amount of sound pressure that would have been generated by the same earphone, had the same voltage been applied when the earphone was coupled to a cylindrical volume of 6 cc. Now the purist might say, "But this isn't the 'real' stimulus intensity; this is an equivalent sound pressure. What is the 'real' pressure at the eardrum or at the entrance to the ear canal?" Figure 4.2 shows the results

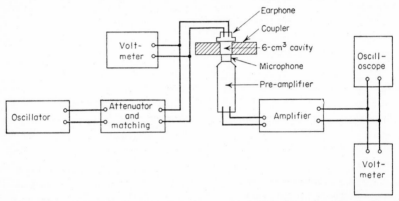

FIG. 4.1. Schematic block diagram of equipment for calibrating an earphone when the voltage output of a standard microphone, for a given sound pressure impinging on its face, is known. A fixed, measured voltage is fed to the earphone at several frequencies. Measuring the voltage output of the microphone permits computation of the sound pressure that the earphone puts out from the calibration curve of the microphone. A typical result from such measurements appears as curve (A) of Fig. 4.2.

of recent measurements that correlate the sound pressure developed in a 6-cc coupler with (1) the sound pressure at the entrance to the ear canal, (2) sound pressures along the ear canal, and, finally, (3) sound pressure measured within a millimeter of the eardrum itself (Wiener and Ross). In other words, given a particular earphone with a known sound pressure as measured in a 6-cc coupler, we can compute any of these sound pressures by referring to the curves of Fig. 4.2.

Another kind of pressure measurement is that of the Minimum Audible Field (MAF) for particular frequencies. Here the quantity measured is not supposed to represent the intensity of the stimulus that actually gets to the ear or the eardrum, but rather is the measure of the intensity of a sound field in which the observer will be placed. The measurement of the intensity of this field is made with a microphone at the place where the observer's head would be. Some interesting discrepancies between the

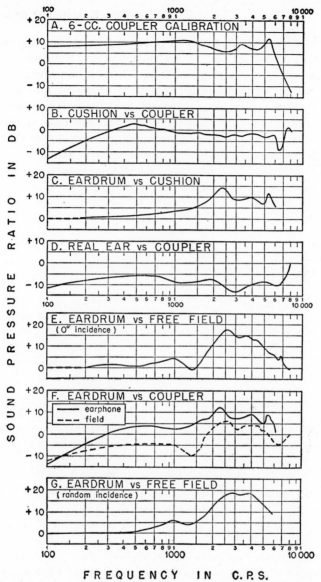

FIG. 4.2. Relations among different kinds of sound-pressure measurements. (A) Sound pressure developed in a 6-cc coupler by a dynamic earphone. (B) Pressure measured with a probe tube under the earphone cushion relative to the coupler pressures in (A). (C) Sound pressures measured at the eardrum with a probe relative to the pressures under the cushion in (B). (D) Field pressures, measured relative to coupler pressures, that sound equal in loudness to the coupler pressures. (E) Eardrum pressures measured with a probe in an open ear canal (no earphone) relative to free-field pressures. (F) Eardrum pressures relative to coupler pressures in both covered and open ear canal. (G) Same measures as in (E), except that the free-field reference is for a sound whose angle of incidence relative to the sagittal plane of the head is random. The free-field reference for curve (E) is that of sounds directly in front, 0° angle of incidence. (*From Pollack,* 1949.)

93

MAF and MAP measures still have not been satisfactorily explained (Rudmose).

These measures of sound pressure in the field, in the ear canal, or at the eardrum are not necessarily the most valid measures of the intensity of an auditory stimulus, but it turns out that they are the most convenient. Electrical and acoustic engineers have developed rather precise techniques for converting electrical measures to measures of sound pressure. Most of the equipment that is used in the course of presenting and measuring auditory stimuli is calibrated very simply in terms of voltage and sound pressure.

There are other measures, certainly, that may be as adequate in particular situations. In discussing the value of the absolute threshold, some experimenters have computed the actual amount of displacement or movement of the eardrum. We can push this measuring process further and further inward and talk about the thresholds for different stages in the auditory system. In order to specify the stimulus for the over-all auditory system, our measure of intensity of the stimulus must be made before, or as, it hits the most peripheral part of the system. If one wanted to determine the threshold of excitation for the end organ within the *cochlea*, one might very well use as a measure of the stimulus the displacement of the *stapes*. If one wanted to measure the threshold for excitation of first-order neurons in the auditory nerve, one might very well use the amplitude of movement of the basilar membrane as a measure of the stimulus to neural excitation.

We are concerned, however, with some measure of the stimulus that is presented to the auditory system as a whole, and we restrict ourselves to a physical measure of the sound wave before, or as, it enters the ear canal or impinges on the eardrum. This convenient external site sometimes leads us astray, as we shall see when we come to discuss recruitment (Chap. 8).

Description of the Response

In our introduction to this chapter we said that the basic problem for the measurement of an absolute threshold is to specify what is the weakest sound that will just yield a specified response. We have now specified how we shall measure the quantity of the physical stimulus—*i.e.*, in terms of sound pressure. But now we come to an equally important problem: what do we mean by saying that a person can hear a tone?

We can never know whether or not the person 'really hears' a tone— whatever that means. We can only observe some response and experimentally establish a relation between that response and the threshold that we are trying to measure. Usually we accept a verbal response as a good indication that a person is perceiving a stimulus. If we want to infer from the observation of this verbal response that the person is actually hearing a tone, we must make the assumption that the observer can and does tell us what he experiences. If we are to be precise, however, we must specify any threshold measurement as a threshold for a particular response.

In clinical audiometry it has been customary to use the pressing of a signal button or the extension of a finger as the threshold response. The threshold that we would measure in this case would be that value of the stimulus that just yields a response, such as extending the finger or pressing the button. But there are many responses in the behavior of the human organism that could be used as indicators for the perception of a tone. Most of them are made only in so far as the observer wants to make them. The voluntary nature of this type of response leads us to call such a class of responses *subjective*.

There have been attempts recently to get around the necessity for taking an observer's word that he hears a tone. Some investigators seek an *objective* measure of the auditory threshold (Kobrak; Doerfler; Bordley and Hardy). This kind of measure utilizes certain responses that may be reflexly connected with auditory stimuli and certain others that may easily be conditioned to auditory stimuli. One may raise some rather serious objections to the interpretation of such measurement as equivalent to the measurement of the threshold for perceiving a tone. Indeed, it is not necessary to assume that an observer perceives a tone simply because his pupils contract when we present a tone. Perception probably involves the highest levels of the nervous system, whereas objective responses such as have been listed in recent literature might very well be functions of lower levels in the nervous system. On an intuitive basis we are loath to describe perception in terms of involuntary responses or reflexes. Rather we tie the concept of perception to that of voluntary behavior. We shall return to this problem in Chap. 10.

We must proceed on the assumption that measurement of a threshold depends, at least in part, on the choice of response to be observed. We do not know whether the variability associated with the choice of response is of the order of 1 to 2 db or 10 to 20 db, because the data on this particular relation are meager.

Psychophysical Procedure

The measurement of an auditory threshold on any particular individual might be a very simple task were it not for the fact that any particular individual's sensitivity to auditory stimuli varies from time to time. We may on one day find that a certain intensity of tone is sufficient to cause the observer to extend his finger, and on another day we may well present the same stimulus intensity and find no such response on the part of the observer. Such considerations as these lead us to the notion that a measurement of threshold on an individual is a statistical measurement, *e.g.*, an average. This means that a meaningful threshold measurement cannot be made with any single presentation of a stimulus but rather involves many presentations at several points in time. If we were to say that a reliable and meaningful threshold for auditory stimuli could not be determined unless we had presented a particular stimulus 100 times, to what percentage of these 100 presentations must an observer successfully respond in order for us to specify a threshold?

In classic psychophysical experiments the shape of the curve that relates the percentage of stimuli to which an observer responds to the intensity of the stimulus (cf. Fig. 4.4) has seemed so similar to that of the normal ogive (*i.e.*, the cumulative normal-distribution curve) that statistical concepts, based on the theoretical normal-distribution curve, have been applied to these psychophysical functions. We might, of course, specify any frequency of response between 0 and 100 as a criterion of threshold, but since we have a distribution of such frequencies, we prefer to use the single value that best characterizes the distribution. This is the *mean* or *median* of the distribution, which usually corresponds to 50 per cent.

Another feature that we would look for in any threshold criterion is that of *test sensitivity*, by which we mean the ability of the test to specify very precisely the particular threshold value. Now, if we are to define threshold in terms of a certain percentage of response on the part of an observer, we should like to use that percentage that changes most rapidly as a function of intensity. Suppose we were to say that a threshold intensity of a stimulus would be defined as that intensity to which the subject responds 100 per cent of the time. Obviously, there is almost no intensity that will yield exactly a 100-per-cent response from an observer if the experiment is carried out long enough. The same is true of a threshold defined as 0 per cent. We might reduce our criterion a bit and say that we would call threshold that intensity of the stimulus at which a person responds 75 per cent of the time. Indeed this would be quite satisfactory, and presumably could be achieved within one experimental session. If we look at our curve in Fig. 4.4, however, we note that the percentage of response is changing most rapidly as a function of intensity around 50 per cent. On this practical count, as well as the theoretical one mentioned above, 50 per cent has considerable advantage, and since it has no obvious disadvantages except for the fact that we cannot hit it exactly in every session, it is ordinarily used in a definition of threshold.

In a preceding discussion of psychophysics (Chap. 1) we have outlined the three most commonly used classic psychophysical procedures for measuring sensory thresholds. These were the methods of *adjustment, limits,* and *constant stimuli.* The measurement of an absolute auditory threshold may also use any one or all of these procedures. In certain respects, however, some procedures have considerable advantage over others.

Method of Adjustment. Perhaps the easiest and quickest way to obtain a threshold measurement with an intelligent observer involves the method of adjustment. In order to measure a threshold for any given frequency,

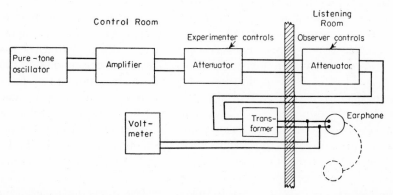

FIG. 4.3. Schematic block diagram of apparatus used to measure the auditory absolute threshold by the method of adjustment. After the experimenter sets a certain level with his attenuator, the observer controls the intensity of the sound with his attenuator in the listening room. The experimenter records setting on both attenuators and computes the Sound Pressure Level from the earphone's response curve and the actual voltage readings across the earphone.

we must provide the observer with some control over the intensity of the tonal stimulus. We must have at hand a source of sinusoidal voltage of adjustable frequency (*e.g.,* a vacuum-tube oscillator), a means of controlling the voltage [*e.g.,* a resistive attenuation network adjustable in decibel (or some multiple of decibel) steps], a voltmeter that measures voltage across the transducer, and, finally, a transducer (*e.g.,* earphone), which converts voltage to sound pressure and is calibrated, *i.e.,* whose SPL at different frequencies for a given amount of voltage applied is known. A block diagram of a typical setup is given in Fig. 4.3.

The instructions given to the observer are extremely important. We must ask our observer to adjust the intensity of the tone that is presented to him so that it is "just audible." We might tell him to begin with the intensity of the tone high enough to be clearly audible and then to decrease

it until the tone disappears. Then he should increase it again until it becomes just audible. Repetition of such a procedure should enable the
observer to bracket a region of uncertainty within which there will be a
point that he may judge to be at threshold. Of course, the rate at which
the intensity is changed, as well as the distance above and below threshold
that marks off the operating range of intensities, is left entirely up to the
observer. The tone that the observer controls may be continuous or
periodically interrupted. If it is continuous, the threshold will be higher
than if it is interrupted, especially for high frequencies. Somehow, the
organism seems to attend more readily and perhaps is more sensitive to
stimuli that change than to stimuli that do not change (see Fig. 4.5).

After a brief experimental period we will have obtained several intensities that the observer has judged to be thresholds for one frequency.
Unless he is a very unusual observer, he will not have repeated the same
intensity for each adjustment. Therefore we shall have to infer the 'true'
threshold from the group of measures obtained. These points will become
clearer if we go through a typical procedure briefly with the apparatus of
Fig. 4.3.

The particular frequency to be used will be selected on the oscillator.
Let us say that we shall attempt to find an observer's sensitivity to a
2000-cps tone. We set the oscillator frequency at 2000 cps and impress
the output voltage across the attenuator. The output of the attenuator
is coupled to a matching device (either a network or a transformer) whose
function it is to match the impedance of the earphone to that of the preceding component of the circuit. A vacuum-tube voltmeter across the
earphone terminals will tell us how much voltage is applied. If we have 0
db of attenuation in the circuit, we may adjust the oscillator output so
that a particular voltage will appear across the phone. Let us say that
this reference voltage is 0.01 volt. Then all measurements during the
experiment may be expressed as decibels of attenuation relative to 0.01
volt across the earphone. If the calibration curve of the earphone tells us
that an applied voltage of 0.01 volt will put out 85 db SPL at 2000 cps,
then our attenuation measures are also relative to 85 db SPL. If a particular threshold setting is 63 db (in attenuation), we may say that the
threshold is 63 db below 0.01 volt applied to a particular earphone, or that
it is 22 db SPL (85–63).

We should have our earphone suspended in a spring-type headband
along with a dummy earphone for the ear opposite to the one under test.
The observer is seated comfortably and is instructed to adjust the intensity of the tone until it is just audible. He should be told that he will, no
doubt, have to go above that point to the clearly audible and below that
point to the definitely inaudible several times before he will be able to

bracket a region that is narrow enough to be called "just audible." The headset should be adjusted so that the cushions of the earphones fit snugly around the ears, without any leaks whereby some of the sound could escape from the ear canal.

The observer now proceeds to measure his own threshold, and the experimenter merely records the results. We should prevent the observer from returning successively to the same dial position on the attenuator (and thus from giving results more consistent than an actual series of thresholds would be) by placing another attenuator in series with the one that the observer uses. The experimenter may then introduce different amounts of attenuation into this second one and thus force the observer to use different amounts on his own attenuator for repeated thresholds.

Let us say that we shall ask our observer to make 10 judgments. Suppose that he gives us the following SPL's as thresholds for each of the 10 settings: 71, 65, 64, 73, 62, 62, 62, 63, 61, 63. What is his threshold? First we may set up a small frequency distribution as follows:

SPL(x)	f	xf
61	1	61
62	3 ($Mode = 62$)	186
63	2 ($Median = 63$)	126
64	1	64
65	1	65
66	0	0
67	0	0
68	0	0
69	0	0
70	0	0
71	1	71
72	0	0
73	1	73

$$\Sigma xf = 646$$
$$\frac{\Sigma xf}{N(= 10)} = Mean = 64.6$$

We have three measures of central tendency from this distribution of individual thresholds. The *mode*, the SPL that was set most frequently, is 62. The *median*, the SPL above which or below which 50 per cent of the settings lie, is 63. The *mean*, or average, is 64.6. Which one of these best represents the threshold? Obviously our decision is arbitrary. We note, however, that the 71 and 73 look like spurious settings that occurred early in the session. They are responsible for the mean's being so much higher than the median. The median (as well as the mode) is unaffected by the magnitude of scores at the extremes of the distribution and hence sometimes turns out to be a more reliable measure than the mean.

Method of Limits.   The apparatus diagramed in Fig. 4.3 will serve to illustrate the use of the method of limits in determining the auditory threshold for a 2000-cps tone. The procedure is not very different from the method of adjustment except that (1) the experimenter, not the observer, controls the intensity, and (2) the approaches from above and below are accomplished at a fixed rate within fixed limits.

We shall instruct the observer to raise his finger whenever he hears the tone and to drop it as soon as the tone disappears. We begin with a tone that is well above threshold and gradually, uniformly reduce the intensity (increase the attenuation) until the observer's finger drops, indicating that he no longer hears. We continue decreasing the intensity for about 10 more decibels below this change-over point and then begin increasing the intensity until the observer signifies that he hears it again. Increasing another 10 db, we repeat this process perhaps ten times. The rate at which the intensity is changed as well as the limits within which it is changed may affect the results.

We obtain a set of measures very much like those that were obtained under the method of adjustment. Half these measures will have been obtained when the intensity was increased from below threshold, and half will have been obtained when the intensity was decreased from above threshold. The same considerations that were given to the data of the method of adjustment may be given here. Extreme spurious measures do not affect the median too drastically. On the other hand, a sufficiently large distribution of scores will yield a mean and median that are very close to each other.

Method of Constant Stimuli.   Although it is time-consuming and unwieldy for a simple determination of the pure-tone threshold, the method of constant stimuli constitutes the model for most of the speech tests with which we shall be concerned in the next chapter. It is also basic for several of the clinical pulse-tone techniques that have been suggested recently (Harris, 1945; Gardner, 1947b; Reger and Newby).

Into the circuit of Fig. 4.3 we must introduce some kind of noiseless interrupter. It may be an automatic switch, mechanical or electronic, or a simple manual interrupting key. We shall present groups of tones to the observer and ask him to record (or indicate to the experimenter, who will record) the number of stimuli heard at each of several fixed intensities. In the classic method of constant stimuli, the intensities of successive tones are ordered at random, and the observer is asked to respond "yes" or "no" to each tone. In either case the data obtained take the form of a graph that relates the percentage of presented tones that are heard to the

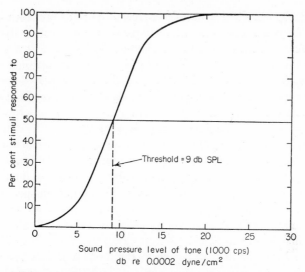

FIG. 4.4. An idealized relation between the number of stimuli to which an observer responds and the Sound Pressure Level at which the stimuli are presented. The threshold is defined as the Sound Pressure Level that corresponds to responses being made to 50 per cent of the stimuli presented.

intensity at which they were presented. Such a graph would ideally take the form shown in Fig. 4.4. The intensity at which the value of the ordinate is 50 per cent is arbitrarily taken as the threshold.

Review of Parameters Affecting Thresholds

In the previous pages of this chapter we have said that the threshold would be different according as the response, the psychophysical technique, and the measurement of the stimulus were of different kinds. Unfortunately, there are not many data that can clearly demonstrate these relations. To be sure, the clinical literature is filled with interesting reports of different thresholds measured on the same patient by two operators, by the same operator with different audiometers, etc. But the majority of these involve too many sources of variability at once. We can mention some few experiments that have attempted to single out some of the factors that influence thresholds.

Continuous vs. Interrupted Tones. One of the results of studies on the physiology of the auditory nervous system is that neural responses are more easily elicited by changing stimuli than by continuous ones. We should expect, therefore, that the threshold for a tone that is continuous over an appreciable time (more than about 1 sec) will be different from the threshold for an interrupted tone or short bursts of tone. DeVries has shown that the absolute threshold increases as the duration of a tone is shortened from 2 sec to 0.04 sec. His results are given in terms of an arbitrary voltage reference across a loud-speaker, and we have, therefore, no way of knowing what the absolute thresholds are in terms of sound pressure or energy. DeVries also showed that the slope of the function relating frequency of response to duration decreases as the duration is made less than 0.25 sec. An experiment by Rosenblith and Miller involving the use of the method of limits shows that the difference in threshold between continuous and slowly interrupted tones increases as the frequency of the tone is increased, reaching a maximum difference at about 4000 cps. At this frequency the threshold for a slowly interrupted tone is approximately 15 db lower than the threshold for a continuous tone. We shall have to take such differences into account when we compare continuous-tone audiometry with the recently suggested pulse-tone audiometry to be discussed presently.

Repetition Rate. When we use short bursts of tone as the stimulus for measurement of the absolute threshold, we find that the threshold varies inversely with the duration. This relation cannot be determined precisely for the general case because it will depend upon the rate at which the pulses, or short tones, follow each other. We should expect, for example, that if we had tones of constant duration, they would be more easily heard if we presented them very rapidly one after the other than if we waited for several seconds. Garner has shown, for example, that the absolute threshold (in terms of energy per sine wave) decreases as the repetition rate (number of tone bursts per second) increases from 1/4 (1 tone every 4 sec) to 33 tones per second. This relation holds for tones of 250, 1000, and 4000 cps. When the individual bursts are of 15 msec duration, the decrease in threshold from 1/4 to 33 tones per second is of the order of 5 or 6 db. If we have such a burst of tone of constant duration, then the higher the rate of repetition, the greater the percentage of the time the tone is on. In the experiments of Rosenblith and Miller, on the other hand, the "duty cycle"—or percentage of time in each cycle that the tone is on—was kept constant at 0.5, *i.e.*, the tone was on for half the time and off for half the time. Particularly for frequencies of 1000, 2000, and 4000 cps, the threshold decreases by about 8 db as the repetitions per second increase from 1 to 256.

Ascending vs. Descending Intensity. You may recall from the discussion of the method of limits that two distributions of threshold measures are obtained. One distribution describes the intensity required for the observer to just hear a tone emerge from silence as the intensity is increased. The other describes the intensity at which the observer reports that the tone disappears from the zone of audibility as the intensity is decreased.

As we shall see presently, the method of limits is basic to what we may call the traditional clinical technique in audiometry. It seems safe to say that most of us have the notion that the threshold is measurably lower when we decrease the intensity from above than when we increase the intensity from below the threshold. The experiment of Rosenblith and Miller quantifies some of these relations. The curves in Figs. 4.5 and 4.6 relate the cumulative percentage of positive response in a method of limits to the SPL of a 4000-cps tone. Figure 4.5 shows three curves obtained from data on *interrupted* tones. Here we observe what our clinical

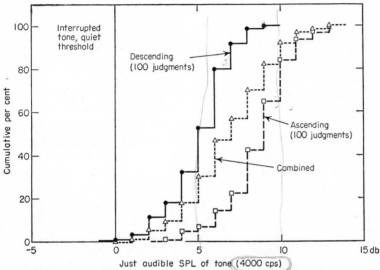

FIG. 4.5. Absolute thresholds for interrupted tones. Ordinate shows cumulative percentage of positive responses in a method of limits as a function of the SPL of the tone. (*From Rosenblith and Miller, unpublished data.*)

experience would have predicted, namely, that the threshold (50 per cent) for the descending series is lower (by about 4 db) than that for the ascending series. Figure 4.6, however, shows us that for *continuous tones* the descending series yield consistently *higher* thresholds than those of the ascending series. Note that the threshold decreases as the level from which the descent is made is decreased. If we begin descending from an SPL as low as 20 db, the thresholds for the ascending and descending series are almost exactly the same. Such a level would be difficult to use in a clinical situation, since we would begin descending at a level just barely above the point where the observer just begins to respond 100 per cent of the time.

Criterion of a 'Tone.' Some very interesting questions are brought to light when we consider the nature of the instructions that we give to an

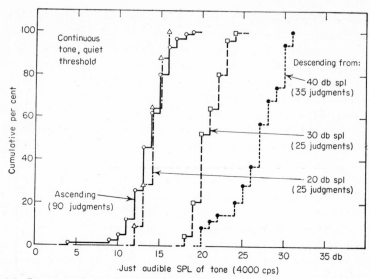

Fig. 4.6. Same relations as shown in Fig. 4.5 for a continuous tone. The three "descending" curves show responses for descents made from three different levels. (*From Rosenblith and Miller, unpublished data.*)

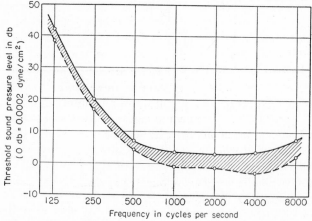

Fig. 4.7. Thresholds of tonality (solid line) and audibility (dashed line) as a function of frequency. (*From Pollack, 1948b.*)

observer, especially in regard to what he is to listen for. Do we ask him to signal when he hears a tone that is definitely a tone with characteristic pitch, or do we ask him to signal when he hears something that is different from silence? Pollack (1948b) addressed himself to this problem and produced results that are shown in Fig. 4.7. Two threshold curves, plotted as a function of frequency, are shown. The upper curve represents the threshold of tonality, obtained from the observer's response to tones that had tonal quality with characteristic pitch. The lower curve represents the threshold of audibility for the same tones, but in this case the observer listened only for 'something,' of any quality whatsoever so long as it was different from silence. Note that, again in the vicinity of 4000 cps, the two thresholds differ by about 7 db, depending upon which of these listening criteria is used. Pollack mentions another interesting finding that we might tuck away for clinical reference, namely, that the variabilities for the two different kinds of thresholds are the same.

Variability in Threshold Measurements. It is quite clear from the discussions so far that if we measure successive thresholds of a given observer several times, either in a single experimental session or at intervals separated by several days, we shall not obtain exactly the same threshold each time. The sources of such threshold variability are numerous and are not necessarily related to the variability of the observer's physiological threshold. For example, Steinberg and Munson report that variations in the fit of the earphone to the ear might account for standard deviations as large as 5 to 7 db. Munson and Wiener attribute a good portion of threshold variability to the method and place of measuring the sound pressure. Under very carefully controlled experimental conditions, however, Myers and Harris report that "the typical short-term fluctuation was less than a decibel." These investigators used a system whose output was varied in 1-db steps according to the method of limits.

Variability among repeated threshold measurements of clinical patients would, no doubt, be higher than some of these laboratory investigations would indicate. Gardner (1947b) reports, for example, standard deviations between 2.4 and 4.25 db in repeated measurements with what he calls the "standard clinical audiometric test." These individual variabilities are, of course, multiplied when we try to estimate the variability in threshold measurements made on a large group of individuals. In this case much of the variability can be assigned to purely physical factors such as the fit of earphones, variations in the size and consequent acoustic properties of ear canals, etc. (Steinberg and Munson, Munson and Wiener).

The Normal Threshold

There are many practical and theoretical reasons for knowing what the normal human auditory threshold is. Meaningful diagnoses in clinical practice are dependent upon a reasonable estimate of the "normal" with which the "abnormal" is contrasted. The importance of the precise determination of the sensitivity of the human auditory system for the physiology and psychology of hearing cannot be overestimated. In spite of the great importance that is attached to this concept, and even after many years of experimental work on small groups in the laboratory and on large groups in surveys, a univocal result has not been found.

There is no single threshold curve that represents *the* normal human auditory system. Certainly there is no single value that obtains under all psychophysical procedures. There will be at least one curve for each psychophysical method that is used. It is also possible that there is more than one value for a single psychophysical method. There are at least three measures of central tendency, any one of which might be used to represent the threshold of a sample of individuals. Figure 4.8 shows two distribution curves: one a normal distribution curve and the other a typical distribution of the auditory thresholds of individuals tested at the New York World's Fair.

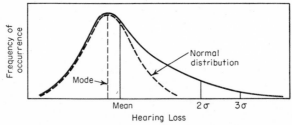

Fig. 4.8. Distribution of hearing loss in a large population. (*From Steinberg, Montgomery, and Gardner.*) The broken lines show a normal distribution curve, and the suggestion is made that the difference between this normal distribution and the actual distribution constitutes pathological cases.

If we draw our sample of persons at random from the population at large, we must anticipate a distribution curve that is skewed in the direction of subnormal hearing simply because pathologic factors that contribute to hearing loss exert influence over a much wider range of intensities than do those factors that contribute to supernormal hearing. Of course, if we had a way of sampling only normal listeners we might anticipate a result much more like the normal curve. But this would involve a prior assumption of normal so that the abnormal listeners might be eliminated—an assumption of the end result in order to produce the result.

Of course, we can take any measure of central tendency for an arbitrary definition of the normal threshold. It would be better, however, to temper our arbitrariness with a consideration of what measure would be most useful to those who would use it as a standard for comparison and a further consideration of what measure will best describe the sample of measurements at hand. The *mean* of the distribution in Fig. 4.8 includes some of the pathologic members of the sample, if we assume that the area that represents the difference between the obtained and normal curves indicates the abnormal or pathologic portion of the sample. The *mode* is a meaningful descriptive measure, but its disadvantage lies in the fact that there are very few statistical manipulations that can be performed on it. The *median* seems to be the best single descriptive measure of central tendency. But perhaps a better description of the sample would be given by a specification of both mean and median, since, in addition to measures of central tendency, a measure of skewness of the distribution may be derived from them.

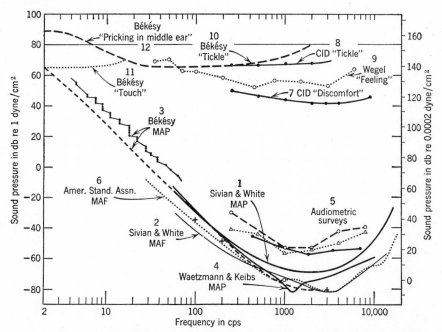

FIG. 4.9. Absolute thresholds for hearing (lower limit) and threshold for feeling (upper limit) as determined by various investigators. (*Reproduction by permission from Licklider, J. C. R., Chapter 25, in S. S. Stevens (Ed.), Handbook of Experimental Psychology, published by John Wiley and Sons, Inc.,* 1951: *after* [1, 2] *Sivian and White;* [3] *Békésy,* 1936a, b; [4] *Waetzmann and Keibs;* [5] *Steinberg, Montgomery, and Gardner; Montgomery; and Beasley;* [7, 8] *Silverman, Harrison, and Lane;* [9] *Wegel;* [10, 11, 12] *Békésy,* 1936b.)

In the experimental work that has been published, there seem to be gross differences between two types of studies. The experimental measurements that have been made in laboratories on relatively small groups have generally employed quite sensitive, experienced listeners and consequently yield thresholds that are very low. Examples are curves 1, 2, 3, and 4 in Fig. 4.9. Less rigorously controlled procedures have been used on much larger samples in surveys like the U.S. Public Health Survey and the

Bell Telephone Laboratories' World's Fair survey. The results of such surveys are shown in curve 5 of Fig. 4.9. Curves 7, 8, 9, 10, 11, and 12 show experimental measurements of thresholds of discomfort, feeling, tickle, etc. These curves represent the upper limit of the audible range, while the absolute thresholds represent the lower limit.

Before concluding this section, we must point out that the situation for the clinician is not too bad. Even though the experimental psychologist and physiologist are still without the threshold curve of *the normal human auditory system*, the clinician can make meaningful measurements by assuming almost any norm, so long as it remains constant through his series of measurements. As a matter of fact, this is already done for him by the manufacturer of the audiometer. The trouble comes when a patient leaves one clinician, goes to another, and finds that his Hearing Loss has changed. This change is not always the result of a favorable therapeutic effect of the clinician or progression of the deafness—the change might be accounted for wholly in terms of the change in audiometric technique, testing environment, or clinical standard.

CLINICAL AUDIOMETRY

This section will deal with measuring the difference between a particular individual's threshold and a normal threshold. In spite of the lack of precision that has attended the attempts to derive a general estimate of the normal threshold, we are faced with certain practical problems. We should like to evaluate the hearing of different individuals for the purpose of determining their fitness for certain occupations. Specific measures of auditory deficiency permit certain diagnostic conclusions on which therapy may be based. We must arbitrarily assume a normal threshold and make our clinical measurements with reference to it. If we use commercial audiometers, we rely on the normal threshold[1] that the manufacturer has used in calibrating his instrument.

We shall discuss first the use of equipment that is generally available to clinical personnel. A further discussion of improvements in method and equipment will allow us to consider how current clinical audiometric procedures may be modified with a view toward more precision, less time consumption, and the possibility of more general agreement in results from one clinic to another or from one audiometrist to another. We may begin by considering the following practical problem: We are faced with a standard commercial audiometer, a patient whose hearing loss for pure

---

[1] This standard is set by the National Bureau of Standards and the American Standards Association (see Appendix A). The manufacturer must conform to the NBS standard in order to have his instrument approved by the American Medical Association's Council on Physical Medicine and Rehabilitation.

tones is to be measured, and a blank audiogram card. How do we obtain this patient's audiogram?

The Audiogram

Figure 4.10 shows an assumed threshold curve for a normal individual (curve A) and a measured threshold curve for a certain patient (curve B).

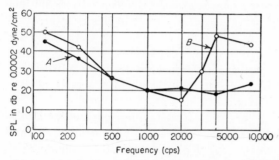

Fig. 4.10. Two absolute threshold curves. (A) represents the threshold for a normal listener (Western Electric 2A Audiometer), while (B) is a threshold of a particular patient.

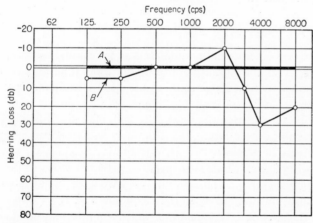

Fig. 4.11. The same two curves as in Fig. 4.10, plotted on the audiogram. The 0-db Hearing Loss is (A) of Fig. 4.10 (if this audiometer has been calibrated according to the Western Electric 2A standard). The differences between (A) and (B) in Fig. 4.10 appear as the ordinate scale (Hearing Loss) for Fig. 4.11.

These curves show what SPL is necessary at the various frequencies for threshold response. Both the ordinate and the abscissa scales represent purely physical dimensions of the stimulus. Figure 4.11 is a reproduction of a typical audiogram card that is provided with audiometers. There are two audiograms plotted on it, one of an individual with normal hearing (curve A) and the other of the patient whose threshold was plotted in Fig. 4.10 (curve B). It is important to note that the units of the ordinate or Hearing Loss scale are decibels, representing purely physical ratios. The audiometer's units of attenuation (or Hearing Loss) are decibels, and hence this scale must represent a physical dimension, albeit one that is dependent upon an assumed threshold norm.[1] We should note that the dimension *Hearing Loss* is exactly the same, by definition, as *Sensation Level*, which we have discussed earlier in this chapter.

Curve A in Fig. 4.10 is the same as curve A in Fig. 4.11. They both represent the same threshold, one expressed in physical units of SPL and the other expressed as a difference (in decibels) between certain measured SPL's and SPL's of the normal threshold. Curve B, of course, is also the same in Fig. 4.10 and in Fig. 4.11.

The "normal" or "0-db Hearing Loss" line of the audiogram is, then, the normal threshold curve after it has been straightened and flipped over. We should note that moving upward on the ordinate of Fig. 4.10 corresponds to increasing the intensity of the tone, whereas moving upward on the ordinate (Hearing Loss) of the audiogram (Fig. 4.11) corresponds to decreasing the intensity of the tone.

Use of the Audiometer

One of several commercial audiometers is shown in Fig. 4.12. We have already described the operating parts and their functions in Chap. 3. The frequency of the oscillator that is built into the audiometer is adjusted on the "frequency" dial. Some audiometers provide for adjustment to only certain fixed frequencies (*e.g.*, 125, 250, 500, 1000, 2000, 4000, and 8000 cps), while others have a continuously variable frequency adjustment. Intensity is controlled by the attenuator marked, on the audiometer, "Hearing Loss." The Hearing Loss attenuator subtracts constant numbers of decibels from voltages that vary with frequency in accordance with the input-output curve of the earphone and the assumed normal threshold. Had we varied frequency with 0 db of attenuation in the circuit of Fig. 4.3, the output would have looked like the calibration curve of the earphone for a constant voltage applied (Fig. 4.2A). If we vary frequency

---

[1] This scale of Hearing Loss has sometimes been unfortunately labeled *Sensation Units*, as if the audiometer were calibrated in steps that were equivalent to equal units on some sensory scale, such as loudness. The fact that the physically defined decibel is approximately equal to the difference limen for intensity within a small range (*see* Fig. 7.2), and, in addition, the assumption that equal successive DL's, or jnd's, were equal units of a sensory scale of loudness (see Chap. 8), led to this untenable notion (cf. Fowler, 1947), which has contributed a good share of confusion to clinical audiometry.

in the audiometer, however, the voltage does not remain constant but rather changes according to the normal threshold. With the Hearing Loss control at 0 db, the output would look like the assumed threshold curve of hearing (Fig. 4.10*A*).

Most audiometers are also equipped with a manual interrupting key (lower left in Fig. 4.12), which allows the audiometrist to turn the tone on and off without making an audible click.

There are many additional features of the newest audiometers, most of which contribute to increased ease of measurement. Many manufacturers

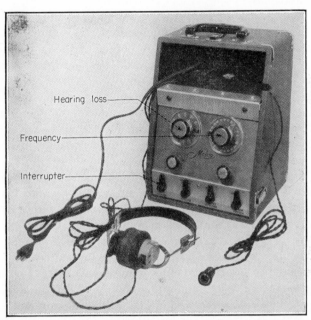

FIG. 4.12. A portable, pure-tone audiometer. The frequency selector is shown at the upper left; the Hearing Loss attenuator is seen at the upper right. (*Photograph courtesy of The Maico Company, Inc., Minneapolis.*)

supply a headband with two earphones (as in Fig. 4.12) to replace the older hand-held type. In spite of the objections of some female patients, a headband-held earphone is preferable to one that is held in the patient's hand. Hand movement transmitted to an earphone constitutes a serious source of noise (Brogden and Miller).

We cannot discuss the full range of possibilities for audiometric procedures because of certain limitations that are imposed by present-day audiometers. For one thing, the Hearing Loss attenuators move in 5-db steps, and some of these attenuators are still so imperfect that, if a change is made while the tone is on, an audible click is produced, especially when the intensity of the tone itself is near threshold. This implies that a strict method of limits with a continuous tone that gradually changes in intensity is virtually impossible. The audiometers with fixed octave and semi-octave frequencies limit the number and regions of frequencies used.

Traditional Audiometric Technique

Most of the technique that will be presented briefly here is drawn from Bunch's *Clinical Audiometry* and the instruction booklets that are supplied with Maico, Sonotone, Audio Development Company, and Audivox audiometers. (See also Chap. 11.)

Before the test is begun, the audiometer should be allowed to warm up for a reasonable time and should be prechecked by the audiometrist (if he is a normal listener) to be sure that 0 db Hearing Loss at several frequencies is just audible. The patient should be seated comfortably in a quiet room (see Chap. 6, Masking) in such a position that he can see neither the control panel of the audiometer nor the operator's hands, which will manipulate the controls. If he has had no practice in listening to pure tones, the patient should be given the opportunity to hear several of the frequencies at reasonably high intensity (*e.g.*, 40 db Hearing Loss; see also Chap. 6, Auditory Fatigue) to gain some acquaintance with this new sensory experience. He should be instructed to raise his finger or press a signal button whenever he hears a tone and to withdraw his finger or release the button whenever the tone disappears.

The order in which the several frequencies are tested is somewhat arbitrary. It is quite generally agreed that the measurement on any one frequency should be completed before going on to another. In other words, in this technique we hold frequency constant while we vary intensity. The experiment of Witting and Hughson indicates that a patient's variability is less at 1024 cps[1] than at other frequencies on the audiometer. Gardner's data (1947*b*) confirm this finding. Most clinicians have taken this result as justification for beginning a test at 1000 cps, testing frequencies in increasing order up to the highest, and then testing frequencies below 1000 cps in decreasing order.

Bunch discusses first the procedure of starting with a tone that is well

---

[1] Older audiometers that use octave frequencies base the octave on a middle C of 256 cps. Recently, probably due to pressure from acoustic physicists and engineers, audiometers are either changing to a 125, 250-cps base or are providing both sets of numbers on the frequency dial. The stability of most oscillators, especially during the warm-up period, is such that either set of numbers describes the actual frequency equally well. Accuracy of frequency would probably be better represented in terms of significant figures by stating frequency thus: $25 \times 10^1, 5 \times 10^2, 10^3, 2 \times 10^3, 4 \times 10^3$, etc.

above threshold (*i.e.*, is easily heard by the patient) and gradually reducing its intensity until the patient indicates that he no longer hears it. An alternative, or supplementary, procedure is to start with a tone that is well below threshold and to increase its intensity until it is heard. Clearly, this is a case of the method of limits in which we gradually approach the threshold from above and below and average (or take some other measure of central tendency of) the results, which will be different for the two directions of approach.

Bunch goes on to mention a well-known clinical fact, namely, that a tone that does not change in either amplitude or frequency is more difficult to listen to, to attend to, than a tone that is changed in at least one dimension. It was for this reason that some workers in the field introduced a warbling tone for testing (Burr and Mortimer). This was simply a tone whose frequency was changed slightly about a mean frequency and was thus more easily heard, or at least better attended to.

Another way of avoiding a completely steady tone is to change, not the frequency, but the intensity. One simple way to do this is to turn the tone on and off. The use of an interrupted tone in a sense modifies the method of limits by bringing in certain experimental features of the method of constant stimuli. The computations involved can still be made as they would be in a strict method of limits except for the fact that the clinician must establish criteria for the number of times that a person must respond to pulses of tone at a threshold intensity. We must remember that these modifications—namely, interruptions, approaches from above and below, etc.—change the threshold. We have already discussed some of these dependencies in the preceding section.

In this regard, we have discussed only regular interruptions. Some teachers of clinical audiometry caution their students to avoid a regular rate of interruption in order to prevent the patient from catching on to a rhythm. Actually there is no reason why a patient should not be given the aid to attention that would be provided by a regular rate of interruption, even though the threshold that would be obtained might be lower than that for a random interruption. Certainly the case for regular periodic interruption is made much stronger when we consider how much more easily quantified the results may be.

When we can specify a threshold intensity as being the least amount of Hearing Loss at which the patient can follow our tone interruptions with his signals, we enter the amount of Hearing Loss on the audiogram by placing a symbol at the intersection of the appropriate frequency line and the measured Hearing Loss line. This procedure is repeated for all frequencies to be tested. The patient's "audiogram" is the line connecting the symbols, each of which represents his Hearing Loss at a single frequency. A different symbol and type of line for each ear will facilitate the distinction between the two on the card.[1]

Pulse-tone Technique

A regular rate of interruption is more easily provided by a mechanical or electrical device than by a manually operated switch. Such devices in conjunction with clinical audiometers are utilized in the pulse-tone technique. The tests that were conducted by the Bell Telephone Laboratories at the New York World's Fair in 1939 (see Steinberg, Montgomery, and Gardner) used this technique, and it has since been suggested, by Gardner (1947b), as an appropriate technique for individual tests. Certainly its advantage for group audiometry has been shown clearly by the World's Fair group; by Harris (1945) and his coworkers at the U.S. Naval Submarine Base, New London; and by Reger and Newby.

The psychophysical basis for the *pulse-tone technique* is a bit complicated. At first glance, it looks like a method of constant stimuli. If so, it is a much modified form in which the levels at which individual stimuli are presented are not ordered at random. The pulse-tone technique is much more like the method of limits with an interrupted stimulus. We present to the patient a group of, let us say, five tones. We ask him how many tones he hears. For groups presented at intensities well above threshold, the patient will respond, "Five." For groups of tones at intensities well below threshold, the patient will respond "Zero." At intermediate intensities he may respond with any number between zero and five. In one variation that has been introduced, a group of stimuli is presented during an interval of time that is usually required for the presentation of five tones, but there is actually presented any number of tones from one to five. It is the patient's task to recognize how many tones were presented each time. The computational procedures used in this method are much more like those of the method of constant stimuli than like those of the method of limits.

The use of a strict method of constant stimuli in a clinical situation is almost impossible, since it requires a random presentation of individual stimuli at intensities that are randomly ordered. Meaningful measures from such a procedure cannot be produced unless 50 or 100 stimuli are presented at each of the intensities to be investigated. Although the classic method of constant stimuli lends itself well to certain types of statistical treatment, it is not very feasible for the clinic.

[1] The standardization of specific symbols for air conduction, bone conduction, right ear, left ear, masking, and no masking was one of the matters under consideration by the Second International Conference on Audiology, London, July, 1949. Final decisions are in the process of being made (see Fowler, Jr.).

The specific procedure that Gardner (1947*b*) describes employs an ordinary Western Electric 6-PB audiometer (no longer manufactured) with the associated equipment for producing the tonal pulses or bursts. Two lights are used as indicators. One light, within view of the patient, is on as long as there is any possibility of a tone's being presented. The other, within the view of the operator only, flashes each time there is a tone. This second light allows the operator to monitor the system visually. The operator selects any number of tones to be presented at a particular level, and the threshold is defined as the lowest intensity (Hearing Loss) at which the patient can *report correctly* the number of tones presented.

From a psychophysical viewpoint, this definition of a threshold is highly questionable. It is really a threshold whose criterion for response frequency is 100 per cent. You remember that a strict use of the method of constant stimuli asks the question at each intensity, How often does he hear the tone or how correctly does he report the number of tones presented? The fact that Gardner's technique differs further from the formal method, in that a different number of tones is presented at each intensity, is not so serious an objection (except by a purist) as the difficulty encountered in attempting to measure the response, "reports correctly." A general use of the pulse-tone technique must await the unraveling of this statistical knot.

A Clinical "Adjustment Method"

The classic method of adjustment has not yet been applied generally in the clinic. Actually it is a very simple and rapid method for the measurement of a threshold and has been found extremely useful in experimental laboratories. The clinician's objection to this method has been that it requires, on the part of the observer, a certain amount of sophistication which is not characteristic of the inexperienced patient. The clinician must give the patient the perhaps difficult task of adjusting the intensity of the tone until he is just able to hear it or, sometimes, just not able to hear it. Again, one measure is not sufficient for a meaningful threshold, but at least we do not have to present many stimuli in order to get a single estimate of threshold. In this method, a single estimate of threshold is given each time the observer adjusts to a setting. The objection of the clinician that this type of procedure is too difficult for patients has been challenged by several experimenters, the most recent of whom is Békésy (1947).

Békésy's discussion of a new audiometer presents evidence that hard-of-hearing patients can make these adjustments not only for a single frequency but also for a slowly changing frequency. Békésy's audiometer produces a single auditory stimulus whose frequency is automatically increased slowly and whose intensity is controlled by the patient. It is so constructed that the patient's adjustments are automatically recorded by a small pen on an audiogram card that moves with the changing frequency. In this way the patient traces out his own audiogram. He is instructed to press a button whenever he hears the tone. This button automatically engages a motor-driven attenuator which reduces the intensity of the tone until it disappears below the patient's threshold. When the patient releases the button, the tone is automatically increased. This method gives us an estimate not only of the patient's threshold but also of the variability in his threshold; that is, the number of decibels between button pressings and releases tells us how wide is the patient's region of uncertainty about the average threshold. Indeed, Békésy has found that the measures of variability which are given on this automatic audiometer are useful in distinguishing between conductive and nerve deafness (See Fig. 8.10.) We shall have more to say about this when we come to discuss the measurement of the difference limen for intensity and its relation to recruitment (Chap. 8).

Screening Tests

The kinds of clinical audiometer that we have discussed so far are designed to obtain individual audiograms primarily for diagnostic purposes. There are many situations, e.g., in the public schools, where the ordinary kind of clinical individual audiometry is too time-consuming for the specific job to be done. In the public school, we are interested in whether or not a particular child hears all the tones above a particular intensity. Having established a criterion, we must know only that the child does or does not meet it. If he does, his case is no longer interesting; whereas if he does not, we must then recommend that a detailed individual audiogram be made (see Newhart and Reger for details).

Traditional audiometry differs from the screening technique only in that in the former we hold each frequency constant while we manipulate the intensity, whereas in the latter we fix a certain intensity (Hearing Loss) and vary the frequency (e.g., see Johnston). For example, suppose we say that we shall refer all children to an otologist for an audiogram and an examination who do not hear all frequencies on the audiometer when the Hearing-Loss dial is set at 20 db. We simply set the dial at 20 and sweep through the frequency range, asking only for a "yes" or "no" at each frequency. The purpose of this kind of test is, of course, to screen a large population for potential pathologic cases. The name sometimes used for this screening technique is the "sweep test," which comes from the actual operations used.

The use of similar techniques in individual diagnostic audiometry has been suggested by van Dishoeck and van Gool. They describe a continuous-frequency audiometer. Instead of measuring the intensity that is just heard at a particular frequency, one measures the frequency range that is audible at a particular Sensation Level. In this way an audiogram is produced that is more detailed in the dimension of frequency.

SUMMARY

We have described the classic psychophysical methods in the specific application of measuring the absolute threshold for hearing pure tones. The absolute threshold must be seen as a statistical concept rather than as some fixed figure above which the observer hears and below which he does not hear. The value of threshold will be determined by the kind and the locus of measurement of the stimulus, the response that is used, the psychophysical technique employed, and other specific parameters such as continuity or intermittence of the tone, frequency of repetition of pulses of tone, and the criterion for listening that is suggested to the observer.

Although the basic operations of measurement are the same, it is suggested that, at least at the conceptual level, a dichotomy exists between experimental and clinical pure-tone audiometry. The former has to do with the measurement of auditory thresholds in terms of physical dimensions of the stimulus. Clinical audiometry is concerned with the measurement of an individual's threshold in dimensions that are relative to the threshold for a standard observer.

Several kinds of technique have been described for clinical audiometry. Their several proponents have recommended their general use on the basis of advantages that are specific to each type. Since there is still no accepted standard technique, the clinician must be warned that the differences among these techniques may be responsible for differences among the thresholds that result from their use.

References for Further Study

Beranek, L. L. (1949) *Acoustic Measurements.* New York: Wiley. Chapter 8, The Audiometer, presents a readable technical discussion of the audiometer and its use. The text for this chapter was prepared by R. H. Nichols, of the Bell Telephone Laboratories.

Bunch, C. C. (1943) *Clinical Audiometry.* St. Louis: Mosby.

Fowler, E. P. (1947) Tests for hearing. In E. P. Fowler, Jr. (Ed.), *Loose-leaf Medicine of the Ear.* New York: Nelson. This and the preceding reference may be considered the classical references for clinical audiometry. Both present rather complete descriptions of the tuning-fork tests as well as of the clinical use of audiometers. Much information on pure-tone audiometry has been accumulated since these works were published, and they are now, therefore, incomplete.

Stevens, S. S., and H. Davis. (1938) *Hearing*. New York: Wiley. Chapter 2 contains a fairly complete account of the experimental parameters on which the absolute auditory threshold depends.

Watson, L. A., and T. Tolan. (1949) *Hearing Tests and Hearing Instruments*. Baltimore: Williams & Wilkins. This book is addressed primarily to practical problems in audiometry. The discussions of the component parts of audiometers, problems of standardization, and audiometric technique are quite complete. Some of the fundamental material on hearing contains errors.

CHAPTER 5

THE INTELLIGIBILITY OF SPEECH

IN THE preceding chapter we discussed methods of measuring the sensitivity of an individual to pure tones. Since it is possible to control the few physical dimensions of a stimulus as simple as a pure tone, we were able to discuss the basic physical and psychophysical concepts in relatively simple terms. But the hearing of pure tones constitutes a very small and insignificant part of the ordinary auditory experience of most individuals. By far the most important sounds to which we listen in civilized life are the sounds of speech—the signals that travel from person to person and so permit the complex communicative society that we have evolved. Although a measure of a person's sensitivity to pure tones of different frequencies tells us a good deal about the characteristics of his auditory system, such measurement is too limited to describe the same individual's ability to understand the speech of his fellow communicators. A second major type of measurement with which we shall concern ourselves is, then, a direct measurement of the person's ability to hear speech.

The last twenty-five years have seen the development of precise techniques for the measurement of speech sounds as physical phenomena and also for the measurement of a person's ability to distinguish the sounds of speech one from another. Such measurement, pioneered by Fletcher and his colleagues at the Bell Telephone Laboratories, has added considerably to our knowledge of speech, of the component sounds of the language, of the dependence of the intelligibility of speech on certain physical parameters, and of the properties of the auditory system that seem to have to do with the understanding of speech.

In addition to supplying basic information, these procedures can be applied to practical clinical situations. The clinician has felt insecure for many decades in his diagnoses and prognoses that have to do with a patient's communicative adequacy in his own society. The extrapolation from the tuning-fork and audiometer tests to the hearing of everyday speech was at best tenuous. The clinician has, therefore, for some time supplemented the pure-tone results with the whispered- or spoken-word tests. Although there were inherent inaccuracies due to the change in the level of the tester's voice and the varying testing conditions in a room with hard walls, we see here a genuine attempt to fill the gap between the information on pure tones and the desired information about an individual's ability to get along. At the present time, the speech part of the testing program that is available for clinical use can be quantified as reliably and easily as can the pure-tone tests.

We have said a little about the physical nature of the sounds of speech in Chap. 2, and, you may remember, we noted that the speech sound differs from a pure tone in that (1) a speech sound contains more than one frequency, and (2) its complicated spectrum changes quite rapidly with time. We have now to examine some of the fundamentals of speech. In particular we shall describe the sounds of the English language as it is spoken in America. We shall show, in a crude way, how each of these sounds is made by referring to the parts of the chest, throat, mouth, nose, and lips that are involved. Having seen what the speech sounds are and a little of how they are made, we can then proceed to examine how the speech sounds are physically different from one another and how the auditory system of a listener provides him with information that allows him to discriminate among sounds within words and among words within sentences. This discussion will lead us to the concept of intelligibility, which is a measure of a person's response to spoken words. Having described the formal procedures that are followed in testing the hearing for different kinds of speech, we shall turn to a discussion of the kinds of tests that have been made available to and have been found useful for the clinician.

SOME FUNDAMENTALS OF SPEECH

The word *speech* is difficult to define precisely, and yet one is sure that everyone knows what is meant when the word is used. We shall restrict ourselves to the kind of speech that involves sound. The case can be made, of course, that two deaf people who converse with one another by watching the lips, eyes, etc., are using speech, but this case is not considered here because we are interested only in phenomena that have to do with hearing and in those physical events that we have heretofore called *sounds*. There are as many different speech sounds as there are methods and mechanisms for producing them. This is in one way fortunate, for if our communication were limited to, let us say, two speech sounds, it would take an extremely long time to say anything. Morse code, for example, employs only three symbols—a dot, a dash, and a pause. Each of the 26 letters of the alphabet is represented by a pattern of dots and dashes, of one, two, three, or four symbols. The time for speaking a single letter (out of 26) is very short compared to the time necessary for three or four Morse symbols. Consequently it takes a long time to transmit a message in Morse code—but, as this example demonstrates, communication is perfectly possible with only three symbols. The multiplicity of the sounds of speech allows us to say more things in less time.

The sounds of speech are traditionally divided into two classes, *vowels* and *consonants*. For our present purposes, we may define a vowel as a sound that originates with the vibration of the vocal folds in the larynx by air from the lungs and is sustained over an appreciable length of time. This fundamental sound is modified by being passed through several cavities before it reaches a point (*e.g.*, the lips) from which it is radiated into the surrounding air. Each of these cavities acts as a resonator (see Chap. 2) and reinforces those components in the complex spectrum of the vocal sound to which it is tuned. If we lift any part of the tongue within the mouth cavity, we find that we have divided the mouth cavity into two smaller cavities. The size of each of the smaller cavities is changed as we move the tongue back and forth. By such tongue movement, and resultant changes in cavity size, we change the resonant frequencies of these cavities and thus change those components of the complex vocal sounds that will be reinforced by these cavities. Other structures besides the tongue contribute to differences among the vowel sounds. The tongue movements, however, are fundamental and provide the most convenient basis for description. Note, for example, that the front cavity can be enlarged not only by moving the tongue back but also by rounding and protruding the lips.

The vowels of English are the sustained sounds of the words listed below. In square brackets beside each word is a symbol for that particular vowel sound. The symbols are those of the International Phonetic Alphabet (IPA).[1]

beat	[i]		put	[ʊ]
b*i*t	[ɪ]		boot	[u]
	[e]		but	[ʌ]
bet	[ɛ]		*Diphthongs*	
bat	[æ]		ba*i*t	[eɪ]
bath	[a][1]		b*i*te	[aɪ]
balm	[ɑ]		bout	[aʊ]
p*o*t	[ɒ][1]		boat	[oʊ]
bought	[ɔ]		boy	[ɔɪ]
	[o]		pew	[ɪu]

[1] Eastern pronunciation.

We rarely use the [e] and [o] alone in English, but usually couple them with [ɪ] and [ʊ], respectively, to make diphthongs. As you have already noted from the examples, a diphthong is a continuous sound that is made by a transition from one simple vowel sound to another.

[1] Hereafter a symbol written in square brackets is from the IPA.

The easiest way to describe the method of producing these different vowels is first to think of the tongue as having two parts, a back part and a front part. We can then describe each of the vowel sounds generally in terms of the height to which either the front or the back of the

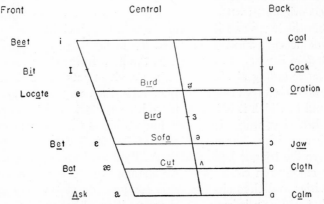

FIG. 5.1. Diagram showing the vowels of American English. The position of the IPA symbols relates the individual vowel to the part of the tongue and the height of the tongue during articulation of the vowel. (*From Miller*, 1951, *p.* 24.)

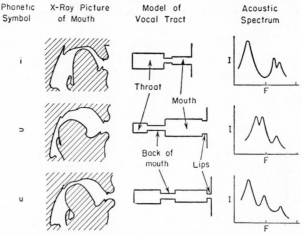

FIG. 5.2. Illustration of the relation between positions of the speech organs, sizes of the resonating cavities, and the resulting acoustic spectra. (*From Miller*, 1951, *p.* 40.)

tongue is raised to produce the sound. Important changes are also brought about by changing the positions of the lips and throat. We can arrange the vowels according to the tongue position, as is shown in Fig. 5.1. The influence of the other parts besides the tongue is shown in Fig. 5.2.

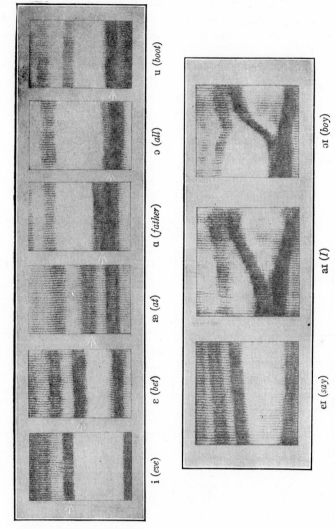

Fig. 5.3. Visible speech spectrograms of English vowels. The dark bars indicate the formants or resonant frequencies of the vocal cavities. Note how these formants change during the articulation of a diphthong. (*From Potter, Kopp, and Green.*)

So that you can be sure that the different vowel sounds are characterized by different spectra, the "visible speech" patterns for these vowels are presented in Fig. 5.3.[1] The pattern that is shown on the visible-speech machine is the spectrum turned on its side. Frequency is shown on the ordinate (the vertical scale), the lowest frequency being nearest the bottom. Instead of showing amplitude or intensity as the height of a line, as we did in the ordinary spectra (Fig. 2.8), intensity is represented on the visible-speech diagram by the amount of blackness. A very black space opposite a particular frequency indicates a very high intensity at that particular frequency component. The white or blank space opposite the frequency indicates that that frequency does not make any significant

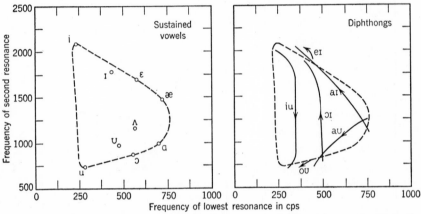

FIG. 5.4. Relation between first and second formants in English vowels. Note the similarity of the spatial arrangement of the individual vowels on these acoustic axes to the positions, shown in Fig. 5.1, illustrating the position of the tongue during articulation. (*From Potter and Peterson.*)

contribution to the total energy. You will note that these blacknesses and whitenesses change in time—time being represented from left to right on the abscissa.

This device, then, gives us a visual indication of the spectrum of a sound and, more than that, gives a moving indication as the sound changes in time. You will note that the representations of the vowel sounds have characteristic "bars" of blackness. Presumably these bars are uniquely related to the formants, or resonant frequencies of the speech cavities. The lowest bar, of course, represents the fundamental frequency of vibration of the vocal folds. The first and second formants above this fundamental are presumably attributable to the back and front cavities in the mouth, respectively. Figure 5.4 shows a plot of the

[1] For a review of the concept of spectrum, you should return to Chap. 2.

intersection of the frequency of bar 1 and that of bar 2 for each of the vowel sounds. The similarity between the diagram thus generated and the one describing the tongue positions of the vowels in Fig. 5.1 is so striking as to bolster one's faith in the notion that the spectra of the vowel sounds are indeed different because of tongue and lip positions and different cavity resonances.

The *consonants* of English seem to be responsible for most of the intelligibility carried by individual English words. There are more consonants

TABLE 5.1. ENGLISH CONSONANTS

Manner of articulation	Place of articulation					
	Bilabial	Labio-dental	Linguo-dental	Linguo-alveolar	Velar	Glottal
Plosive: Voiced	[b]			[d]	[g]	[ʔ]
Unvoiced	[p]			[t]	[k]	
Nasal	[m]			[n]	[ŋ] (si*ng*)	
Lateral				[l][r]		
Fricative: Voiced		[v]	[ð] (*then*)	[z] [ʒ] (a*z*ure)		
Unvoiced	[ʌ] (*wh*en)	[f]	[θ] (*th*in)	[s] [ʃ] (*sh*e)		[h]
Continuants	[w]			[j] (*y*es)		

than vowels, the consonants being made in more different places in more different ways than the vowels. We can best summarize the consonant sounds of English by pigeonholing each of them according to the place where it is made and the manner in which it is made. Table 5.1 shows such a summary. Columns from left to right represent the places or parts of the mouth that are articulated (brought together) to produce the consonants. For example, a *bilabial* consonant is produced by an articulation between the upper and lower lips; *labiodental*, by the articulation of a lip with the teeth; *linguodental*, by the articulation of the tongue with the teeth; *linguoalveolar*, by the articulation of the tongue with the alveolar ridge, which is a hard, bumpy little ridge just above and behind the upper teeth; *velar*, by the articulation of the back of the tongue with the velum (soft palate); *glottal*, by articulation of the two vocal folds.

The rows of Table 5.1 are labeled according to the manner in which the consonant is made. A *plosive* consonant is made when the two points of articulation (described by the proper column) are firmly brought together so that the air stream is temporarily shut off and then is released explosively. The *nasal* continuants are peculiar in that the air column, vibrating with the vocal tone, passes out through the nasal cavity while the articulating surfaces of the oral cavity are approximated. *Lateral* sounds are made when two surfaces are articulated closely enough to modify the voiced sound passing through but not so close as to produce friction. *Fricative* consonants are made by approximating two of these articulating surfaces, not so firmly as to stop the air stream, but just close enough so that a friction or turbulence is produced by the relatively large volume of air being passed through a very small opening.

You will notice that there are two rows of plosive and fricative sounds, one called *voiced* and the other *unvoiced*. Consonants can be made in the places and manner indicated either when air is rushing up from between open vocal folds (unvoiced) or when the vocal folds are in vibration at the same time (voiced).

Measurements made with the visible-speech spectrograph (Potter, Kopp, and Green), as well as the older measurements of Sacia and Beck, show that the physical characteristics of vowels and consonants are quite different. Generally speaking, the vowels have higher intensities (usually from 12 to 20 db higher) than the consonants. The vowels have spectral components that are lower in frequency than those of the consonants. Vowels achieve a steady state for a longer time than do consonants. In other words, the consonants are more transient than the longer, sustained vowels. These physical characteristics are the kinds of things that are detected by a microphone and an oscillograph. We shall see later how some of these physical parameters also affect the intelligibility of speech.

We have described some of the parts that, when put together, make up speech. The individual phonetic units are put together in certain ways to make up spoken words and sentences. Teaching a child a language is essentially the establishing of relations between patterns of these phonetic units and arbitrary *meanings*. It would be presumptuous of the author to embark upon a linguistic approach to the relations between words or linguistic symbols and the things, events, or states that they symbolize. And, in fact, it is doubtful that such an approach is necessary for the present purposes. We shall discover that our concern with the measurement of a person's ability to hear the sounds of speech or whole spoken words does not require that we investigate the meanings of words.

Intelligibility

Suppose that we have a phonographic recording of a relatively long passage of spoken English, so monotonous that the intensity of the individual words does not vary much. This might represent one sample of English speech. We wish to know whether or not an individual can hear that speech. How is this situation different from the case that we have discussed earlier, namely, the one in which we present a pure tone and wish to know whether or not the person can hear the tone? You remember that we had to specify, in the case of a pure tone, the response that the observer would make in the presence of the tone. We shall be concerned in this section with the specification of such a response to the presence of speech.

If we play different phonograph records through an amplifier and feed the output to an earphone, we can simply ask the observer, as we did in the case of a pure tone, to judge whether or not he hears anything. We do not care whether he recognizes the speech sounds as speech sounds but rather ask only for his judgment relative to the presence of a sound. Having found the intensity (of speech) at which the observer reports that he hears something 50 per cent of the time, we shall have measured a *threshold of detectability*. This threshold, however, gives us very little more information than we might have obtained had we used a combination of tones, a buzzer, or any one of a number of different kinds of sound. It is clear that we want to know more about the individual's ability to recognize and differentiate the sounds of speech.

We must proceed, then, from the concept of *detectability* to the concept of *intelligibility*. We shall ask one or both of the following questions: (1) How intense must a particular sample of speech be in order that it be just intelligible to a listener? (2) At a given intensity, how intelligible is a given sample of speech? You will recognize that the first question has to do with a measurement of a *threshold of intelligibility* in which we specify a certain amount of intelligibility as threshold response and use the intensity of speech as the dependent variable. The second question has to do with the measurement of the amount of intelligibility in a sample of speech that is presented at a fixed intensity.

When is speech intelligible? Clearly our criterion of intelligibility must be more exacting than that for detectability. Must a person be able to define each of the words that is presented? Or must he only recognize the words as words of, for example, the English language? A workable criterion for intelligibility seems to lie somewhere in between these two. We want the observer to be able to differentiate sounds or words from one another, but we probably do not care whether or not he understands the meanings of the words that he recognizes. This concept of intelligibility may be readily quantified if we adopt the following definition: a given sample of speech is intelligible if and only if the observer repeats, either by writing or by speaking aloud, the speech sample that is presented to him. Of course, each sample must be short enough so that we are measuring only the intelligibility of the units and not the memory of the observer. The threshold of intelligibility is, from this definition, the *intensity of the speech* at which an observer can *repeat 50 per cent of the speech* that is presented.

Using this criterion, we may now proceed to describe methods of measuring intelligibility. The formal methods that have been evolved have enabled investigators to relate the intelligibility of speech to such physical parameters as intensity, frequency, distortion, and noise backgrounds. Before going to these formal tests, however, we must describe the different ways in which speech may be sampled for the acquisition of materials for such tests. Test results are critically dependent upon the kinds of sample used.

Representative Types of Speech

One of the reasons for considering the measurement of a person's ability to hear speech is to fill in the gap between the audiogram and the person's ability to communicate with his fellows in everyday life. Having thus justified the discussion of hearing for speech, we might simply gather up some good examples of everyday speech and measure their intelligibility. Everyday speech, however, is not easily quantified and therefore does not lend itself well to measurement. If we could produce smaller sampling units we could set up more precise relations between intelligibility and the physical dimensions of the test units. We might, for example, use sentences and ask the observer either to answer a simple interrogative sentence or to repeat a declarative sentence. More than this, we might present lists of words and ask the observer to repeat each of the individual words. As a matter of fact, we could list the individual phonetic elements of the language and prepare lists of nonsense syllables whose repetition would require that an observer hear each of the individual speech sounds. The experimental literature on the intelligibility of speech is full of examples of all these types of speech sample. We must now describe them a little more fully and show how each might be used in the measurement of intelligibility.

Nonsense Syllables.   Information about a person's ability to recognize the individual phonetic elements of English could be obtained simply by presenting these individual phonemes and asking the observer to repeat what he hears. The consonants of English, however, are difficult to recite alone. It is hard to say d, which is not the symbol for *dee* but rather for *d*, which usually comes out *duh*. The most usual spoken units are combinations of (1) a consonant followed by a vowel, (2) a vowel followed by a consonant, or (3) a vowel between two consonants. Any of these three combinations constitutes what we may call a syllable. Although there is not much agreement among phoneticians about the definition of a syllable, we may understand it to be any unit of speech that contains one vowel. If we want to find out whether or not a person can discriminate the consonants one from another, we might make a list of nonsense syllables using different consonants but retaining the same vowel. If, on the other hand, we wish to know whether the person can discriminate the vowels, we should construct a list of syllables using the same consonants before, after, or surrounding different vowels. The use of nonsense syllables in the study of intelligibility represents an analytic approach in which our interest is focused on the intelligibility or repeatability of specific phonetic elements.

Lists of nonsense syllables have limitations in any testing program because of the difficulty encountered in eliciting appropriate responses from the observers. If one had at his disposal observers who were trained in the use of the IPA, it would not be difficult for these observers to write down, in phonetic transcription, the syllables that they hear. If we attempt to avoid the difficulties of written repetition by using oral repetition, we find ourselves doing a double test: we are testing the ability of the observer to hear the phonetic elements and at the same time the ability of the tester to hear the phonetic elements as they are repeated by the observer.

The advantage of using nonsense syllables lies in the fact that they are devoid of meaning and hence their intelligibility is in no way dependent upon the vocabulary of the observer. Early in the development of testing techniques, the group at the Bell Telephone Laboratories selected their nonsense syllables by drawing cards at random from three bins. The first of these supplied the initial consonant, the second the vowel, and the third the final consonant. This provided a pool of nonsense syllables, but a great many of the units thus drawn were words in the English language. As we shall see presently, however, it is possible to make up whole lists of words that will test at least indirectly the ability to hear spoken speech sounds. The convenience of using words rather than nonsense syllables is probably responsible for their more general use.

Monosyllabic Words. After nonsense syllables, the next least analytic unit of speech is the one-syllable word. There is a surprisingly large number of English words of one syllable, constituting a pool from which we can draw. Most of the possible combinations of consonants and vowels have been taken into the language as words. Such words seem to be more easily repeated than nonsense syllables, particularly by untrained observers.

In the course of setting up a program for the measurement of intelligibility, members of the Psycho-Acoustic Laboratory at Harvard (see Egan) attempted to construct lists of monosyllabic words, each of which lists would represent the different phonetic elements in frequencies of occurrence that were roughly the same as those that obtained in normal conversational English. If, for example, the sound [i] occurs twice as often as the sound [a] in normal conversational English, then we should find that each of the 50-word lists contains twice as many [i]'s as [a]'s. This attempt to balance the sounds in any one list according to their normal frequency in everyday use has given these lists the name *Phonetically Balanced Lists* or *PB lists.*

The PB lists have been found to be extremely useful in studying the amount of intelligibility carried by different pieces of communications equipment and, more recently, in measuring hearing deficiency. We shall have more to say about such lists when we discuss the formal articulation test.

Dissyllabic Words. Still less analytic than the monosyllabic word is the word that consists of two syllables. The situation is not very different from the preceding one, in that the listener must hear both syllables in order to repeat the word correctly. The exception to this requirement is found, of course, in the fact that not all the combinations of two syllables constitute words in English. For example, the two monosyllables *horse* and *fly* when put together in one way yield the perfectly respectable word *horsefly*, but put together in reverse order, they give the word *flyhorse*, which is not used in English. You will see that as we become less analytic in choosing the units of speech to be used in our speech samples, we cut down the number of possibilities that are available to the listener. Syllables can be made up of any combination of consonant and vowel. Only certain of these combinations, however, produce single syllables that are English words. And then only certain combinations of two monosyllables constitute dissyllables that are English words.

We must remember that in the case of words with two or more syllables, there are additional cues for intelligibility. In order to repeat a monosyllabic word correctly we must hear each of the phonetic elements. A word of two syllables, however, can be distinguished from other two-syllable words not only on the basis of phonetic elements but also on the basis of stress pattern. You may remember something about these stress patterns from your high-school study of poetry. There we learned about iambic, trochaic, spondaic, and other kinds of feet. Certain kinds of feet consist of only two syllables: iambic with stress on the second syllable, trochaic with stress on the first syllable, and spondaic with equal stress on both syllables. Examples of these three in words are *again, farmer,* and *football.*

Words that employ these different kinds of stress patterns are not all equally intelligible. If all the words for a particular test have the same stress pattern, a listener cannot respond correctly to a test word on the basis of stress pattern. Such a list is homogeneous with respect to intelligibility (Hudgins *et al.*). Choosing all the words of a spondaic pattern, for example, yielded the list of words that has come to be known as the *Spondee Test.* Again, we shall have more to say about this when we discuss the tests.

Sentences. We usually like to work with words in measuring intelligibility, because we can construct a list of words and present each word to a listener at a given intensity. To be sure, the relation between such lists and the continuous flow of words that we encounter in conversation is not very clear. Instead, therefore, we may attempt to devise a more valid test by using groups of words that might appear in conversation. One such group is, of course, the sentence.

Sentences were used by the Bell Telephone Laboratories in their early work (Fletcher and Steinberg). These early lists consisted of interrogative sentences that were not to be repeated by the observer but were rather to be answered. Some examples are "Why is it dangerous to put gasoline on a coal fire?" "What happens to a punctured tire?" The sentences were presented to the observer as they would be spoken normally, although some attempt was made to minimize the variation in intensity within the sentence. These earlier lists were not found so useful for the clinician as had been anticipated, because the test demanded not only that the observer hear the words of the sentence, but also that he provide answers to some fairly difficult questions. Typical examples, from these earlier lists, are "Why is silk preferred to cotton for umbrellas?" "Why are fresh eggs necessary for invalids?" "Explain the advantages of a checking account." Another disadvantage of these earlier lists was that they required some knowledge of New York City and environs. For the purpose of the Bell Telephone Laboratories' group, the sentences were undoubtedly suitable.

Simpler lists of sentences were constructed at the Psycho-Acoustic Laboratory (Hudgins *et al.*) during the course of its testing program.

Again questions are used, but they are so simple as to require of most listeners only that they hear the words of the question. These, too, will be described in a section on Clinical Tests.

Continuous Discourse. Although difficult to quantify with respect to the response of the observer, the most valid sample of English speech is, of course, a whole paragraph or several paragraphs of continuous discourse. There is available material that is so uniformly monotonous and uninteresting that a speaker can repeat the material with remarkably little variability in intensity. Recordings have been made, for example, of passages from Adam Smith's *The Wealth of Nations* and of certain news broadcasts. When one puts a meter across the output of a phonograph that is playing back these recordings, one notes that the indicator does not vary much as the passage progresses. The use of such continuous passages employs a kind of method of adjustment in which the listener may change whatever physical dimension of the stimulus is being studied. He must maintain his own criterion for what is just intelligible.

Having described very briefly some of the materials that can be used in tests for the intelligibility of speech, we must now proceed to discuss the properties of such tests and some of the relations, especially in regard to physical parameters, that have been obtained in their employment.

ARTICULATION TESTS

We are bowing to tradition in the use of the term "articulation test." When such tests were originally designed, the primary goal was an evaluation of the ability of a telephone system to transmit speech. This was an indirect test of the ability of the parts of the telephone system to articulate properly. More recent writers have preferred such terms as "speech-reception tests" or "speech-perception tests" or "speech-hearing tests." The articulation test discussed here has no relation to the articulation test given by a speech teacher to evaluate the ability of an individual to speak particular sounds.

An articulation test is simply a method of measuring the intelligibility of a sample of speech as a function of some variable dimension of the stimulus. The typical procedure involves lists of test items that the listener is to repeat. If he can repeat 45 out of 50 items in a given list, his *articulation score* is 90 per cent. We can measure the articulation score as a function of many different dimensions of the stimulus. We have already described, for example, different kinds of material from which we might choose our test items. The articulation score obtained for a given set of physical parameters will be different for different test materials. Using any one kind of test material, we can change the intensity at which the speech is presented, we can hold the intensity constant and change the band of frequencies that is passed by our reproducing system, or we can change the amount of distortion introduced by the system.

The particular procedure for a given articulation test depends to a large extent upon the purpose for which the test is designed. To determine the threshold of intelligibility (see below) we would use a particular kind of test material as well as a certain test procedure. For other measures of intelligibility we would use different test material.

Factors That Determine the Articulation Score

Now we are ready to study some of the data that have been reported on the measurement of intelligibility as a function of several physical dimensions of the stimulus. We may gain two different kinds of information from this discussion: (1) the physical dimensions of speech that are important for its intelligibility and (2) the physical dimensions that must be controlled in any experiment or test that we may set up to determine an individual's ability to hear or repeat speech.

Role of Intensity. It is almost too obvious to say that as we increase the intensity of speech from a very low value (for example, so low that it cannot be heard) toward a very high level, the articulation score, or percentage of items that a listener will repeat, will increase. A systematic relation between the intelligibility of speech and the intensity at which speech is presented is shown by the articulation-gain function: the ordinate is articulation score, and the abscissa is intensity, SPL, or the gain of an amplifying system. The necessary experimental equipment for obtaining such a gain function consists of a series of test lists and a system by which speech is presented at controlled intensities. The speech may be recorded and then presented through a phonograph, or the speech may be presented "live" through a microphone whose output can be monitored.[1] The experimental procedure is essentially the psychophysical method of constant stimuli modified in two ways: (1) a number of speech items to be presented at any one level may be presented as a group; (2) the individual stimuli in any group are not necessarily identical but usually represent speech items that are thought to be roughly equivalent with respect to intelligibility. Strictly speaking, the method of constant stimuli would be utilized only if we presented one word over and over

[1] Suppose you are seated before a microphone, prepared to recite a list of words that will either be presented to a listener directly or will be recorded on a phonograph disc. Your ear gives you the only indication of the intensity of your voice, which you want to keep as constant as possible. If, however, a voltmeter is inserted across the output of the microphone amplifier, you can 'see' your intensity and adjust it according as the meter readings are above or below a monitoring target.

again 50 times at each level and asked the subject to repeat the word each time he heard it. There are some practical difficulties here, however, which may be overcome if the successive words are different.

Speech Materials. The articulation curves for different kinds of speech material differ in shape and average slope. Figure 5.5 shows the relation between *articulation score* and *relative intensity* for three different types of words: spondees, unselected dissyllables, and PB monosyllables. The abscissas for the three curves are scaled in decibels relative to the intensity at an articulation score of 0 per cent. On an absolute intensity scale the three curves would be pulled apart only slightly more. In later sections when we talk about specific measures of intelligibility that are

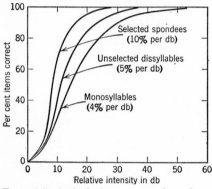

FIG. 5.5. Articulation score for three different types of speech material plotted as a function of relative intensity. (*Hudgins et al.*)

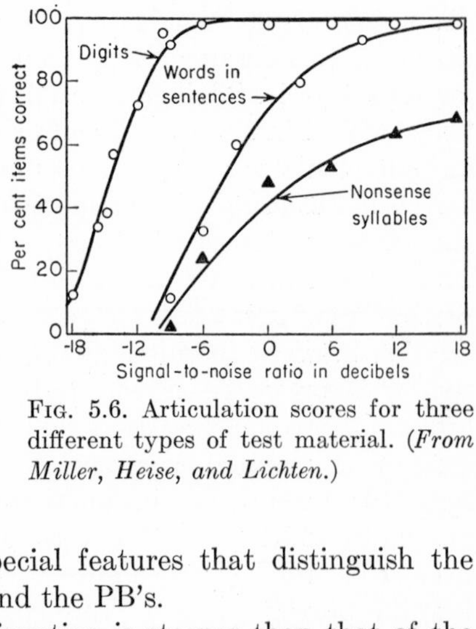

FIG. 5.6. Articulation scores for three different types of test material. (*From Miller, Heise, and Lichten.*)

used clinically, we shall refer to special features that distinguish the articulation curves of the spondees and the PB's.

We note that the spondees' gain function is steeper than that of the PB's. Its average slope between 20 and 80 per cent is about 10 per cent per decibel. This is a graphic correlate of the homogeneity of spondees contrasted with the relative heterogeneity of PB's. Ideally, of course, the most sensitive gain function would be that of lists of words that were so homogeneous that all words would become just intelligible at the same intensity. The steepness of these curves represents the homogeneity of the words, or lack of it, as they are normally presented in constant monitoring.

It is possible to change the steepness of a gain function by manipulating the homogeneity of a list with respect to intelligibility. Harris (1948*b*), for example, attempted to homogenize lists of PB words so as to make their gain functions more nearly as steep as those of the spondees. Figure

5.7 shows the results for PB words recorded in three different ways. The middle curve represents the normal recording with a constantly monitored carrier. The flat curve represents a re-recording of the normal list in which compensations were introduced for differences in intensity (*i.e.*, variability in monitoring) among the individual words. The steepest of the three curves represents another kind of recording in which compensations were introduced for differences in intelligibility among the individual words. This steepest curve of homogenized PB's is almost as steep as the curve for spondees, which is shown for comparison.

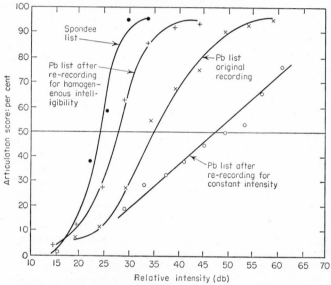

FIG. 5.7. Articulation curves for three different recordings of a PB list compared to that of a list of spondees. The steepness of the curve is increased by re-recording according to differences in intelligibility among the different words. Re-recording by making the words more alike with respect to intensity decreases the steepness. (*From Harris*, 1948*b*.)

If the unit of our articulation test were the sentence, we should find that the gain function would be about as steep as that for the spondees, if not a little steeper. We have some evidence available that gives us a few clues about why some items are easier to hear than others. We define "easy" in terms of how little intensity is needed for a particular criterion of intelligibility. Figure 5.8 shows the articulation score at a given intensity for lists of words that differ in respect of the number of syllables in each word. At a given intensity, the more syllables there are per word, the more intelligible the word and the higher the articulation score for a list of such words. It is not surprising, therefore, that at a given intensity a listener hears a higher percentage of a list of spondees than of a list of monosyllabic words. To be sure, the spondee words and the monosyllables of the PB lists are not the only sampling units of speech that can be used to make up articulation tests, but a considerable amount of data has already been accumulated on these two types of words.

One very important concept that must be considered in comparing the intelligibility of different kinds of speech material is the amount of context that is present in the sample. Each word in a list of words is presented by itself. The listener is given no additional cues about what the word might be from either preceding or succeeding words. When

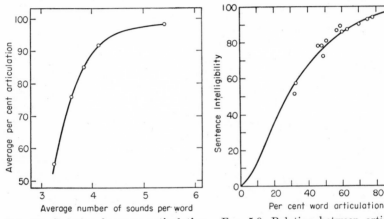

FIG. 5.8. Relation between articulation score for a list of words and the average number of sounds per word. (*From Egan.*)

FIG. 5.9. Relation between articulation score for sentences and the score for words. Note that, when a listener can repeat 50 per cent of the list of words, he can repeat almost 80 per cent of the list of sentences. (*From Egan.*)

the test material consists of sentences, the many interactions among the words in a given sentence yield more information about what the individual words might be than is contained in the words themselves. Figure 5.9 compares the articulation score for sentences with that for words when both kinds of material are presented at the same intensity. We note that the comparable intelligibility of sentences is always higher than that of words, and that 50 per cent of a list of sentences will be repeated correctly at an intensity where only 30 per cent of a list of words would be repeated correctly.

Another interesting comparison is made in Fig. 5.10. Here we see two articulation curves for the same set of words: in one test (lower curve) the words were presented as individual items of a list, while in another test (upper curve) articulation scores were obtained for the same words at comparable intensities when they appeared as key words in English sentences. Articulation scores are shown as a function of the intensity of the speech relative to the intensity of a background noise. If we compare the relative intensity of the speech at 50 per cent on each of these curves, we note that we push the *threshold of intelligibility* (see below) down by about 6 db simply by putting the word into a sentence. This is an important fact, particularly for the clinician. Suppose we ask a patient to repeat the word *horseshoe*. He does not seem to hear it and so we might repeat the word by saying "You know, the horse wears a *horseshoe* on his hoof." Such a repeti-

tion constitutes a different test. We should be measuring two kinds of thresholds, one for the isolated word and one for the word as it appears in a sentence, and if we extrapolate from the curves of Fig. 5.10, we might account for a difference as large as 10 db.

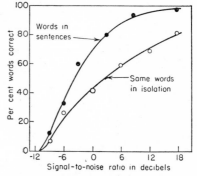

FIG. 5.10. Two articulation curves for a single list of words. In one case the words were presented singly in a list; in the other case the words appeared as parts of sentences. (*From Miller, Heise, and Lichten.*)

This problem of context is a bothersome one, particularly when we consider that a man's ability to understand speech in ordinary communication is aided constantly by the context among the words of conversation. We sometimes wonder about the relation between articulation scores for lists of isolated words and the "score" a person would obtain for his ability to understand conversational speech. We should like to know the latter, but we can quantify only the former.

A notion that is basic to this problem of context involves the number of possibilities for choice that are available to a listener to whom a given item of speech is presented. The word is more distinguishable when it appears as a member of a sentence than when in isolation, presumably because the surrounding words cut down the number of possibilities that are available for choice.

Miller, Heise, and Lichten attacked this problem experimentally and produced the curves of Fig. 5.11. Articulation scores as a function of the intensity of the speech (relative to that of the noise) are shown for lists of words whose total vocabulary was known and available to the listener. The uppermost curve represents the articulation curve for a list of only two words. The listener knew what the two words were and had only to guess between them for the selection of each item. As we move farther down we note that the vocabulary for the test list increases. The third curve from the bottom, for example, represents a series of articulation scores for a test list of 32 words. The listener knew what the 32 words were and had only to choose among them to make his response. Suppose the only word on the list ending in *at* is *pat*. Our listener hears something that sounds like *bat*—or maybe it was *mat* or *hat*—but he knows that *pat* is the only possibility, so he rules out all the others. Just so, a patient who listens to numbers in the clinical testing room does not have a difficult job in choosing among combinations of only ten words (digits), which are known to be the only possibilities for the test items.

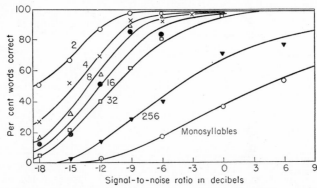

FIG. 5.11. Relation between articulation score and intensity of the speech relative to that of a background noise for test lists of different size. The vocabulary for each test list was known to the listener. (*From Miller, Heise, and Lichten.*)

Distortion. In the process of transmitting speech sounds through various kinds of electrical and electronic gear, certain kinds of distortion, imposed by the properties of the systems, may be encountered (see Chap. 3). We wish to examine the effect of the two basic types of such distortion, which we have already discussed in Chap. 3, on intelligibility for two reasons: (1) we wish to be able to predict what effect an imperfect system with known amounts of distortion will have upon the intelligibility of a given sample of speech, and (2) by controlling the distortion we can determine the limits of certain physical dimensions that are crucial for the intelligibility of speech.

Some amplifying systems through which we transmit speech may be nonlinear with respect to intensity. This is simply another way of saying that as the intensity of the input signal increases, the output of the amplifier does not increase proportionally, particularly at the higher levels. Such a defect in an amplifying system will produce *amplitude distortion.* One example of this process, symmetrical *peak clipping,* is shown in Fig. 5.12. The *transfer characteristic* (a graphic representation of the relation between the output and the input of a system) of a linear amplifier with a gain of 1 would be a straight line that makes an angle of 45° with the abscissa. The transfer characteristic of the amplifier that is represented in Fig. 5.12, however, is nonlinear, as is shown by the breaks at the upper and lower ends of the solid line, which indicate a

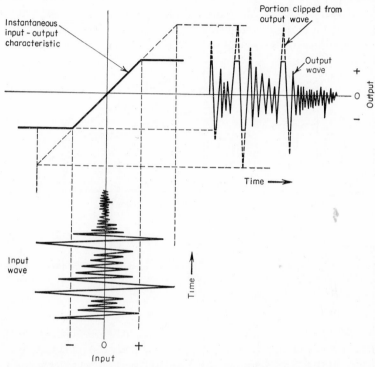

Fig. 5.12. The effect of the peak-clipping type of amplitude distortion on a speech wave. A linear transfer characteristic would show an output wave that would look like the input wave. Since the linearity of this transfer characteristic stops at the indicated limits, the output wave shows that the wide excursions of the input wave have been cut off or clipped. (*From Licklider, 1944.*)

limitation beyond which the output signal cannot go. We see below the transfer characteristic the waveform of a particular sample of speech. To the right of the transfer characteristic is a waveform of the output of this amplifier, which shows that the peaks of the input wave have been cut off at the limits imposed by the system. Amplitude distortion is quite common in amplifiers and transducers, particularly when they are operated with input or output levels higher than those for which the amplifier

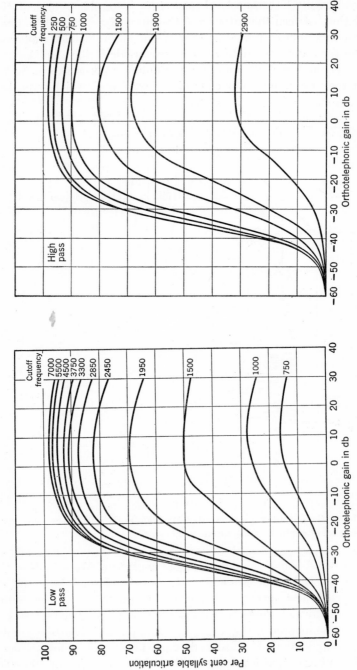

FIG. 5.13. Articulation score (syllables) as a function of relative intensity for speech passed through low-pass and high-pass filters. The parameter is the cutoff frequency of the filter. (*From French and Steinberg.*)

was designed. Although the effects of amplitude distortion on the waveform of the speech appear to be quite severe, the experiments of Licklider (1944, 1946) have shown that the effects of this type of amplitude distortion, or peak clipping, on intelligibility are relatively small.

Frequency is another dimension of the stimulus in respect of which an amplifying system or any component of a system may not be linear. If a system passes, let us say, all frequencies between 100 and 5000 cps equally well (*e.g.*, within ±2 db) we say that the system is *flat* as a function of frequency between the specified limits. If, however, the system favors some frequencies and suppresses others, we say that the system introduces *frequency distortion*.

With the aid of a set of filters we may control the width of a band of frequencies that a system will pass. Using such filters to suppress the high and low frequencies of a system, experimenters at the Bell Telephone Laboratories have shown the relative importance of different frequencies for the intelligibility of speech. Figure 5.13 shows the results of one of these studies. The *low-pass*[1] curves show the relation between articulation score (syllables) and gain for different low-pass-filter cutoff frequencies. The curve marked 1500, for example, shows how the articulation score rises to a maximum of 50 per cent as gain increases when *only those frequencies in the speech below 1500 cps are passed*. The *high-pass* curves show similar relations when only those frequencies *above* the indicated cutoff frequency are passed.

If we now take all points at, for example, a gain of 10, we may plot the articulation score as a function of the cutoff frequency for both the low-pass and the high-pass filters. The results of such a plot are shown in Fig. 5.14. The superposition of these two curves indicates that the most important frequencies for the over-all intelligibility of monosyllabic words lie in a range between 1500 and 2500 cps. This is an interesting fact, particularly when compared with the over-all power spectrum of speech that was shown in Fig. 2.9. Whereas most of our speech energy is concentrated in the low frequencies, the frequencies that contribute most to the intelligibility of speech lie in a higher frequency region. It is also interesting to note, from the biological point of view, that the frequencies that are most important for the intelligibility of speech lie in the range where the human ear is most sensitive (see. Fig. 4.9).

Recorded vs. "Live" Speech. It is clear that if we want to present controlled intensities of speech to our listeners, we should use electroacoustic combinations of equipment that permit measurement of speech

[1] An *n-cps low-pass filter* is a device that transmits (or passes) all frequencies below *n* cps and rejects, or blocks, all frequencies above that frequency. An *n-cps high-pass filter* passes all frequencies above *n* and rejects all below.

voltage and its mechanical analogue, sound pressure. The sound will be delivered through either an earphone (or earphones) or a loud-speaker. It will be fed to one of these by an amplifying system with appropriate attenuation controls. But what about the input to the amplifier? Speaking the items of an articulation test into a microphone constitutes one method of which a great many clinical workers approve (Carhart, 1946a). But the words must be repeated each time we give the test. On the other hand, suppose that we speak items once and for all into a system that will put our speech on a phonograph record or strip of magnetic tape. Then we can conduct our articulation test simply by using this recorded version of the test as the input for the amplifier above.

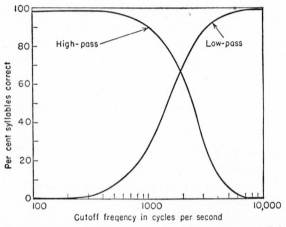

Fig. 5.14. Articulation score (syllables) as a function of the cutoff frequency of a low-pass and a high-pass filter for speech at a constant intensity. At this intensity, for example, when all frequencies above 1000 cps are passed, the score is about 90 per cent, whereas speech that contains only frequencies below 1000 cps is only 27-per-cent intelligible. (*After French and Steinberg; from Miller, 1951, p. 64.*)

Unfortunately, we do not have reliable data that compare the intelligibility of live and recorded speech on a large enough sample of listeners. If the monitoring is kept at a constant level in the *live-voice* technique and if the physical characteristics of the microphone and phonograph systems are the same, there is no reason to assume different results. The clinician sometimes favors the live-voice technique because it permits a good bit of flexibility in his clinical procedure: he can wait between items, etc. The recorded tests, on the other hand, can be better standardized. The talker error is eliminated, since the talker is the same on all the records, and successive tests at one place or tests conducted at many places can be known to be the same.

CLINICAL SPEECH AUDIOMETRY

Threshold of Intelligibility and Hearing Loss for Speech

We must return now to the concept of threshold and attempt to establish a reasonable method for measuring the *threshold of intelligibility for speech*. We have already defined intelligibility in terms of a person's ability to repeat words that are presented at a certain level. The 50-percent criterion was chosen for the threshold for pure tones because it is the most representative statistic about the distribution of responses. There is also the fact that the frequency of response is rising most steeply when it passes through the 50-per-cent point.

Can we not further apply this criterion to the choice of material to use for measuring the threshold of intelligibility? To be sure, this threshold will be different for different kinds of speech, but it can be measured most reliably with lists of words that yield a very steep articulation curve (articulation-*vs.*-gain function). The steeper the gain function, the more easily the threshold can be determined. The spondees or digits seem to be likely candidates for such a measurement because their great homogeneity is associated with steep curves. Indeed, recorded tests for measuring the threshold of intelligibility have employed both digits and spondee words (Western Electric 4-A,B, and C audiometers and Psycho-Acoustic Laboratory Auditory Test No. 9).[1] If we refer again to Fig. 5.5, we see that there is a spread of at most about 6 db between 20 and 80 per cent on the spondee curve, so that if a person gets any reasonable number of spondees at all short of 100 per cent at a particular level, one is already within a very few db of threshold.

Something further should be said about the use of spondees for measuring the threshold of intelligibility. Homogeneity seems to be most useful in providing the steepness for a gain function that is required for threshold measurements. There is no a priori reason why the steepest curve of Fig. 5.5 or 5.6 should also be the curve of the most intelligible material. Spondees are relatively intelligible even when transmitted by a system that passes only low frequencies, whereas a comparable amount of intelligibility for PB's is achieved only with a system with a fairly wide range of frequencies. It has been known for some time that persons with high-frequency Hearing Loss may have a normal threshold of intelligibility when these thresholds are measured with lists of spondees or numbers. Harris's (1948b) re-recording techniques for PB lists were prompted by his desire to use, for threshold measurements, material whose intelligibility depended more upon the higher frequencies than do

[1] PAL Auditory Test No. 9 has been replaced, for clinical use, by Central Institute for the Deaf (CID) Auditory Test No. W-2.

the spondees. His demonstration that PB words can be presented in a way that makes them appear almost as homogeneous as normally recorded spondees seems to imply that a more valid measurement of the threshold of intelligibility might be made with PB lists.

Hearing Loss. When a clinician stands 20 ft away from a patient and speaks numbers or words for the patient to repeat, he is attempting to estimate the patient's *Hearing Loss for Speech.* The traditional way of presenting the results of such a test has been in terms of the distance fraction. If a patient can repeat all the words or numbers satisfactorily and the clinician is 20 ft away, the patient is said to have 20/20 hearing. If the clinician must come, let us say, to within 10 ft of the patient in order for him to repeat the words and the numbers satisfactorily, he is said to have 10/20 hearing.

This kind of testing has certainly been useful to the clinician in the past and is still in use in most private offices and even in some larger installations. The difficulties of interpretation of such tests are numerous. The term "10/20 hearing" should mean that the patient has a 6-db Hearing Loss for Speech. That is, if we must halve the distance between the speaker and listener, we are multiplying the energy at the listener's ear by 4 (inverse square law), and a fourfold increase equals 6 db. But the usual testing situation does not permit this simple interpretation. For one thing, it is extremely difficult, even for a well-trained speaker, to keep the intensity of the voice really constant as one approaches or goes away from the patient. Imagine, then, the variability from speaker to speaker! Harris (1948*b*) has recommended the use of a sound-level meter as a minimum aid for such a test, so that the clinician can remain aware of the level of his speech.

Another difficulty lies in the fact that most of these tests are given in rooms with hard walls. This means that even if the speaker's voice is kept at a constant intensity as he changes his position in the room relative to that of the patient, the distribution of sound energies at the patient's ear will vary. For example, if the clinician is very close to the patient, the patient will hear sounds that come directly from the lips of the speaker. If, however, the speaker is quite far away, the patient will hear not only the sounds that come directly from the speaker's lips but also the sounds that are reflected from the hard walls. This situation can be helped, of course, by the use of heavy draperies or other appropriate deadening materials.

One other difficulty lies in the lack of specification of the response. Some clinicians demand that the patient hear all the numbers or all the words at a particular distance, while others demand that he hear only 50 per cent of the words or numbers. Finally, interpretation of the distance fraction is difficult, particularly when a comparison is to be made between the results of such a test and the pure-tone audiogram. If the test were given in an acoustically dead room (*i.e.*, one that had no reflections), the intensity of the speech at the ear of the patient would vary inversely as the square of the distance between patient and clinician. Since, however, the inverse square law holds only in a dead room, it has been difficult to relate the results of these two tests.

It is possible to measure the threshold of intelligibility for a particular kind of speech on a sufficient number of observers to obtain an average or normal threshold. Table 5.2 shows the absolute thresholds of intelligibility

TABLE 5.2. THRESHOLDS FOR SPEECH TESTS ON NORMAL EARS
(Monaural listening with earphone. Data from Davis, 1948)*

Test	Number of ears	Experimenter	Db re 0.0002 dyne/cm²	SD	PB equivalent, per cent
No. 9.........	50	Falconer and Davis	22.46	±2.63	8
No. 12........	20	Breakey	26.65	3.89	23
Continuous discourse	50	Falconer and Davis	23.23	3.77	12
PB...........	14	CID (unpublished)	33.2	?	50
Detectability .	14	CID (unpublished)	15.0		
	?	Miller (1947a)	10.0 (approx.)		
Intelligibility .	?	Miller (1947a)	22.0 (approx.)		

* Thresholds for the new (1952) Auditory Tests W-1, W-2, and W-22 of the Central Institute for the Deaf are lower: spondees, about 18 to 20 db; PB's about 25 db.

for several different kinds of speech material. These measurements were made on normal populations at the Central Institute for the Deaf. Thresholds of intelligibility for spondees center around an SPL of about 25 db when the words are presented in the quiet. If we now find a person who hears 50 per cent of a list of spondees that is presented at, for example, 55 db SPL, we have a person who is not so sensitive to these words as a normal person, that is to say, one whose threshold of intelligibility is 30 db higher than normal. This difference between an individual's threshold and a given normal threshold is his *Hearing Loss for Speech*, in this case hearing loss for spondees. This particular measure of hearing loss is analogous to the audiogram in the sense that both are thresholds. We still know nothing about how fine a distinction such a person could make among very difficult speech items at supraliminal intensities. We know only that in order for him to hear as many words in a list of spondees as does a normal person we must present the list at a higher intensity.

In a clinical situation the measurement of this threshold would be too time-consuming if we had to present long lists of words over and over again until we found an intensity at which a person just heard 50 per cent of the words, and so specific tests have been developed to allow the clinician to measure this threshold fairly quickly. One of the first tests designed to measure the threshold of intelligibility was incorporated in the Western Electric 4A audiometer. This device employed phonograph records on which were recorded series of two-digit groups at decreasing levels. For purposes of screening, especially with large groups, this test has been found to be quite satisfactory. The monitoring on the records, however, is somewhat erratic, and not enough is known about the relative intelligibility of digits.

Auditory Tests No. 9 and No. 12, developed at the Psycho-Acoustic Laboratory, are designed to obtain thresholds of intelligibility for spondees and short sentences, respectively. Auditory Test No. 9 consists of 12 records, on each of which are recorded 42 spondee words. The level on each record decreases 4 db at the end of each successive group of six words, so that each record covers a range of 28 db. The experimenter starts a record well above a patient's threshold, so that he can repeat accurately at least the first one or two groups. The next problem is to specify the level at which a person would hear three out of six words. If a 4-db decrement is given to every six words, we can assume that on the average each single word is equivalent to a decrease of about ⅔ db. This assumption allows one to draw up a table that permits easy computation of the threshold (see Hudgins *et al.*). A similar scheme for the test on the intelligibility of short sentences is used in Auditory Test No. 12. Auditory Tests No. 9 and No. 12 have both been described in detail by Hudgins *et al.*

At the time of writing, Auditory Test No. W-2, adapted from Auditory Test No. 9 by the Central Institute for the Deaf, is being distributed.

Articulation Score and Discrimination Loss

It is apparent from the articulation-vs.-gain functions that the articulation score increases as the intensity of the speech increases. Normally it rises to 100 per cent if the intensity is made great enough. We have already said that the intensity at which this function crosses the 50-per-cent line is the threshold of intelligibility. A person who requires a higher intensity than does a group of normal individuals in order to repeat 50 per cent of a list of words has a Hearing Loss for Speech that is equal, in decibels, to the difference between his threshold and that of the normal.

Now we wish to measure intelligibility at a particular intensity instead of measuring the intensity required for a particular amount of intelligibility (namely, 50 per cent). We are no longer concerned with the threshold. In experimental situations that are set up to evaluate the effective transmission of speech afforded by a particular piece of equipment, this articulation score is a useful evaluative measure for a given set of physical input conditions. We have already said that spondees are very intelligible, and it is a poor system indeed that will not yield an articulation score of 100 per cent for spondees if they are presented at a sufficiently high intensity. Systems that are limited in, for example, frequency response impose a limitation on the maximum articulation score that will be obtained with the relatively difficult PB words no matter how high the intensity (see Fig. 5.13).

Measuring intelligibility at high intensity is important in the clinical situation, because this measure provides additional information that cannot be predicted from threshold measurements. It is very well to say that a person has a 30-db Hearing Loss for spondees, but we do not know from this information alone how much speech would be intelligible if the intensity were made sufficiently great. It is not uncommon to find two individuals who have the same Hearing Loss for Speech in decibels but whose articulation scores are very different at intensities so high that further increase in intensity would not improve the articulation score. Ideally the ceiling that could be reached by increasing the intensity of speech is 100 per cent, but some persons can never get more than 40 or 50 per cent no matter how intense the speech.

Specifically, let us consider individuals A and B, whose audiograms are presented in Fig. 5.15. Individual A has a Hearing Loss of 45 db that is fairly constant as a function of frequency, while individual B has a Hearing Loss that increases as frequency increases and is apparently not at all sensitive to frequencies above 4000 cps, at least within the limitations of the audiometer. Both these individuals show about the same 40-db Hearing Loss for Speech (A, 45 db; B, 37 db) when this Hearing Loss is measured with spondee words. When PB's are presented at 100 db SPL, individual A has an articulation score of 96 per cent, whereas individual B gets only 60 per cent. This apparent ceiling on B's intelligibility may be converted to the clinical term *Discrimination Loss* by subtracting the maximum articulation score from 100 per cent. B's Discrimination Loss is therefore 40 per cent, while A's is only 4 per cent. The articulation-gain functions for these two individuals are shown as curves *A* and *B* in Fig. 5.16. Presumably the adequate discrimination of a high percentage of PB words depends upon the recognition of phonetic patterns that involve fairly high frequencies. These frequencies come into play for individual

A when speech is made intense, but they seem to be absent from the response system of individual B. (See Recruitment and Diagnosis, Chap. 8.)

We may note in passing that the function of a hearing aid even at its best is to provide amplification (*i.e.*, more intensity) for speech sounds. Amplification of 40 db would give individuals A and B both approximately normal thresholds for spondees and further would provide individual A with almost 100 per cent intelligibility for sounds at a conversational level. A hearing aid by amplification alone, however, can never push individual B's ceiling above 60 per cent. This demonstrates the impor-

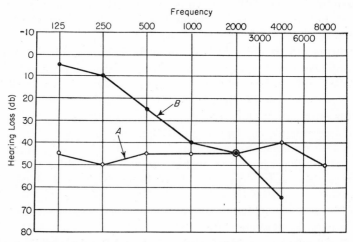

Fig. 5.15. Audiograms of two patients, A and B, whose articulation curves are shown as curves *A* and *B* in Fig. 5.16.

tance of measuring the intelligibility of difficult material at a high intensity in clinical routine and also emphasizes the relative unimportance of measuring a Hearing Loss for spondees that can be predicted fairly accurately from the audiogram (Carhart, 1946b; Harris, 1946).

Relation between Speech and Pure-tone Audiometry

In spite of this seeming unimportance of measuring the threshold of intelligibility or the Hearing Loss for Speech, the very fact that this Hearing Loss can be predicted so well from the audiogram suggests that we may profitably use a measurement of the Hearing Loss for Speech as a check on the accuracy of the pure-tone audiogram. Inconsistency between the Hearing Loss for Speech and the average Hearing Loss for frequencies of 500, 1000, and 2000 cps should make the clinician suspicious of one or the other of these measurements. Carhart (1946b) has tested the correlations between Hearing Loss for Speech and different estimates of the audiogram. The three-tone average mentioned above seems to correlate best with the Hearing Loss for Speech in a large number of clinical observations. More recently Fletcher (1950) has suggested an even simpler formula. He reports that Hearing Loss for Speech is best predicted by noting the Hearing Loss for the middle three frequencies and then taking the average of the smallest two. In most cases the average three-tone and this two-tone average are almost the same.

Another favorable result of the close relation between the audiogram and Hearing Loss for Speech has to do with children. The difficulty in obtaining reliable responses to pure tones from most children is well known to most clinicians. Children who have acquired some language can, however, give reliable responses (*i.e.*, can repeat words) when a simple speech test is used. An example of such a test, in which a child points to an object that is symbolized by the test word, is reported by Keaster.

So far as the relation between the audiogram and Discrimination Loss is concerned, we can only point out that here lies one of the greatest points of ignorance in contemporary clinical audiology.

INTELLIGIBILITY AND COMMUNICATION

This chapter has been concerned with the measurement of intelligibility of speech. We have seen that such measurement is facilitated when we break down what we consider normal continuous speech into small analytic units. Methods for measuring the intelligibility of sentences, words, and syllables have been described. We have seen that it is possible to estimate the threshold of intelligibility even for continuous discourse, but this particular measurement was shown to be inadequate because of the difficulty of quantifying the intelligibility. Rather we had to depend upon the listener's setting up his own criterion of "just intelligible." The many persons who are concerned with the estimate of an individual's ability to hear speech are interested, in a very practical way, not in the intelligibility of words and syllables but rather in the intelligibility of speech as it flows in everyday life.

We can approach an estimate of this general ability from the results of some of our articulation tests. We know, for example, that if spondees are presented at a level where an individual can repeat 50 per cent of them, he will be able to understand speech in normal context perfectly. (Only a small number of such relations can be obtained from data such as those in Table 5.2.) It would be better, however, for the patient, the doctor, the insurance claim adjudicator, and the industrial hygienist if this estimate could be more precise and at the same time offer a reasonable amount of face validity.

It is possible that Davis (1948) and his collaborators have approached an answer to this knotty problem. They have attempted to combine information on the threshold of intelligibility for sentences, spondees, or numbers with information on the articulation score at several critical levels for the PB lists. The resultant datum has been called the *Social Adequacy Index* (SAI). Because the adjective "social" may appear too ambitious, it should be pointed out that "social adequacy" refers to communicative adequacy or *social adequacy for hearing.*

The speech that we hear every day covers a wide range of intensities. We cannot predict a man's performance throughout this range if we make a measurement at only one intensity. Roughly speaking, SPL's of 55, 70, and 85 db correspond respectively to faint, average, and loud conversational speech. At these levels a person with normal hearing obtains articulation scores of 94, 100, and 100 per cent, respectively, with PB lists. The average of these three is 98 per cent, and it is this average that is called the Social Adequacy Index.

The normal articulation curve with an SAI of 98 is shown as the leftmost curve in Fig. 5.16. An individual with a purely conductive hearing loss of 50 db would typically give an articulation curve like the rightmost curve in Fig. 5.16. It is simply the normal curve shifted horizontally by 50 db. Note that this curve crosses the everyday levels of 55, 70, and 85 db SPL at 0, 3, and 58 per cent. The SAI would be 20.

It would be very time-consuming to generate an entire articulation curve for each patient who comes into the clinic or even to get three stable articulation scores at 55, 70, and 85 db. Let us assume instead that the articulation curves of all individuals—normal as well as those with conductive and perceptive hearing losses—have the same shape. We know that we could find the SAI of a man with purely conductive hearing loss by shifting the normal articulation curve horizontally by the amount of his *Hearing Loss for Speech.* Having said that his loss is conductive only, we know that the maximum articulation score reaches nearly 100 per cent. This datum tells us that in order to find the SAI, we need only move the normal curve horizontally, because the maximum scores of the normal and the conductive-loss patient approach the same value.

But what about our man with the perceptive loss who may not have such a severe Hearing Loss for Speech but does not seem to be able to get an articulation score of more than 60 or 70 per cent no matter how intense we make the speech? Davis (1948) and his coworkers have submitted the notion that the articulation curve for such patients is shifted downward on the scale of *articulation score* rather than horizontally on the scale of *Hearing Loss.* The leveling off at a lower than perfect articulation score that characterizes these perceptive hearing losses should not be

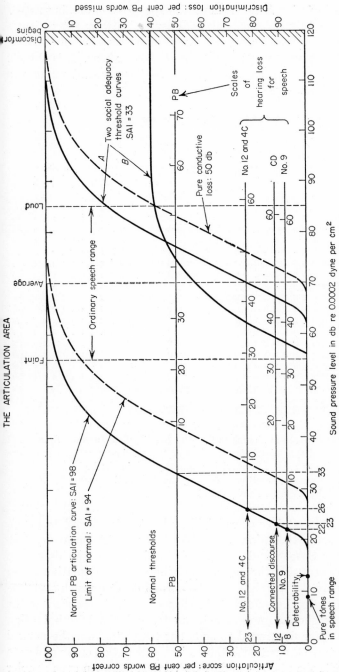

FIG. 5.16. Articulation scores for PB lists as a function of Sound Pressure Level. The leftmost solid curve shows a normal articulation curve for PB lists. The vertical broken lines at the left of the figure show the Sound Pressure Levels that correspond to 50-percent scores for different kinds of articulation tests. The numbered horizontal lines show the Hearing Loss for Speech relative to the several thresholds of intelligibility. The lines at 55, 70, and 85 db SPL show estimates of faint, average, and loud speech, respectively. The articulation curves marked A and B might have been obtained from patients A and B whose audiograms were shown in Fig. 5.15. Note that these two quite different-looking curves have the same Social Adequacy Index, the average articulation scores at 55, 70, and 85 db SPL. (*From Davis*, 1948.)

interpreted as a deviation from the normal shape of the curve, but rather as a shift downward that is equal to the difference between the patient's maximum articulation score (the one that is so high that a further increase in intensity will not increase the score) and 100 per cent. This shift is called the *Discrimination Loss* and is equal to 100 per cent minus the maximum articulation score.

SOCIAL ADEQUACY INDEX

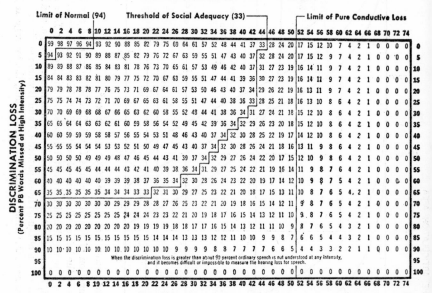

Fig. 5.17. A chart of Social Adequacy Index which permits one to obtain an SAI from two measures of speech audiometry: first the *Hearing Loss for Speech* measured in decibels, and second the *Discrimination Loss* or the maximum articulation score subtracted from 100 per cent. The resulting figures given in the body of the chart are those that have been obtained by averaging the articulation scores for PB lists at 55, 70, and 85 db SPL. (*From Davis*, 1948.)

We can then take a piece of celluloid and cut out a template in the form of the normal articulation curve. We need only two measures: the Hearing Loss for Speech and the Discrimination Loss, the difference between 100 per cent and the person's maximum PB articulation score. The basic tools are the template and the normal curve on such a plot as Fig. 5.16. The Hearing Loss for Speech tells us how far to the right of the normal curve we should move our template, and the Discrimination Loss tells us how far downward to shift our template from the normal curve. We then trace the patient's theoretical articulation curve and note where it intersects the 55-, 70-, and 85-db vertical lines. An even simpler calculation of the SAI is afforded by the numerical chart of the SAI (Fig. 5.17).

The SAI is not a new measurement, and it does not require a new clinical test. It is simply a combination of data already being obtained on all patients in many clinics. A general concept is needed for expressing a hearing impairment in terms of what a man can or cannot do. Having noted some basic invariances (namely, the shape of the curve) in the data on a large population of patients, Davis and his group may well have found a descriptive quantity that is practically useful.

References for Further Study

Egan, J. P. (1948) Articulation testing methods. *Laryngoscope, St. Louis,* **58,** 955–991. A somewhat abbreviated report of a basic study on articulation tests. The basic principles for choosing words and making up lists, as well as other practical matters, are described.

Fletcher, H. (1929) *Speech and Hearing.* New York: Van Nostrand. Basic information on the physical characteristics of speech. Some of this material is dated. The speech analysis, in particular, has been superseded by Potter, Kopp, and Green.

Licklider, J. C. R., and G. A. Miller. (1951) The perception of speech. Chap. 26 in S. S. Stevens (Ed.), *Handbook of Experimental Psychology.* New York: Wiley. This chapter summarizes most of the present-day information on the physical and psychological factors that have to do with the perception of spoken language.

Miller, G. A. (1951) *Language and Communication.* New York: McGraw-Hill. This new text, written by a psychologist, about the production and the perception of spoken language provides an excellent background for the serious student.

Potter, R. K., G. A. Kopp, and H. C. Green. (1947) *Visible Speech.* New York: Van Nostrand. This book is a summary of the early development of instrumental and teaching techniques in visible speech.

CHAPTER 6

AUDITORY MASKING AND FATIGUE

EVERYDAY listening goes on in a fairly complex acoustic environment. We usually listen to speech or music against a background of noise or of other voices. Remarkably enough, we seem to be able to single out the *signal*, which we wish to hear, and to suppress the effects of the *noise*, or unwanted extraneous sound. We can understand the speech of our fellows when it is submerged in the noise of a factory or of traffic, and indeed, it is quite necessary that we do this in order to get along in our noisy culture. The measurements that were discussed in the last two chapters, however, were concerned with the absolute thresholds for sounds that were turned on one at a time. In other words, we measured the absolute thresholds for pure tones and for speech in the quiet; or at least as quiet as one can get in spite of the presence of the internal noises of blood vessels, etc.

Now we must ask about the effects of other sounds on these thresholds. We cannot always hear the voice of our neighbor in the subway; at some point the noise becomes too great and *masks* the voice. *Masking* is, then, a kind of exception to our ability to analyze out of a complex of sounds the one to which we wish to attend. It is one way in which a sound affects the audibility of another sound. *Auditory fatigue* is another, differing from masking in that a sound has an effect on the audibility of another sound that follows it in time.

INTRODUCTION

Why do we wish to know about the influence of one sound on the audibility of another? For one thing, having measured a man's ability to hear only in the quiet, we cannot be sure about his ability to hear speech or other sounds in the presence of everyday noise. In other words, these further measurements permit us to extend the *validity* of clinical and experimental audiometry.

A second purpose of this discussion is to provide a fairly rigorous definition of the term *quiet*. What do we mean when we say that we have measured a person's threshold *in the quiet*. Clearly we cannot mean that there is no molecular motion in the air, for this would require a room temperature of absolute zero—a rather chilly testing environment. Rather we mean only that there is a certain amount of noise present and that this amount has been shown not to influence the absolute threshold that was measured in the presence of a lesser amount of noise.

Finally, there are certain specifically clinical relations to be found in the experimental work on masking and fatigue. The problems of acoustic trauma and hearing losses incurred in connection with industrial and military noise are bound up with these same phenomena. In addition, tests of masking and fatigue have provided predictive information about the presence of the phenomenon of *recruitment*, to be discussed in Chap. 8. Our topic is as complicated as it is important, and the present level of our knowledge will allow us only to scratch the surface.

General Definitions

By way of introduction, let us define our two main terms generally. One sound may influence the audibility of a second sound in several ways, two of which are of primary interest here. When one sound causes a second sound to become less audible by coexisting with it, the phenomenon demonstrated is called *masking*. The sound that was audible and is now less audible is called the *masked sound*, while the sound that renders this masked sound less audible is called the *masking sound*. If a sound renders a second sound less audible by preceding it in time, we speak of *auditory fatigue*. Depending on (1) the amount of stimulation provided by the first sound, (2) the interval of time between the cessation of the fatiguing sound and the test sound, and (3) the amount of fatigue, other terms are used: *after-effect masking* (deMaré, 1937), *adaptation* (Lüscher and Zwislocki, 1947, 1949*b*), *residual masking* (Munson and Gardner), *acoustic trauma*, and *temporary hearing loss*.

Suppose that we have two sounds, *A* and *B*. We first measure the absolute threshold for sound *A* in the quiet. Then we turn on sound *B*, and, while *B* is presented to the same ear, we again measure the threshold of *A*. We have done a simple masking experiment and have measured the amount of masking that is produced by *B* on *A*. This amount of masking is the difference, in decibels, between the threshold of *A* in the quiet and the threshold of *A* in the presence of *B*. Now suppose that we turn on *B* alone for a certain period of time, turn it off, and *then* measure the threshold of *A*. The difference between this new threshold and the previous threshold of *A* in the quiet is the amount of auditory fatigue produced by a certain exposure to *B* and measured at a particular time after the cessation of *B*.

Masking vs. Fatigue

There is an important difference between the measurement of masking and the measurement of fatigue with respect to time. Under usual conditions, the *masking* remains fairly constant so long as the masking sound is constant. *Fatigue*, on the other hand, changes in time after the fatiguing sound is turned off. Immediately after exposure to the fatiguing sound the amount of fatigue will be maximum, and it will then decrease in time until recovery is indicated by a return to the prefatigue threshold. Fatigue measurements must, therefore, either be specified for a particular interval of time or else be measured as a function of time, whereas the data on masking do not need to be so specified.

There are many combinations of sounds that could be studied with respect to either masking or fatigue. We shall restrict ourselves, however, to only a few that involve three different kinds of sounds: tones, speech, and noise. Tones and speech have been described in Chap. 2 and have been discussed in Chaps. 4 and 5, respectively. We have only to think of the everyday circumstances in which we listen to tones and speech to realize the necessity for introducing the third type of sound, namely, noise (see Chap. 2).

The first and second main sections of this chapter will deal, respectively, with masking and fatigue. In the discussion of masking, we shall consider first the masking effects of noise. An idealized "white" noise has been used in the experiments that we shall discuss, and we shall attempt to extrapolate from these data to the more usual noises that are found in factories, offices, etc. The presence of a noise affects not only the audibility of pure tones but also the intelligibility of speech, and we shall be concerned with effects on both.

Of slightly more academic interest are the masking effects produced by pure tones. Pure tones have been shown to mask speech as well as other pure tones. Some of these experimental measurements have been applied to clinical audiometry, while others remain simply interesting results.

In the discussion of auditory fatigue we shall find less generality among the experiments, because there are more parameters to be controlled.

MASKING

It must be made clear at the outset that our use of the term *masking* refers to a particular phenomenon that may be demonstrated in different ways. We do *not* use *masking* to mean a method by which one 'blocks the other ear.' That particular clinical use of the term will emerge later as an application of more general considerations.

We shall restrict our discussion of masking to those aspects that are particularly germane to clinical problems. The main problems that we shall keep in mind are (1) the disturbing effects of noise on the measurement of the absolute threshold, (2) the use of masking in measuring the hearing of one ear at a time, and (3) the relation between masking and the phenomenon of *recruitment*. The specific application of this third relation will be postponed until the discussion on recruitment in Chap. 8.

A typical experiment on masking is designed to measure the effect of the presence of one sound upon the audibility of a second, simultaneous sound. Suppose that we wish to determine the effect of a certain type of

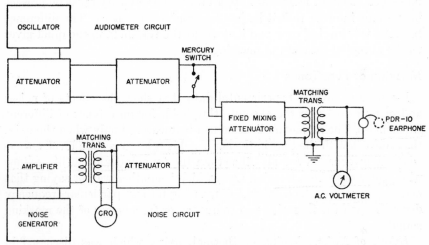

Fig. 6.1. Schematic block diagram of apparatus used for the measurement of pure-tone thresholds, both in the quiet and in the presence of white masking noise. (*From Hawkins and Stevens.*)

noise upon the audibility of a pure tone. The procedure will require first that we measure the absolute threshold of the pure tone. Next we introduce a specified level of noise *into the same ear* and remeasure the threshold for the pure tone in the presence of the noise.

One example of an array of equipment for such measurement is given in Fig. 6.1. The oscillator at the top of this diagram is the source for pure tones whose level is computed by conversion of the voltage across the earphone to SPL by means of the frequency-response curve for the particular earphone. The tone and the noise are made available simultaneously to the same earphone by means of the mixing attenuator. The level of the noise can also be obtained by measuring its voltage across the earphone. The switch permits the listener to interrupt the tone so that he may listen for an intermittent signal in a continuous noise.

We may wish to make these measurements to obtain one or both of the following relations: masking, by a given amount of noise, as a function of the frequency of the pure tone whose threshold is measured; or masking of a pure tone at a given frequency as a function of the level of the masking noise.

There are logically two ways to obtain a measure of masking. First, we may sound a tone at a threshold intensity and measure the amount of noise that will just obliterate the tone. This measure tells us that a noise of such a measured level or more will mask a tone at its threshold value. A second method is more generally used. This involves setting the noise at a constant level and noting how much intensity must be present in the tone in order that it be just heard above the noise. The difference between this level of tone and its level at the threshold in the quiet gives us the accepted measure of masking.

Masking of Pure Tones

Let us turn now to experimental data that show the effects of noises and of pure tones on the absolute thresholds for pure tones of different frequencies. The *normal* audiogram can be measured only when the noise that coexists with the tone in the ear canal is below a certain level. Otherwise the presence of sounds other than the tone under test will produce what appears to be a Hearing Loss, which is another way of saying that masking is present. The amount of masking for any particular frequency depends upon the intensity and frequency or frequencies of the masking sound.

Effects of Noise. White, or thermal, noise, which was discussed in Chap. 2, constitutes a very convenient source for masking because of its uniform spectrum—*i.e.*, all frequencies are represented in such a noise at equal average energies. The acoustic noise that actually comes from the transducer (earphone or loud-speaker) has a more limited spectrum, because the response of the transducer usually falls off after a certain frequency in the audible range. The spectrum of thermal-noise *voltage* coming from an electronic noise generator may be flat up to a few hundred kilocycles per second, but if this voltage is applied to an earphone, such as the PDR-10 of the Permoflux Corporation, the *acoustic spectrum* will be flat up to only about 7000 cps because the earphone does not respond so well above that frequency.

We must consider how we specify the Intensity Level of such a noise in an experiment on masking. If the noise voltage is measured at the input to the earphone, we note that the needle of the voltmeter quivers a little in response to the random fluctuations that are characteristic of thermal noise, but an approximate reading can be taken. If we read, for example, a voltage of 1 volt, we cannot say that the over-all SPL of the noise is 128 db, even if we know that the response of the earphone to 1 volt is 128 db throughout a considerable portion of the frequency range. The reason is, of course, that a great part of the electrical energy lies in frequencies above the cutoff frequency of the earphone and hence in frequencies that never get transduced.

A precaution that should be followed, then, in making such measurements is to insert a sharp, low-pass filter ahead of the earphone. The cutoff frequency of the filter should be at or below the cutoff frequency of the earphone. If we now make voltage measurements at the earphone (after the filter), we may be sure that all the voltage that we read gets transduced.

There is still another problem in specifying the level of noise. The ideal flat spectrum of thermal noise is relatively easy to specify either in terms of over-all pressure or in terms of pressure per small band of frequencies. The *over-all SPL* of a noise with a flat spectrum is easily computed from the type of measurement described in the previous paragraph. Perhaps more important for masking, however, is the *Pressure Spectrum Level*, or *Sound Pressure Level per cycle*. In the case of a flat-spectrum noise, we simply divide the over-all intensity by the frequency range (in cycles per second) to obtain the intensity in each 1-cps band. In the case discussed above, the frequency range is 7000 cps. If we have a noise whose over-all SPL is 100 db relative to 0.0002 dyne/cm^2, then the Pressure Spectrum Level, or SPL per cycle, is the over-all energy divided by 7000. Dividing a number by 7000 is the same as subtracting from the logarithm of that number the logarithm of 7000. Since 100 db is already logarithmic, we have only to subtract about 38 db (10 $\log_{10}$ 7000 = 38).

Thus the SPL per cycle in a 7000-cps band of noise whose over-all SPL is 100 db is about 62 db. In most of the data that follow we shall be concerned with a 7000-cps band of noise (PDR-10 earphone), and therefore we can use either over-all SPL in the band or SPL per cycle, which will be about 40 db less.

Now we are ready to see what happens to the threshold of a pure tone when different amounts of white noise are presented simultaneously to the same ear. Figure 6.2 shows the effect of increasing the intensity of white noise on the threshold for several pure tones of different frequency.[1] In terms of the over-all SPL of the noise, we note that the noise must be at least 20 or 30 db before any appreciable masking for pure tones takes place. The masking of lower frequencies does not appear until the noise reaches even higher levels. In other words, in the presence of any

---

[1] Each presentation of the tone has a duration of at least 1 sec. For shorter durations the thresholds will be higher (Garner and Miller).

more or less random noise up to an over-all SPL of 30 db, the absolute
threshold for pure tones will be the same as in the quiet. In audiometry,
as a matter of fact, we tend to define *quiet* as any level of noise less than
30 db. Another important generality, which is shown in Fig. 6.2, is that
the relation between masking and the intensity of the noise is linear. That
is, after the initial acceleration of the curve, each additional decibel of
noise produces an additional decibel of masking. Another way of stating

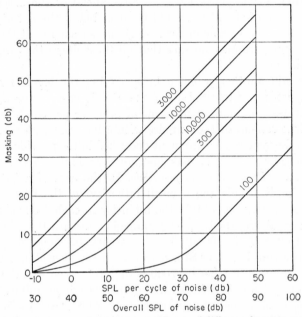

Fig. 6.2. Relation between masking for pure tones of different frequency and the level
of the masking noise. Two abscissas are shown, the upper for the Sound Pressure Level
per cycle of the noise, the lower for the over-all Sound Pressure Level in a 7000-cycle
band. These curves appear to be linear above about 10 db of masking. (*After Hawkins
and Stevens.*)

this linearity is that the signal-to-noise ratio at the masked threshold is
constant. We shall return to this relation in the following chapter.

The effect of white noise on the audibility of pure tones is shown as a
function of frequency in Fig. 6.3. The bottom curve is the normal threshold, measured in the quiet. A small amount of noise affects the thresholds
of only the most audible frequencies. Tones below 400 cps, for example,
are relatively undisturbed by low levels of noise. Eventually, however, as
the intensity of noise is made high enough, the masked thresholds for
pure tones at all frequencies lie on an almost straight line. We may
summarize this figure by saying that a given amount of white noise will

always mask pure tones in the middle range of frequencies more (in decibels) than it will mask tones at either end of the frequency range; and further, that the masked thresholds for pure tones at all frequencies measured in the presence of very intense noise will be approximately equal, whereas in the quiet the absolute thresholds for tones of middle frequencies are much lower (in decibels) than those for either very high or very low frequencies.

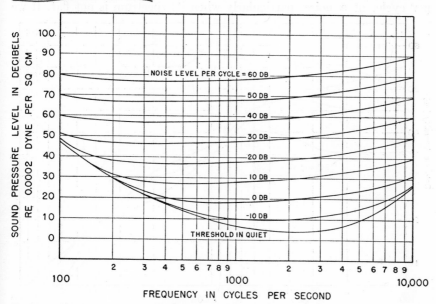

FIG. 6.3. Absolute and masked thresholds for pure tones as a function of frequency measured in the presence of different background noises. The parameter is Sound Pressure Level per cycle of the masking noise. Parametric values may be converted to approximate over-all Sound Pressure Level in a 7000-cycle band by adding 40 db. (*From Hawkins and Stevens.*)

Although white noise is convenient to use in experiments on masking. it is not particularly representative of the noises that we commonly encounter. Figure 6.4 shows, for example, some spectra of noises in which we are very likely to find ourselves listening to speech or other signals. How can we generalize from the somewhat idealized situation represented by white noise to these practical cases? The particular effects on speech will appear later. For now, let us consider the threshold for pure tones in relation to the spectrum of the masking noise.

Fletcher has provided a unifying concept in such matters known as the *critical band* (see Licklider, 1951). It is derived from two assumptions: first, the only important frequencies for masking in a given noise are those frequencies that lie within a small band centering around the frequency of the pure tone being masked; second, when a tone is just audible in a given noise, the total energy in this critical band of frequencies is equal to the energy of the tone. The width of the critical band is not the same at all frequencies. Figure 6.5, for example, shows how the width of the critical band varies with frequency. Perhaps now we can see how important it is to specify the Spectrum Level, or SPL per cycle, of a noise, particularly when its spectrum is not flat. If we

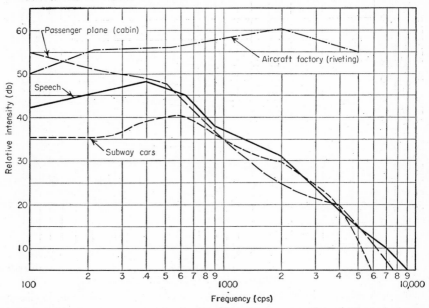

Fig. 6.4. Spectra of various kinds of noise. The measurements for speech are in terms of intensity per cycle, while the others are in terms of intensity per octave. These curves should not be interpreted as having the same ordinate scale. (*After data from Miller, Wiener, and Stevens; and Bonvallet.*)

know, for example, the SPL per cycle around 1000 cps for a given noise, we have only to multiply this figure by the width of the critical band whose center is 1000 cps to predict the masked threshold for a 1000-cps tone in that noise. Thus we can calculate the masking on pure tones that will result from a noise of any specifiable spectrum.

In general, a noise will mask most effectively those frequencies that correspond to peaks of energy in the noise. When the noise spectrum is more or less flat, the masking will be greatest for the most audible (in the quiet) frequencies.

In order to show the unifying property of this notion of a critical band, we may replot the data of Fig. 6.2. In our new plot the abscissa will represent neither the over-all SPL nor the Spectrum Level of the noise, but rather will represent the *effective level*, or the number of decibels in a critical band above the absolute threshold (Sensation Level) for that critical band (or for its center-frequency tone). The results are shown in Fig. 6.6. Here the relation between the masking and the Sensation Level of the critical band is the same for all frequencies.

Suppose we wish to know how much noise is permissible in a room in which we do pure-tone audiometry. We can see that a single figure

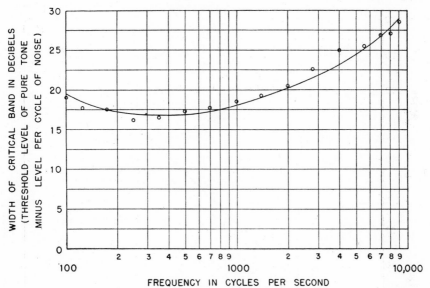

FIG. 6.5. Width of a critical band as a function of frequency. The width, in decibels, is equal to $10 \log_{10} W$, where W is the width of the critical band in cycles per second. The smooth curve is from data obtained at the Bell Telephone Laboratories. (*From Hawkins and Stevens.*)

representing the noise is meaningless unless the spectrum of the noise is flat. If the spectrum is flat, we say, according to Fig. 6.3, that the over-all SPL of the flat-spectrum noise should not exceed 30 db. But if the noise spectrum is not flat, as is usually the case, we must measure the amount of energy in the critical band of each frequency that we plan to test. In order to obtain normal absolute thresholds, the energy in each of the critical bands must not exceed the energy (or SPL) of the corresponding pure tone at threshold. If such measurements are impossible, we must make the masking measurements directly, noting the significant differences between the thresholds for a group of listeners in the room under consideration with the thresholds for the same listeners in a room known to be quiet.

If we make both the measurements of noise in critical bands and the actual threshold measurements, we may find a discrepancy that tells us that we were too strict in our interpretation of the data on critical bands. This is due to the fact that a sound-level meter measures the noise in the room, while the threshold tells us about the effect of the noise in the ear canal. Practically speaking, we should subtract the

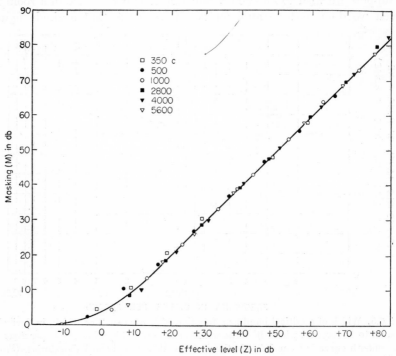

Fig. 6.6. Relation between masking and the effective level of the masking noise. The *effective level* (db) is the difference between the total energy in a critical band and the threshold energy for a pure tone whose frequency is at the center of the band. Experimental results indicate that effective level may also be interpreted as the Sensation Level of the critical band of noise. (*From Hawkins and Stevens.*)

attenuation afforded by the earphone cushions or sockets from the noise measurements (Miller, Wiener, and Stevens, p. 157).

To make such a subtraction, we must look into the attenuation characteristics of earphone cushions and sockets. The usual earphone cushion cuts out about 20 db of the externally produced noise. Figure 6.7 shows photographs and the amount of acoustic insulation of two generally used earphone cushions. The MX-41/AR, used in many experimental studies, is made of Neoprene and fits on the ear. The chamois-lined M-301, found in many clinical instruments, fits around the ear and is generally favored for patients and young children because it is comfortable to wear. Note that the acoustic insulation is small for frequencies below 1000 cps but becomes appreciable for higher frequencies. These measures of acoustic

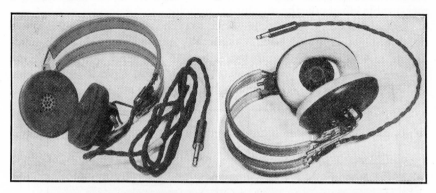

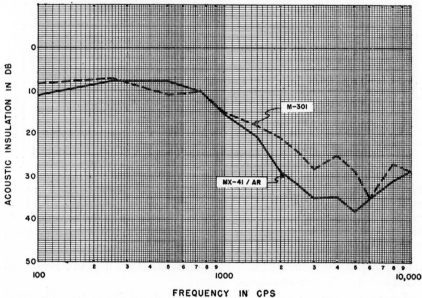

FIG. 6.7. Acoustic insulation afforded by two typical earphone sockets. Left above, Permoflux PDR-10 earphone in HB-7 headband with MX-41/AR earphone socket. Right above, HS-33 with M-301 earphone socket. (*From Shaw.*)

insulation represent the difference between free-field absolute thresholds measured with and without the earphone over the ears.

Now, to take the effect of earphone-cushion attenuation into account, we must modify our previous statements about how much room noise to allow in the case where the noise has a flat spectrum (white noise). We have said that the over-all SPL (in a 7000-cps band) should not be greater than 30 db. But with some of this noise attenuated by the earphone cushions, we may now allow perhaps 40 or 50 db without anticipating measurable effects on the absolute thresholds.

It should be borne in mind, however, that these earphone cushions have disadvantages as well as advantages. For example, a tight-fitting earphone, and in particular one that is held in the hand, can provide the circumstances for the production of enough *physiologic noise* (Brogden and Miller) in the ear canal to offset the favorable attenuation effects on

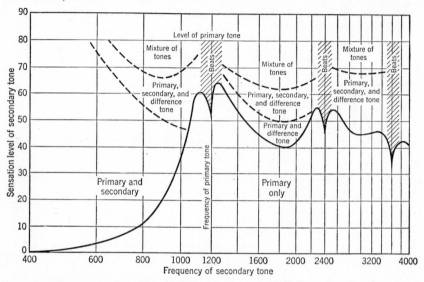

FIG. 6.8. Masking produced by a 1200-cycle tone at 80-db Sensation Level on tones at various frequencies. The various sensations produced by interactions of the 1200-cycle tone with the other tones are shown. (*After Wegel and Lane; reproduction by permission from Hearing: Its Psychology and Physiology by S. S. Stevens and H. Davis, published by John Wiley and Sons, Inc., 1938, p. 211.*)

room noise. Noise generated under earphones that are held in a headband is only slightly less troublesome.

Effects of Tones. Because of the physical simplicity of the pure tone, it is not surprising that there are early data available on the masking of one pure tone by another. The masking of tones by tones has also appeared in certain types of clinical measurement (Huizing, 1942) where the only controlled stimuli available are the pure tones of audiometers.

The first experimental measurements of this phenomenon were made by Wegel and Lane in 1924. The results of one of their experiments are shown in Fig. 6.8. These results show the masking effects of a 1200-cps tone at a Sensation Level of 80 db upon tones of various frequencies from 400 to 4000 cps. The 1200-cps tone remained constant and the intensity of each secondary tone was varied until the masked threshold was obtained. This graph shows the extent to which a single pure tone can influence the hearing of another tone as a function of the frequency of the second tone.

Above moderate intensities the ear seems to introduce amplitude distortion, and a tone at a Sensation Level of 80 db is sufficiently intense so that aural harmonics are produced. The influence of these harmonics may be seen in the second and third dips at 2400 and 3600 cps. These

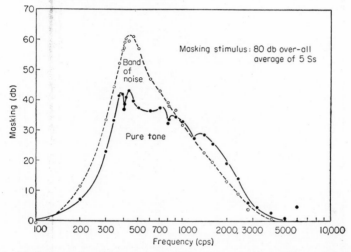

FIG. 6.9. Masking produced by two stimuli, one a pure tone at 400 cps and the other a narrow band of noise, centered at 410 cps, as a function of the frequency of the tone being masked. (*From Egan and Hake.*)

dips remind us that the masking experiment becomes an experiment on the detection of beats for frequencies that are near the frequency of the primary or masking tone or its harmonics. Whereas at most regions within the frequency range shown, the listener reports the presence or absence of a second tone, in these beat regions the listener reports whether or not the primary tone sounds constant in loudness or whether its loudness changes periodically in the manner of beats. The extent to which stimulation at one specific region of frequencies affects the hearing at all other frequencies is therefore obscured by these beat phenomena.

This question has been partially resolved by the experiments of Egan and Hake, who used a primary tone at a frequency of 400 cps. Their masking results are shown as a solid line in Fig. 6.9. The dips due to beats are again present. But in a second part of their experiment, Egan and Hake used as the primary or masking stimulus a narrow band of noise whose center frequency was 410 cps and whose width (at the half-power points) was 90 cps. The noise does not interact with the pure tone that is being masked in such a way as to produce pronounced beats. The masking effect, as a function of the frequency of the masked tone, for such a narrow band of noise is shown as the less irregular broken line of Fig. 6.9.

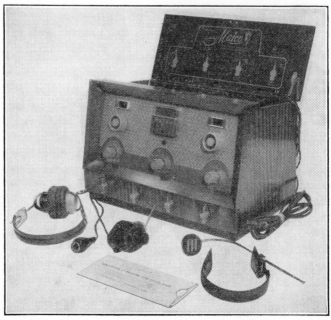

FIG. 6.10. A clinical pure-tone audiometer with a self-contained masking circuit. The control for the masking sound (saw-tooth wave) is seen at the lower right of the instrument panel. (*Photograph courtesy of The Maico Company, Inc., Minneapolis.*)

Masking in Audiometers.   Before going on to discuss the masking of speech, we must point out the relation between certain types of masking stimuli that are generated within commercial audiometers and the two types of masking stimuli that we have discussed above. When either wide-band or narrow-band noise is used to mask pure tones, the relation between the masking and the frequency of the pure tone masked is a smooth continuous function. When pure tones are masked by pure tones, however, there are certain frequencies at which interactions between these two tones produce ambiguity so far as the measurement of masking is concerned.

The spectra of the masking stimuli that are supplied in most commercial audiometers lie physically somewhere between those of pure tones and those of white noise (see pure tone, square wave, and white noise in Fig. 2.8). The waveform of these masking stimuli is usually either a saw-tooth wave or a square wave. The basic repetition rate of this waveform is usually that of the line voltage or a harmonic thereof, namely, 60 or 120 cps. Whereas the white noise contains all frequencies at equal average energy, the saw-tooth wave contains only those frequencies that are multiples of the basic repetition rate, and these appear at decreasing

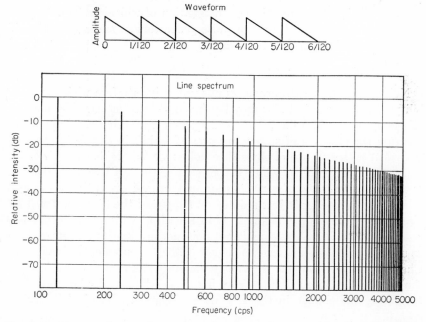

Fig. 6.11. The waveform and spectrum of a saw-tooth wave with a basic repetition rate of 120 per second. Such a wave is typical of those used to produce the masking sound in commercial audiometers.

amplitude. Near 1000 cps, then, the white noise contains all neighboring frequencies at equal amplitudes, whereas this saw-tooth wave contains only frequencies 840, 960, 1080, and 1200 cps. Beats or difference tones may occur between the component at 960 cps and the test tone at 1000 cps.

One can see from Fig. 6.8 that the masked threshold is changing rapidly as a function of frequency in those small regions that show the dips due to beats. The frequency of a pure tone of an audiometer will vary somewhat from day to day, and from minute to minute as the audiometer is warming up, but the frequency of the line voltage remains relatively constant. This means that, whereas our 960-cps component might remain quite stable in frequency, the frequency of the test tone might vary from 1000 cps upward to 1050 or downward to 950 cps, producing very different masked thresholds, as one can see from the steep slope of the curves on either side of the dips. There is a further observation, from experience in different experimental situations, that the interaction of two periodic stimuli yields less reliable psychophysical measurements than the interaction of one periodic with an irregular aperiodic sound (Hirsh and Webster). From the standpoint of reliability and validity, therefore, it would seem that the installation of white- or random-noise generators rather than 'buzz' or pulse generators as masking devices in audiometers might well be encouraged.

Masking of Speech

Noises and other extraneous sounds not only interfere with the audibility of pure tones but also may be shown to have measurable masking effects upon speech. Adhering to the definition of masking given above, we measure the masking of speech in terms of a shift in threshold. And we may deal with any one of three thresholds: *the threshold of intelligibility*, or the level of speech at which 50 per cent of the test items are *repeated correctly; the threshold of perceptibility*, or the level of continuous speech at which the listener is just able to *get the gist* of the discourse; and *the threshold of detectability*, or the level of speech at which the listener *just hears the speech sounds* as sounds but does not necessarily recognize them as units of a spoken language. A review of the measurements discussed in Chap. 5 should allow one to predict the emphasis that we shall give to the threshold of intelligibility. Masking of speech may also be studied by measuring the change in the articulation score at a particular level of speech.

Effects of Noise. Normally, in the quiet, the threshold of detectability for continuous discourse lies about 12 db below the threshold of intelligibility for the same material. If noise is added to the speech in the same ear, both thresholds will be raised, depending upon the amount of noise that is introduced. The relations between the masked thresholds of intelligibility and detectability and the noise level are shown in Fig. 6.12. Note that the normal threshold of intelligibility is not changed until the over-all SPL of the noise reaches about 20 db (0 db per critical band; −20 db per cycle). We may say, on the basis of this observation, that the noise level in the ear canal of a normal listener whose absolute threshold of intelligibility is to be measured must not exceed about 20 db SPL over-all.

The noise used in the experiment discussed above had a flat spectrum extending up to approximately the cutoff frequency of the earphone. If, now, we wish to know whether or not certain frequency regions in the noise are more effective than others in masking speech, we must divide the noise into bands. The results of such an experiment are shown in Fig. 6.13. Each curve shows the relation between the articulation score of the speech at an SPL of 95 db and the SPL of a band of noise.

Ignoring the curve for the broad band (A) we see that, at low intensities, noise in the frequency regions 1300 to 1900 (F) and 1800 to 2500

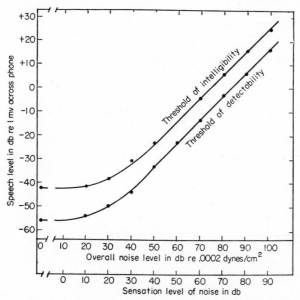

FIG. 6.12. Relation between speech level and the level of a background noise for the threshold of intelligibility and of detectability. Note that after about 10 db of masking, the relation between masking and noise level is linear; the signal-to-noise ratio for either threshold remains constant. (*After Hawkins and Stevens.*)

(G) cps is most effective in masking speech. (We might have predicted this on the basis of the relative contributions of different regions of frequency to the intelligibility of speech in the quiet that were shown in Fig. 5.14.) At higher intensities, however, the most effective bands for masking appear to be from 135 to 400 (B), from 350 to 700 (C), and from 600 to 1100 (D) cps. This shift in the frequency of optimum masking as the intensity increases is presumably due to the spread of masking into harmonics that is produced by distortion in the ear at high intensities.

Effects of Tones. What effect have pure tones or the complex masking tone of an audiometer on the intelligibility of speech? Figure 6.14 shows the amount by which the threshold of perceptibility for continuous dis-

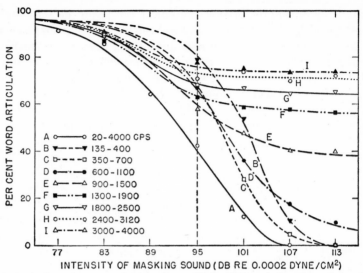

FIG. 6.13. Articulation score for speech at 95 db SPL as a function of the SPL of masking noise. The different curves show this relation for different frequency bands of noise. (*From Miller, 1947a.*)

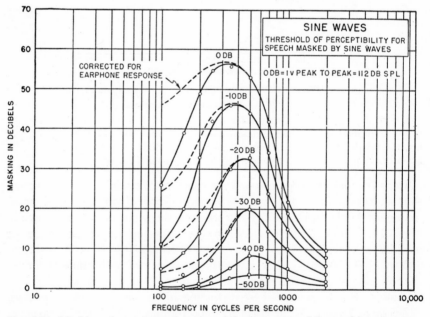

FIG. 6.14. Masking of speech as a function of the frequency of the masking pure tone. This relation is shown for six different levels of the tone: 112, 92, 82, 72, 62, and 52 db SPL. (*From Stevens, Miller, and Truscott.*)

course is changed in the presence of pure tones at various frequencies for six different SPL's. We may note again a shift in the optimum masking frequency from somewhere around 500 or 600 cps to 300 cps as the intensity of the tone is increased. Similar data are given in the same experiment for masking by regularly spaced pulses and by square waves. The masking of speech by these regular stimuli is probably comparable to the masking of speech that would be provided by the saw-tooth or square waves of commercial audiometers. A cursory review of some of these masking data seems to warrant the general statement that regular stimuli such as pure tones or complex tones (square waves, pulses, etc.) are not so efficient in masking as are the more irregular stimuli that are represented by various kinds of noise.

The dependence of the masking of speech, by both complex tones and noise, on frequency indicates that the typical mixtures of noises that are found in factories, offices, and airplanes, with the usual emphasis of low frequencies, are particularly well adapted to give a maximum amount of masking of speech. During World War II this constituted enough of a problem to figure in the designing of aural protective devices to be used in noisy situations. Although the primary purpose of these earplugs was to prevent acoustic trauma (see next main section), it was shown that they also improved the intelligibility of speech in noise if the noise showed low-frequency emphasis and the level of noise was high enough (Kryter, 1946). The V-51R Ear Wardens, for example, attenuated most frequencies throughout the audible range by about 30 db (Miller, Wiener, and Stevens, p. 43) and thus would attenuate speech by that amount. But since the normal articulation score reaches its maximum at about 60 db SPL, any speech at 90 db or more in the quiet would not be impaired by wearing the earplugs.

Now if we reexamine the data in Fig. 6.12, we see that the signal-to-noise ratio for the threshold of intelligibility remains absolutely constant as the intensity of the noise is raised. It should not, therefore, make any difference whether both speech and noise are high (no earplugs) or both speech and noise are low (earplugs); the ratio for the threshold of intelligibility should be the same. Kryter's measurements were of considerably more practical importance, because he used a noise whose spectrum showed more energy in the low frequencies than in the high. For such a noise, we might expect the shift in the relative position of the earplug and no-earplug curves that we see in Fig. 6.15.

Effects of Other Speech.   We can sometimes predict fairly well the amount of masking that will be encountered in certain types of rooms by extrapolating from the data on white noise and on narrow bands of noise. Such noise is qualitatively very different from the speech. When, how-

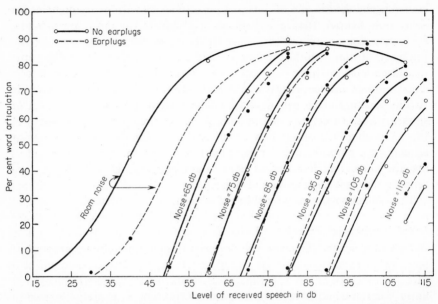

Fig. 6.15. Articulation score as a function of speech level in the presence of different levels of noise. The solid curves show the result of listening without earplugs, whereas the broken curves show similar results for listening with earplugs. The spectrum of the noise used shows an emphasis in the low frequencies. In such a noise, we see that speech is more intelligible when earplugs are used than when they are not, when the noise level exceeds about 90 db. (*From Kryter, 1946.*)

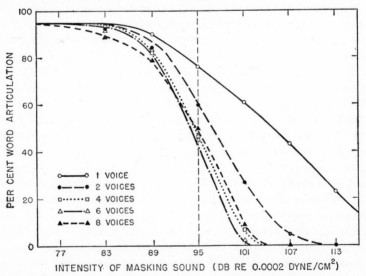

Fig. 6.16. Articulation score for speech at 95 db SPL as a function of the level of different numbers of voices that served as a masking background. (*From Miller, 1947a.*)

ever, speech is masked by other speech, the situation becomes rather more complicated. Figure 6.16 shows the amount by which the articulation score for speech at an Intensity Level of 95 db decreases as the intensity of one or more other voices is increased. Note that when only one other voice is in the background, the intelligibility holds up over a wide range of intensities. By the time we have as many as four voices in the background, the intervals of silence between vowel peaks in the masking sound have become few and far between, and the intelligibility of the desired speech deteriorates rather rapidly. It seems to be the masking spectrum rather than what is said that is crucial in determining the amount of masking. For example, such masking has been shown to be equally effective even when the other voices are speaking a language that the listener does not know (Miller, 1947a).

Clinical Use of Masking

In ordinary clinical usage the term *masking* refers to the introduction of a sound to an ear in order to 'block' that ear while the other ear is being tested. Certain problems arise because of the relatively nonquantitative way in which these masking stimuli are used in a clinical situation. And these problems are not at all helped by the manufacturers of commercial audiometers who advertise that their machines contain a "calibrated masking control," which is only "calibrated" in decibels relative to an unspecified level.

So far it is difficult to connect the experimental data on masking with the kind of masking that is done in the clinic because of the fact that the stimulus that is used for clinical masking is usually a complex tone of a saw-tooth or square waveform with a basic frequency of 60 or 120 cps, and very few experimental data have to do with these masking sounds directly. If, however, we can make some only slightly unreasonable assumptions about the similarity between the line spectrum given by such a complex tone and the continuous spectrum of white noise that has been used in some of the laboratory studies, we may be able to establish, for clinical use, certain general principles that are extrapolated from experimental results.

Elimination of "Cross-hearing." Probably the widest use of masking in clinical audiometry is found in the case of a patient whose hearing in one ear is very different from that in the other. The extreme case is a patient with one normal ear and one ear that is completely deaf. We may first test the good ear in a routine way and obtain a normal audiogram. Then, by applying the tones of the audiometer to the other earphone in the headband, we proceed to test the worse ear. Again using routine procedures, we may obtain an audiogram that shows a 50-db Hearing

Loss that is more or less uniform throughout the frequency range tested. We must then ask the question: Does this 50-db Hearing Loss represent the actual hearing for this ear, or does it represent the loss in transmitted energy from the ear under test to the good ear, which may be presumed to be doing the hearing? One way to answer this question is, of course, to introduce a masking sound into the good ear on the assumption that the masking sound will keep the good ear so busy that it cannot respond to the energy in the pure tone that may be radiated or transmitted through the headband from the other ear.

A further, more difficult question is, How much masking sound do we need? If we refer to the data on masking of pure tones by white noise in Fig. 6.2, we note that the over-all SPL of the noise (between 0 and 7000 cps) must be about 30 db before any appreciable masking is observed for a tone at, for example, 1000 cps. But now we must consider the case in which the tone is introduced, not to the ear to which the noise is introduced, but to the opposite ear. In other words, any sound that is presented to only one ear may affect the other ear, not so much by bone conduction as by radiation through the air around the head or by vibrations transmitted through a headband (Békésy, 1949); but the energy loss across the head is about 50 db. If, therefore, we wish to be sure that the good ear does not hear the tone that is presented to the bad ear, we must present to the good ear at least 30 db SPL of white noise. And we could increase that noise to about 80 db SPL and still be quite sure that it would not start masking the tone presented to the worse ear even if that ear were also normal. With this 80 db of noise, we could be sure of measuring, in the bad ear, as much as 100 db Hearing Loss before any unmasked signal would evoke a response from the good ear. For Hearing Losses of greater than 100 db on the bad ear, the intensity of the masking tone in the good ear would have to be increased proportionately until about 120 db is reached.

If this is accepted as a maximum, then we must assert that the maximum Hearing Loss that we could measure independent of cross-hearing would be about 140 db, a figure greatly in excess of the maximum Hearing Loss that can be measured with most commercial audiometers anyway. Certainly there will be great individual differences among different listeners and particularly among testing situations that differ in respect of type of earphone, earphone cushion, and headband (see Békésy, 1949). The above is not to be taken as a 'cookbook' rule. Let it serve rather as an example of the kind of clinical procedure that can be evolved from results of experimental measurements.

Masking in Bone Conduction. This topic is listed here for the sake of logical order, but it will be considered later in the discussion of bone conduction in Chap. 10. Suffice it to say, by way of foreshadowing, that the application of a bone-conduction vibrator to the skull sets up one of two kinds of vibration that produce hearing almost equally effectively in both cochleas. The only precise way, therefore, of testing the hearing of one ear by bone conduction is to apply a masking sound to the other ear. The general principles that will be applied to determine the amount of masking sound to be used are exactly the same as those that apply to the elimination of cross-hearing, which was discussed in the paragraphs above.

Masking and Recruitment. The work of Huizing (1942) and Langenbeck (1950*a*, *b*, *c*) has pointed to a definite clinical relation between pathologic loudness functions (recruitment) and masking functions. In this case, both the signal and the masking sound are brought to the same ear. Generally speaking, the use of masking in the measurement of recruitment enables one to arrive at the same answers as would be given by the more traditional loudness-balancing methods—methods that are thought by some workers to be considerably more difficult for the naive patient to execute. The basic assumption is that the relation between the growth of masking and the intensity of the masking sound is essentially the same as, or at least is uniquely related to, the relation between the growth of subjective loudness and the intensity of the physical stimulus. We shall return to this argument in the latter sections of Chap. 8.

AUDITORY FATIGUE

The phenomenon of masking is an exception to the auditory system's ability to analyze out of a combination of sounds one sound or signal. But the fact is that we can usually hear several sounds at once and identify them separately. This is only slightly more remarkable than the fact that the auditory system resists fatigue by previous stimulation. There are exceptions, however, to this ability also, and it is with these exceptions that the present section is concerned.

We shall use the term *auditory fatigue* to refer to the elevation of the absolute threshold or the decrease in loudness of a sound that comes as a result of stimulation by a preceding sound. In using the term thus we are not following distinctions that have been made by previous authors among *adaptation* (Lüscher and Zwislocki, 1947; Hallpike and Hood), *stimulation deafness* (Caussé and Chavasse, 1947), *residual masking* (de Maré, 1937; Munson and Gardner) or *acoustic trauma* (Rüedi and Furrer, 1947). These phenomena have been differentiated more on the basis of theoretical aspects concerning the nature and site of fatigue than on clear breaks among the sets of experimental data. When previous stimulation results in a hearing loss that remains quite stable after a reasonable time has elapsed (and thus appears to be irreversible), the use of *permanent hearing loss* or *acoustic trauma* seems justified.

Our use of *auditory fatigue*, then, covers a wide range of experimental conditions. At one extreme we have experiments that show that a sound at a Sensation Level as low as 20 db produces a subsequent rise in absolute threshold for the same frequency if we measure the threshold about 0.4 sec after the cessation of the stimulating tone; but several seconds later the threshold is perfectly normal again. At the other extreme we have very loud sounds at Sensation Levels of 100 db or more to which a listener may be exposed for several minutes, several hours, or, as in the case of industrial noise, several years. In these cases of intense stimulation the absolute threshold is raised considerably and does not recover to normal for several minutes, several hours, several days, or not at all, depending on the conditions of stimulation. All the experimental literature on these various types of auditory fatigue show one common factor: individuals are very different from one another in respect of fatigue, and it is almost impossible to generalize quantitatively about auditory fatigue as a phenomenon or process of the 'normal' auditory system.

If we look for practical reasons for telling the story of auditory fatigue, we find three important ones: (1) certain data on auditory fatigue tell us not to turn the intensity of a tone too high when we first present it to a listener whose audiogram we are about to measure; (2) long-term auditory fatigue, when measured, tells us about the way in which hearing loss occurs as a result of long exposures to intense sounds and may, in the future, lead to an auditory measurement that will predict a given individual's susceptibility to permanent hearing loss after working in a noisy environment; and finally (3) short-term auditory fatigue is characterized differently in cases of normal hearing or conductive hearing loss from what it is in nerve-type or recruiting hearing loss. It seems possible to distinguish these two types of hearing loss on the basis of fatigue measurements (Gardner, 1947a). Although these three applications of the measurement of auditory fatigue are of great practical importance, the data are too vague and insufficient to permit wide immediate application.

Parameters in Auditory Fatigue (Temporary Hearing Loss)

The experimental literature on auditory fatigue is discouragingly large. The size itself is not so discouraging as the disjointed and apparently unrelated nature of the parts. As a matter of fact, in auditory fatigue the unsolved problems greatly outnumber the established facts. We shall attempt to summarize some of the parameters that have appeared to be important in a few experiments on fatigue. We cannot, however, submit general experimental results that may serve as standards against which pathologic behavior relative to fatigue may be measured.

Let us review the general procedure. A *stimulating sound* is turned on for a specified length of time, maybe 2 sec or 30 min. After it is turned off, the absolute threshold for the *test sound* is measured. The amount by which the threshold for the test sound is higher than it was before stimulation is the amount of fatigue. The ear recovers from fatigue, however, and if the absolute threshold is measured at a particular time, the time must be specified. The fatigue will be higher, for example, 10 sec after the stimulating tone has been turned off than it will be 30 min after.

Now what can we vary in this situation? In the stimulating sound we can vary the frequency, intensity, and duration. Then we can vary the interval between the cessation of stimulation and the presentation of the test sound. We can also vary the frequency and duration of the test sound (but not its intensity, since this intensity remains the dependent variable). If all these possible dimensions were to be investigated systematically, we might be able to give an acceptable summary of experiments on auditory fatigue and perhaps even predict the kinds of hearing loss that would result from exposure to various noises. But they have not. Only a few pieces of the jigsaw puzzle are available, and we do not know whether these few pieces even belong to the same puzzle.

Effects of Duration of Stimulation. The range of duration of the stimulating sound in the literature on fatigue extends from about 0.1 sec to 64 min. The relation between fatigue and the duration of stimulation is not the same throughout this range. Although earlier data are available in the studies of de Maré (1939), Lüscher and Zwislocki (1947), and Gardner (1947a) on very short stimulating tones, the short-duration range has been most extensively explored by Harris (1950). When he used a primary or stimulating tone of 1000 cps, a secondary or test tone of 1500 cps, an interval of 20 msec between the two, and a duration of 30 msec of the test tone, fatigue remained constant as duration of the stimulating tone increased from 0.1 to about 5 sec for Sensation Levels ranging from 40 to 80 db.

According to fatigue measurements of Caussé and Chavasse (1947) made about 25 sec after cessation of the stimulating tone, as the durations are further increased from 10 sec to 40 sec, fatigue increases linearly (in db). Their results involve Sensation Levels of the stimulating tone from 10 to 40 db and a frequency of 1000 cps. At a Sensation Level of 100 db (2048 cps), Hood also reports a linear increase of fatigue with increase of duration of the stimulating tone from 10 to 320 sec.

Farther along on the duration dimension, Davis *et al.* (1950) report that at Intensity Levels of 110, 120, and 130 db, the relation between fatigue and durations from 1 to 64 min goes from linearity to positive acceleration.

If we ignore the great differences among these experiments in respect of frequency, intensity, and time interval between stimulation and test, we may summarize the results by saying that fatigue remains small and constant as the duration of the stimulating tone goes up from 0.1 to about 5 sec. As the duration is increased further between 10 and 60 sec, the fatigue increases linearly (in db). Above 1 min, as durations are increased to 64 min, fatigue increases more and more rapidly with duration.

Effects of Intensity of Stimulation. In general, the more intense the stimulating sound, other things being equal, the greater is the auditory fatigue at any instant and the longer it will last. The studies using very short stimulating tones (de Maré, 1939; Lüscher and Zwislocki, 1947; Gardner, 1947a; Harris, Rawnsley, and Kelsey) are all in general agreement on this point, although the shape of the functions is not exactly the same. When the duration is 1 min and fatigue is measured 10 sec after stimulation, Hood reports only slight increases in fatigue as the Sensation Level of the stimulating tone increases from 60 to 90 db, but then the fatigue increases more rapidly as the Sensation Level is further increased to 110 db. When the durations are from 1 to 8 min, Davis *et al.* (1950) report that the temporary hearing loss continues to increase as the intensity of stimulation increases from 110 to 130 db. Exceptions are reported in which the fatigue appears to be maximum at 120 db and a further increase in intensity does not increase the subsequent hearing loss.

Effects of Frequency. In general, temporary auditory fatigue is a phenomenon that involves hearing for frequencies above 1000 cps. There are at least two ways to approach the relation between fatigue and frequency. First, given stimulation by a tone at a particular frequency, how does fatigue vary as a function of the frequency of the test tone? Second, if the stimulating and test tones have the same frequency, how does fatigue vary with frequency?

Among the short-duration studies we find a most thorough exploration of the first question in the results of Munson and Gardner. Figure 6.17 shows the amount of short-duration auditory fatigue that is produced at various frequencies by a 1000-cps tonal impulse. The asymmetry of this curve is not reflected in the results of Caussé and Chavasse (1947), who used slightly longer durations and a longer interval before measurement: at low intensities of stimulation their results show a symmetrical spread of fatigue about the stimulating frequency. Hood also reports such symmetry at low intensities but notes further that as the intensity of stimulation is increased, the fatigue spreads toward the higher frequencies, probably indicating fatigue effects by higher harmonics that are produced at high intensities.

There are many data on this question in the experiments of Davis *et al.* (1950), from which we can make the following generalization: the maximum temporary Hearing Loss after prolonged exposure to loud tones appears at a frequency that lies approximately one-half octave above the stimulating frequency. When noise is used as the stimulating

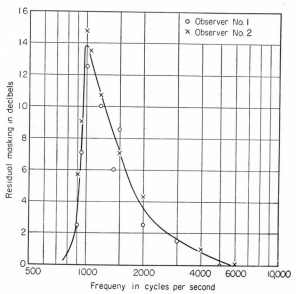

Fig. 6.17. Fatigue (residual masking) produced by a 1000-cycle tone at 70 db Sensation Level as a function of the frequency of the test tone. Fatigue is maximum when the test tone has the same frequency as the stimulating tone, and then falls off more sharply below than above this frequency on a logarithmic frequency scale. The time interval between the cessation of stimulation and the test tone was about 30 msec. *(From Munson and Gardner.)*

sound, frequencies between 2000 and 6000 cps seem to be most vulnerable (Davis *et al.*, 1950; Rüedi and Furrer, 1946, 1947). This observation is corroborated by the many measurements that have been made in connection with deafness resulting from industrial noise (*e.g.*, Rosenblith; Rüedi and Furrer, 1946). Audiograms taken after exposure to white noise at 115 db (over-all SPL) for 20 min are shown in the results of an experiment by Egan in Fig. 6.18.

Information on the second question concerning fatigue as a function of frequency in the case where the stimulating and test tones have the same frequency is provided in part by Caussé and Chavasse (1947). Their

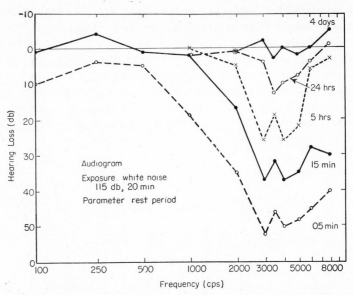

Fɪɢ. 6.18. Audiograms measured at different intervals of time after the cessation of an exposure to white noise at 115 db for 20 min. (*From Postman and Egan, p.* 72.)

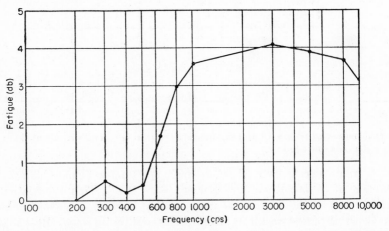

Fɪɢ. 6.19. Relation between fatigue, measured about 25 sec after cessation of stimulation, and frequency. Fatigue is measured for the same frequency as that of the stimulating tone. Sensation Level of the stimulating tone was 30 db. (*After data of Causse and Chavasse,* 1947.)

results, shown in Fig. 6.19, indicate that short-term fatigue is appreciable only above about 500 cps. Figure 6.20 from Lüscher and Zwislocki (1947), shows thresholds for short impulses of tone as a function of frequency for different levels of stimulation. The apparent similarity between the shapes of these curves and those of equal loudness suggests some relations between fatigue and recruitment that have been emphasized by de Maré (1939), Hallpike and Hood, and others. We shall come back to them briefly in Chap. 8.

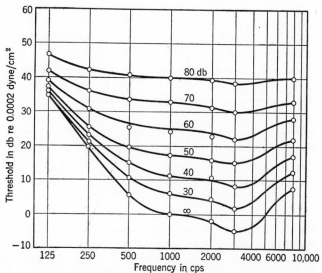

FIG. 6.20. The momentary threshold for tonal impulses 20 msec after stimulating tone of 0.4 sec duration. Both stimulating and test tones have the same frequency. The parameter is Sound Pressure Level of the stimulating tone. The bottom curve shows this momentary threshold measured without any previous stimulation. (*From Lüscher and Zwislocki*, 1947.)

Recovery and Time of Measurement. Still another generalization may be made: the longer one waits before measuring the absolute threshold for a test tone after the cessation of the stimulating sound, the less will be the fatigue. Such monotonic recovery is characteristic of short-duration studies (Lüscher and Zwislocki, 1947; Gardner, 1947a; and Harris, 1950). In the audiograms of Davis et al. (1950), made over a range of much longer delays after more intense and prolonged stimulation, recovery from maximum temporary Hearing Loss is rapid at first and then more gradually approaches normality. Similar to these audiograms is the set in Fig. 6.18 from Egan's work on stimulation by white noise.

The problem of recovery is handled in an interesting way in the studies of Hood. In his experiments, the listener adjusted the intensity of the variable stimulus, and a continuous record of his adjustments was made, so that a recovery curve in time was obtained. But when the observer continuously controls the intensity of a sound with the knob of an attenuator, he tends to make adjustments not only on the basis of what he hears, but also on the basis of how far he feels that he has turned the knob from some average position. This difficulty is overcome by Hirsh and Ward, who use a remotely controlled attenuator—attenuation is increased or decreased by the pushing or releasing of a simple switch (Békésy, 1947). The recovery curves obtained by Hirsh and Ward reveal exceptions to the generalization made at the beginning of this paragraph. That is to say, they report cases in which, after cessation of the stimulating sound, the threshold recovers to normal in from 40 to 60 sec, after which it again rises, reaching a second maximum at about 2 min (see also Bronstein). But such exceptions are not general; some listeners show such a diphasic recovery curve and others do not.

Applications

The preceding discussion of some experimental results on fatigue has been sketchy and pedestrian. We have walked through a mass of data without knowing where to stop and take longer looks. There are many experiments from which many graphs might have been taken, but the generality is always very limited. In a sense, such a discussion has little place in an introductory book. We have not discussed the details of procedure and equipment for measuring auditory fatigue.[1] But to omit any discussion of auditory fatigue would have been to omit a very important area in the measurement of hearing, not so important for the information that we have as for the problems that remain to be solved. At the present time we can see no immediate widespread clinical application of fatigue measurements. We do not know whether the most applicable might be short-time or long-time exposures, for high or low intensity, etc., etc. We should, however, see if there are some statements that can be made relative to the clinical applications that were mentioned in the introduction to this section.

Effect of Fatigue on the Audiogram. There is no doubt that if one presents a tone at 100 db or more for 1 min or more, an effect will be produced on the audiogram that is measured subsequently. On the other hand, it is clear that exposure of the order of 10 sec, which is usual for the beginning of an audiometric test, with moderate intensities will not produce disturbing fatigue effects, provided that the audiogram is measured at least some seconds after the cessation of such an orienting tone.

[1] The interested reader should consult the original articles for details. See also the reviews in Banister; Stevens and Davis; Kryter (1950); Hood; and Licklider (1951).

In audiometry we should be particularly worried about fatigue at the same frequency as that of stimulation. Such fatigue at moderate intensities is important only at frequencies above 800 cps (see Fig. 6.20), and even then, for example at 2000 cps, the effects do not become appreciable until the Sensation Level exceeds about 80 db (Hood). In cases of severe hearing loss, we must present at least the first tones at much higher intensities in order to be sure that the patient knows what to listen for. Although the amount of fatigue from such intensities will, of course, depend on the type of hearing loss, a precautionary pause after such a tone before exploring the threshold would be advisable.

Industrial Deafness. No words need be written to emphasize the importance of this practical problem. It remains a problem that commands the attention of many clinical and experimental workers today. Industry is getting noisier, and hearing losses that result from such noise are becoming more numerous. Very few controlled studies on the relation between permanent hearing loss and the conditions of stimulation are available. This is undoubtedly due to the difficulty in obtaining experimental listeners. The tremendous literature on the nature of permanent hearing loss that is found in actual practice affords little by way of an analysis of the important dimensions of stimulating sounds. Such studies as the one of Davis *et al.* (1950) come close to the objective, but the hearing loss measured was temporary.

Certain stimulus dimensions have been teased out of industrial surveys (*e.g.*, Rosenblith). The relation between Hearing Loss and duration of exposure, for example, was obtained from two groups of workers, one of which had been employed in noisy work for 15 to 20 years and the other for 20 to 25 years. The average Hearing Loss for the latter group was about 10 db more severe above 2000 cps. Rosenblith also measured the average Hearing Loss for three groups of workers, namely, boilermakers, blacksmiths and ironsmiths, and machinists, in order to relate Hearing Loss to intensity of stimulation. The average noise levels to which these groups were exposed for more than 15 years were 90, 80, and 75 db, respectively. The results in Fig. 6.21 show how Hearing Loss increases as the intensity increases.

Work on prophylaxis goes on in several directions. First, many attempts are being made to find an appropriate test to determine a man's susceptibility to permanent hearing loss as a result of prolonged exposure to noise (Wheeler). Many such tests are based on measurements from short-time low-intensity stimulation. What is not as yet clear is the relation, if any, between short-time auditory fatigue or adaptation and the more permanent hearing loss that comes as a result of more prolonged, more intense stimulation. A reasonable degree of validation of stimulation for 5 min by tones has been achieved by Wilson (1943, 1944), who successfully extended the work of Peyser. Even if such a test were found, it is difficult to see how it would be used in view of the large number of people who would be found to be "susceptible."

A second attack on the problem has to do with the use of earplugs. It is now possible to obtain as much as 30 db attenuation with an inserted

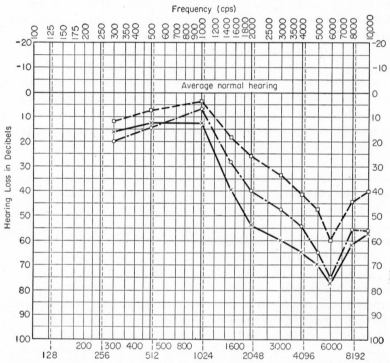

Fig. 6.21. Average Hearing Loss for three different groups of workers after 15 years of employment. Each type of work was associated with a different average noise level: boilermakers, 90 db × (solid); blacksmiths and ironsmiths, 80 db ○ (dot-dash); and machinists, 75 db □ (dashes). (*From Rosenblith.*)

earplug and perhaps 20 db more with an over-the-ear device. This amount of attenuation, although not sufficient to eliminate the problem in all industrial cases, is important enough that industrial health officers might well establish measures for enforcing the use of such safety devices in a way similar to that used for eye goggles and other devices in connection with industrial safety hazards.

A third direction has to do with the engineering aspects of making working environments more quiet. This has obvious limitations in terms of the size and power of modern machinery, but improvements can still be made in many industrial and military establishments where noise levels are dangerously high.

Fatigue and Diagnosis. It has been observed that persons with nerve-type hearing loss are more susceptible to further hearing loss from loud sounds than are persons with normal hearing or conductive hearing loss. Extrapolating downward toward short-time fatigue, we might assume, then, that in order to diagnose this type of nerve deafness we might measure a person's fatigue after a tone of short duration to determine whether or not he is abnormally fatigable. De Maré (1939), Gardner (1947a), Hallpike and Hood, and others have reported the use of measurements of auditory fatigue for the indirect determination of the presence of recruitment, which serves as evidence for certain kinds of nerve deafness (see Chap. 8). The complications in measuring auditory fatigue are considerable and probably impede widespread clinical use of this technique at the present time. But the connection between fatigue and recruitment or loudness seems to be well established both clinically and experimentally.

Another relation between fatigue and diagnosis is found in the fact that the type of hearing loss produced by prolonged exposure to intense sounds is the type that involves recruitment. The method of loudness balancing has shown this to be true for temporary hearing losses (Davis *et al.*, 1950) as well as for permanent hearing losses (Rüedi and Furrer, 1947).

References for Further Study

Kryter, K. D. (1950) The effects of noise on man. *J. Speech & Hearing Disorders,* Monogr. Suppl. 1. Parts II and III summarize an extensive literature on masking and fatigue by noise. Particular emphasis is placed on the masking of speech and the deafening effects of industrial and military noise.

Licklider, J. C. R. (1951) Basic correlates of the auditory stimulus. Chap. 25 in S. S. Stevens (Ed.), *Handbook of Experimental Psychology.* New York: Wiley. The section on Masking and Fatigue (pp. 1005–1015) summarizes recent data on these subjects.

Stevens, S. S., and H. Davis. (1938) *Hearing.* New York: Wiley. Chapter 8, Auditory Masking, Fatigue and Persistence, summarizes the important experimental data on masking and fatigue up to 1938.

CHAPTER 7

DIFFERENTIAL SENSITIVITY

IF, BY hearing, we could tell only whether a signal is present or not, our auditory capacities and experiences would be very limited indeed. The absolute threshold, an interesting experimental measurement, seems a little esoteric so far as our ability to get around every day among ordinary acoustic events is concerned. As a matter of fact, it is doubtful if we are ever called upon to detect the presence of a signal in the quiet. More often the signal is masked, perhaps to only a slight extent. If we were to classify these more general kinds of tasks, we should probably talk about, not our ability to barely hear something, but rather our ability to note that a change has been made against an otherwise constant background. This ability is basic to the auditory part of our ability to *discriminate*, to tell that two different stimuli are different. *Discrimination* has already been exemplified in Chaps. 5 and 6, where the listener was called on either to distinguish one word from a set of possible words or to tell the difference between a noise with a tone sticking out of it and a noise alone. In this chapter we shall attempt to run such auditory capacities down to their limits and to note some of the methods by which these limits are measured.

INTRODUCTION

If one were to survey the kinds of audiometry that are performed in most clinical establishments, one would find very little practical justification for this discussion of the ability to detect a difference in a book that purports to consider topics basic to clinical procedures. But the seeming importance of this ability to detect a difference in telling apart the voices of friends, telling a car horn from a train whistle, telling one word from another, telling a child's laugh from his cry makes one feel that, if clinical audiometry moves toward a prediction of a patient's ability to hear in everyday situations, it must include some of these differential measures.

Acuity

It is interesting that in the field of vision the situation is just the opposite. In most clinical examinations, the ophthalmologist is not

188

interested in the minimum light energy that a patient can just detect; rather he wants to know how far apart he can separate two dark lines on a white background before the patient reports that there are two, no longer one. The minimum separation between two lines (which is a more basic way of saying the "smallest letters that can be seen") constitutes the clinically important measure of *visual acuity*. This acuity tells us about the individual's ability to make fine discriminations.

Now, in hearing, the basic clinical measure appears to have been the minimum acoustic energy that the patient can just detect. The otologist has not been interested, as the ophthalmologist has been, in the ability of the patient to make fine discriminations. In Chap. 4 we stated that the term "acuity" would not be used in reference to this absolute threshold. We can rather use the term consistently, throughout all the senses, by referring to the observer's ability to make a discrimination, or, more simply, to tell that two different stimuli are different.

That *auditory* acuity has not figured so large in clinical measurement as *visual* acuity does not necessarily mean that acuity is any less basic a quantity in hearing than it is in vision. Rather it seems that the otologist's diagnostic problems are solved more readily by his study of the absolute threshold than are the similar problems of the ophthalmologist. Visual acuity can sometimes tell the clinician about how much refraction must be supplied by eyeglasses, but we have no such prosthetic devices in hearing that might be 'fitted' by a similar measure of auditory acuity. On the other hand, the ophthalmologist might well be interested in measuring the absolute threshold for light in the case of cataract or retinitis pigmentosa, which seem to act for the eye as does a conductive impairment for the ear—*i.e.*, some of the energy that is put in is attenuated before it reaches the receptors. In cases of cataract the ophthalmologist infers some properties about this light attenuator from the measurement of visual acuity or the ability of the patient to distinguish between separated lines or letters. In otology, just the opposite is done— we measure the absolute threshold or the loss by attenuation of some of the energy that is put in and then infer certain properties about the patient's ability to make discriminations at above-threshold levels. It seems that more information could be obtained clinically for both vision and hearing if each of these two clinical fields borrowed a little of the other's methods.

Auditory Discrimination

Normal listeners can tell that one sound is different from another if the two sounds are sufficiently different in their physical properties. When we set out to measure *differential sensitivity*, we are actually trying to quantify this sufficient physical difference. We know, in general, what physical dimensions are important for certain everyday discriminations. We can distinguish between the speech sounds [u] and [i] because the spectra of these sounds are different. Different speech sounds are characterized by different frequencies, different durations, different intensities at different frequencies, etc. Spectral differences probably also permit us to distinguish the croak of a frog from the chirp of a bird, the voice of a man from that of a child, the tone of a French horn from that of a violin. Even though the over-all intensity and fundamental frequency of two tones from two different musical instruments are the same, we can distinguish the tones. Also, we can distinguish a *pianissimo* from a *fortissimo* from the same instrument, presumably on the basis of differences in intensity. We can distinguish a high pitch from a low pitch from the same instrument playing two tones at the same over-all intensity, presumably because of different fundamental frequencies.

But these are gross, unquantified physical differences, and we wish to know how small we can make some of these physical differences and still have the listener report that the stimuli are different. Such is the nature of the measurement of differential sensitivity in audition. It is not an entirely new measurement but rather has been anticipated by our discussion of masking in the previous chapter. We shall now turn to this relation between masking and differential sensitivity, not so much for the sake of logical order as for ease in understanding the basic concepts involved.

MASKING AND DIFFERENTIAL SENSITIVITY

Let us review the experiment in which we measure the masked threshold for a pure tone heard against a background of white noise. To measure the masked threshold (not the masking) we present to the observer a constant white noise and then, if we employ the method of adjustment, ask him to adjust the intensity of an interrupted tone until he can just barely detect the tone against the noise background. From Fig. 6.3 we see that the masked threshold for a 1000-cps tone heard in the presence of a white noise whose SPL per cycle is 60 db lies at 78 db SPL. This means that a mixture of white noise (60 db SPL per cycle) and a 1000-cps tone at about 75 db or less is not discriminated by the observer from a white noise mixed with no tone at all. When the tone reaches an SPL of 78 db, however, the mixture of tone and noise is judged to be different from the noise alone. It is in this way that we relate masking to differential sensitivity.

We have already discussed the masking by white noise of speech and of tones, but we have not yet discussed the masking of a white noise by a white noise. This is not an absurd measurement when we think of the actual procedures involved. We turn on a continuous white noise. We then add different amounts of the same noise to itself intermittently and ask the observer when he can just detect these intermittent bursts of white noise. It is only because of tradition that we do not ordinarily refer to such an experiment as one on masking. Rather we call it an experiment on the sensitivity to changes in the intensity of a white noise, because when a noise is added to the same noise, the only thing that we have changed is the over-all intensity. The experiment on differential sensitivity is, then, a special case of the experiment on masking —the case in which both the masked and the masking stimuli are the same.

Difference Limen (DL) for Noise

By how much must we increase the intensity of a white noise in order for a listener to detect the change? This is a restatement of the experimental problem introduced above. The datum that we are seeking is the *difference limen* (DL) for the intensity of white noise. In Chap. 1 we discussed some of the classic methods by which this DL is measured. From that discussion we adopt as a definition of the DL for our present purposes the amount of change that is needed in order that a listener detect the difference 50 per cent of the time. This is also, by definition, the *just noticeable difference* (jnd), or the *differential threshold*. These three terms describing the threshold for detecting a difference are equivalent and are related to differential sensitivity reciprocally, in the same way that the absolute threshold is related to absolute sensitivity.

We can express the DL in several different ways. We have stated that it is a physical change, *e.g.*, in intensity. But a change in intensity can be expressed either as an absolute quantity or as a relative quantity. If to a noise whose sound pressure is 2 dynes/cm^2 we must add 0.5 dyne/cm^2 in order that this increase be detected 50 per cent of the time, we may express this increase either as 0.5 dyne/cm^2 (absolute DL) or as a relative increase of $\frac{1}{4}$ or 25 per cent $\left(\frac{0.5}{2}\right)$. And using decibels, which describe ratios anyway, we could also refer to the relative DL as one of about 2 db $\left(20 \log_{10} \frac{2 + 0.5}{2} = 1.92\right)$. Furthermore, we may state the absolute increment in terms of intensity or sound pressure, ΔI or ΔP. We may state the relative increments, $\Delta I/I$ or $\Delta P/P$. And we may also discuss the absolute and relative increments in decibels: $10 \log_{10} \frac{\Delta I}{I_0}$ and $20 \log_{10} \frac{\Delta P}{P_0}$

or $10 \log_{10} \dfrac{\Delta I + I}{I}$ and $20 \log_{10} \dfrac{\Delta P + P}{P} \cdot$ You may convert from any of these expressions to any other by means of the nomogram (Miller, 1947b) shown in Fig. 7.1.

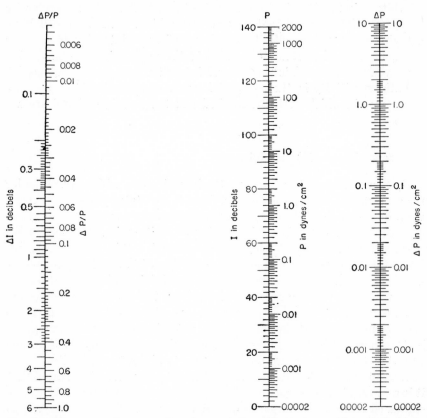

Fig. 7.1. Nomogram for converting from relative DL ($\Delta p/p$ or ΔI in decibels) to absolute DL (Δp) when the Sound Pressure Level at which the measurement is made is known. If we know the relative DL to be 0.5 db or 0.06 (in $\Delta p/p$) at 40 db SPL, then we lay a straightedge so that it intersects these figures on the first two vertical scales. It will then intersect the third scale at 0.0014 dyne/cm² , indicating the absolute pressure increase that was made from 40 db. (*From Miller, 1947b.*)

Now we are ready to discuss some data, derived from an experiment by Miller (1947b), on the differential sensitivity for intensity of white noise. Figure 7.2 shows his results for two observers who were instructed to report when they heard an increase in the loudness of a noise. We see that after the initial acceleration, the function that relates the DL (absolute, in decibels) to the intensity of the noise is a straight line with a slope of 1. The points on this graph come from Miller's data, while the line drawn through them is the function that relates the masking (of pure tones) to the *effective level* (see Chap. 6, Masking of Pure Tones) of white noise obtained by Hawkins and Stevens (Fig. 6.4). The amount of increase in the intensity of noise that a listener is just able to detect goes up as the intensity from which the change is made goes up. In the same way, the intensity of a pure tone that is just heard against a background

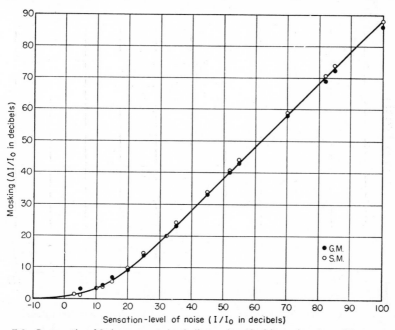

FIG. 7.2. Just-noticeable increments in the intensity of white noise plotted in a manner similar to that of the masking experiment. Ordinate shows absolute DL in decibels $\left(10 \log_{10} \dfrac{\Delta I}{10^{-16} \text{ watts/cm}^2} \right)$ for the data points and masking in decibels for the solid line, which was obtained by Hawkins and Stevens from the masking of tones and speech by white noise. (*From Miller*, 1947b.)

of white noise goes up as the intensity of the noise goes up. But the ratio of the signal to the noise or of the increment to the level from which the increase was made remains quite constant.

Weber's Law in Hearing

It is this constancy of the signal-to-noise ratio in masking or of the relative DL that Weber wrote about in 1834. Weber's Law states that the ratio of a stimulus increment that is just noticeable to the intensity of the stimulus is constant (see Chap. 1). Our previous examples in terms of weights might be repeated or we might also mention a classic example that has to do with light and candles. If to 10 candles we must add just 1 in order that the change in illumination be just noticeable, then to 100 candles we should have to add 10, and to 1000 we should have to add 100. The absolute DL goes up (1, 10, 100) as the illumination goes up (10, 100, 1000). But the ratio of increase to the intensity that was increased remains the same—namely, 1:10.

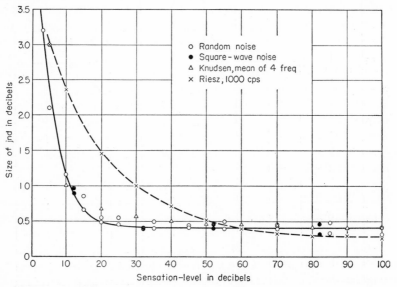

FIG. 7.3. Relative DL in decibels $\left(10 \log_{10} \dfrac{I + \Delta I}{I}\right)$ for changes in the intensity of a white noise as a function of the Sensation Level of the noise. Pure-tone data of Riesz and of Knudsen are shown for comparison. Note that the relative DL remains constant (about 0.5 db) throughout most of the range. (*From Miller*, 1947*b*.)

Now Miller's data show that this relation also holds for increments in the intensity of a white noise. Figure 7.2 shows how the *absolute DL increases* as the intensity increases, but now we can also see how the *relative DL remains constant* as the intensity is increased. Figure 7.3 shows this relation between the relative DL in decibels $\left(10 \log_{10} \dfrac{\Delta I + I}{I}\right)$ and the Sensation Level of the noise. From this graph we conclude that Weber's Law holds (for white noise) from about 20 to 100 db Sensation Level. Within the restrictions of this experiment, the application of Weber's Law covers a very wide range of intensities, allowing one to state that above 20 db Sensation Level, the relative DL is about 0.5 db.

DIFFERENTIAL SENSITIVITY FOR PURE TONES

In order to illustrate some general properties of the DL, we have used an example of sensitivity to changes in the intensity of white noise. But now we wish to use a simpler stimulus in order to find out how much of a physical change needs to be made in order that a listener detect the change. A pure tone can be modified in either of two physical dimensions, namely, frequency and intensity. We can ask, then, two questions. First, holding the intensity of a pure tone constant, what is the smallest change in the frequency of that tone that will be detected 50 per cent of the time? Second, holding the frequency of a pure tone constant, what is the smallest change in the intensity of that tone that will be detected 50 per cent of the time? The answers to these two questions have been said to describe *pitch discrimination* and *loudness discrimination*, respectively. But, as will become clearer in the next chapter, these measures should more accurately be called *frequency discrimination* and *intensity discrimination*, since we measure the physical change in the stimulus that corresponds to a response of "different" and know nothing about the psychological attributes in question.

Intensity Discrimination for Pure Tones

We can distinguish a very weak tone from a very strong tone even though both have the same frequency. But we wish to know the limit of this ability to discriminate. What is the *minimum* change in intensity that can just be detected? It is difficult to give a single general answer to this question for pure tones. The pure tone is simpler than white noise, but changing the intensity (or frequency) of a pure tone is not so simple as changing the intensity of a white noise. If we add a sudden increment to the intensity of a continuous pure tone, not only is the intensity increased, but also energy is spread in the frequency dimension by virtue of the transients involved in an abrupt change. Because of the complications involved in producing the intensitive change that is to be detected, we must discuss the DL for intensity with regard to certain experimental variations.

Method of Change. In an early study of the DL for pure tones, Knudsen obtained values for the intensitive DL that were smaller than those of most subsequent experiments. This was apparently due to the fact that Knudsen changed the intensity of his tones quite abruptly, and therefore the listener could base his response not only on the change in intensity but also on the by-products of the abrupt changes, such as added frequencies.

A more thorough study of the intensitive DL for tones was made by

Riesz. By mixing the outputs of two oscillators, at slightly different frequencies, Riesz obtained a tone of intermediate frequency whose intensity fluctuated at a rate that corresponded to the difference between the two frequencies. The listener was asked to judge whether the tone sounded constant in loudness or whether its loudness fluctuated, that is, whether *beats* were heard. In this way the changes in intensity were made gradually and periodically. The rate at which the changes were

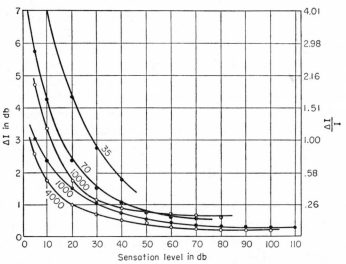

Fig. 7.4. DL for intensity of pure tones as a function of the Sensation Level of the tone. Parameter is frequency. Left-hand scale gives relative DL in decibels; right-hand scale shows relative (linear) DL. (*After Riesz; reproduction by permission from Hearing: Its Psychology and Physiology by S. S. Stevens and H. Davis, published by John Wiley and Sons, Inc., 1938, p. 138.*)

made affected the results considerably, and Riesz determined that the best rate (or beat frequency) was about three beats per second. Figure 7.4 shows the DL for tones of different frequency plotted as a function of the Sensation Level of the tone. The left-hand ordinate shows the relative DL in decibels $\left(10 \log_{10} \dfrac{\Delta I + I}{I}\right)$, and the right-hand ordinate shows the linear relative DL ($\Delta I/I$). Again we see that Weber's Law (that the relative DL remains constant) holds for a considerable part of the range used but not so large a part as for white noise. Riesz's results for 1000 cps and Knudsen's results averaged for four frequencies are shown for comparison with Miller's data on noise in Fig. 7.3.

An Interval of Silence. We have considered the just detectable change that is introduced into an otherwise constant pure tone. This is not quite the same as presenting two tones separately to a listener and asking him to report whether they are the same or different (in respect of loudness). In the first case we listen for a change in a tone that sounds continuous. In the second case we attempt to judge whether the intensities of successive tones are the same or different. It is really this second case that fits the formal methods that were described in Chap. 1.

Now what happens to the DL's that have been specified in the preceding figures if the experimental method is changed to one in which we present first one tone and then another and ask about the smallest difference between their intensities that is necessary for a listener to report that the two tones are different? In the case of the DL for intensity, we find that the results depend upon the interval of time between the two tones. This *auditory time error* comes about because the loudness that we hear when a tone is sounded does not remain fixed in time after the tone has been turned off. Postman has studied this time error for both intensity and frequency discrimination. He reports a relation between the point of judged equality and the time interval between the two successive tones that indicates that the *remembered loudness* of a tone first waxes and then wanes after the tone is turned off. This memory of the loudness of the tone is what we compare with the second tone, and so the time after the first when the second is turned on is crucial for this measurement.

The difference between results on changing-tone and successive-tone methods for measuring the DL is introduced not only for theoretical reasons but also because both appear to be in current use in the clinical applications of the measurement of the DL to be discussed presently. Lüscher and Zwislocki (1949a) and Békésy (1947) employ continuous tones into which changes are introduced, while Denes and Naunton use successive pairs of tones.

Before concluding this section on intensity discrimination for pure tones, we should go back and look at the relation between masking and differential sensitivity, which was discussed in connection with white noise. Does the relation still hold for pure tones? Theoretically, of course, the argument remains the same. The DL for intensity for pure tones is a special case of the masking of one pure tone by another—the case in which the two tones are the same. The bottoms of the sharp dips in Fig. 6.8 represent exactly this case. Let us compare the results of these two different experiments (Wegel and Lane on masking and Riesz on the DL), both about the same phenomenon. The masking data of Fig. 6.8 tell us that to a 1200-cps tone at 80 db Sensation Level we must add a 1200-cps tone at 50 db Sensation Level in order that the addition be noticed. According to Riesz's data in Fig. 7.4, the relative DL for a 1000-cps tone at 80 db Sensation Level is 0.29 db.

Do these observations mean the same thing? Let us assume that at 1000 and 1200 cps the Sensation Level equals the Intensity Level. Now we can put the nomogram in Fig. 7.1 to work. Locate Riesz's relative DL of 0.29 db on the leftmost scale. Lay a straightedge across so that it intersects this point and 80 db Intensity Level, on the left side of the middle scale. The ΔP, or increase in sound pressure from 80 db that is required, is found on the third scale to be 0.07 dyne/cm^2. Now Wegel and Lane state that a 50-db 1200-cps tone must be added to the 80-db 1200-cps tone in order that the increase be detected. And the decibel increase for Riesz's ΔP of 0.07 dyne/cm^2 is $20 \log_{10} \dfrac{0.07}{0.0002}$, which is about 51 db. *q.e.d.*

Frequency Discrimination for Pure Tones

Certainly we can distinguish the highest note on the piano from the lowest. And we know that most people can recognize certain melodies in which changes of only a musical semitone are heard. But what is the limit of this ability to discriminate between two auditory stimuli that are the same in all respects except frequency? How small a difference in frequency can we establish and still have the listener report that the tones are different? Again our answer will depend upon the experimental procedure.

Method of Presentation. Knudsen's early determination of the frequency DL for pure tones was extended more thoroughly by Shower and Biddulph. Again, Knudsen had changed the frequency quite abruptly, whereas Shower and Biddulph periodically changed the frequency more gradually. They found the minimum DL when the frequency change was made from 2 to 3 times per second. Figure 7.5 shows the relative DL for frequency ($\Delta f/f$) as a function of frequency for tones at several Sensation Levels. Above about 40 db Sensation Level, the frequency DL does not depend markedly upon the Sensation Level. Since this ordinate plots the relative DL, we see that for frequencies above about 1000 cps, the absolute DL (Δf) increases linearly as the frequency from which the change is made is increased, because the relative DL ($\Delta f/f$) remains fairly constant.

In discussing the rationale of introducing slow changes in the frequency of a continuous tone, Harris (1948a) has argued that a more valid picture of the frequency discrimination of the human auditory system is given when two tones are separated in time and are compared in respect of pitch. In view of this suggestion, it is interesting to note that the time interval between two such tones does not play a role in determining the DL for frequency. Postman's data on the time error (see above) indicate that although the interval of the time between two successive tones is crucial when they are compared with respect to loudness (by varying intensity), the comparison with respect to pitch (by varying frequency) is independent of the time interval. The differences between these two basic methods for measuring differential sensitivity appear to be much greater for intensity discrimination than for frequency discrimination.

Weber's Law. Perhaps we should not speak of Weber's Law in connection with frequency discrimination, because it was formulated with respect to stimulus intensity. We cannot ignore the fact, however, that the relative DL for frequency remains constant at about 0.003 as the

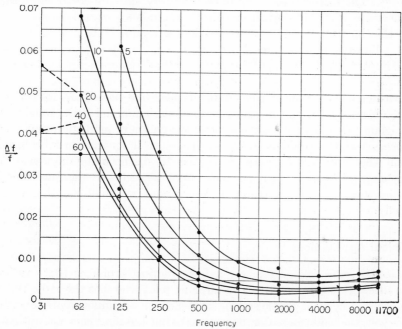

FIG. 7.5. Relative DL ($\Delta f/f$) for frequency as a function of frequency. Parameter is Sensation Level. Above 1000 cps and 40 db Sensation Level, the relative frequency discrimination remains quite constant. (*From Shower and Biddulph.*)

frequency is increased above 1000 cps. This means that at 1000 cps we can detect a change in frequency of about 3 cps, and that at 5000 cps we cannot detect a change of less than 15 cps. Just as in the case of intensity discrimination, so in the case of frequency discrimination, man seems to keep his ability to discriminate stimuli on a relative basis.

AUDITORY DISCRIMINATION

If all the various sounds that we normally encounter sounded the same to us, we should be dull creatures indeed. We could know, by means of hearing, only that a sound was sounding but nothing more. Fortunately, however, we are endowed with capacities that enable us to tell that different sounds are different. Were it not for such capacities, we should be unable to cope with the many auditory discriminations that constitute everyday hearing. The bases of all these discriminations are not clearly understood, but some evidence on simple discriminations, such as frequency and intensity discrimination in pure tones, points to certain fundamental properties. For one thing, the more stimulation there is present, the more of an absolute change is needed for us to detect the change. The fact that so many of our auditory data are written in terms of decibels, which are logarithms of ratios, tends to obscure the necessity for this increase in the amount of change required. As a consequence of the linearity of this increase, we find that our auditory systems respond to constant relative changes, in a manner that was predicted by Weber's Law.

Although there are sufficient data to speak of a *normal DL* for certain stimuli, we do not find measurements of the abnormal being sought by clinicians. This lack persists in spite of the notion or prediction that such processes as the recognition of different speech sounds must be based upon the more fundamental capacities to discriminate different frequencies, different intensities, and different spectra. Some few clinical applications have been made, however, and we shall mention these briefly.

Clinical Applications

DL for Intensity. There are a few practical problems that involve the intensitive DL directly. The airplane pilot who flies the radio range knows that he is on course so long as he hears a continuous pure tone. If, however, the loudness of the tone begins to fluctuate in a certain rhythmic pattern (*A* or *N* in Morse code), he knows that he is either to the right or left of his course. In order for him to recognize the *A* or the *N*, the radio engineers must have built into the radio beams enough of a power increase at certain points so that the added acoustic power is as great as or greater than the normal DL for intensity. Since it does not seem possible to predict exactly a man's DL from a measurement of his absolute threshold or audiogram, it would seem that the intensitive DL of these pilots might well be measured along with their ability to discriminate color, depth, etc.

Pilots, as well as others who use radio equipment, must listen to speech and pure tones in the presence of considerable background noise. A man's ability to pick out a signal from a background of noise is not precisely predictable from the audiogram, either. But since masking and the DL seem to be so well related, perhaps one measurement would test both abilities.

We shall discuss, in some detail, the application of the measurement of the intensitive DL to the detection of the phenomenon of recruitment in the following chapter. Let us mention here a serious problem that arises in connection with this relation. That recruitment can be measured indirectly by measuring the DL for intensity rests upon the fact that certain kinds of hearing loss exhibit abnormally small intensitive DL's relative to their pathologic thresholds. Now it happens that persons with such losses are the same ones, discussed in Chap. 5, whose articulation score for speech will rise to some moderate value and then stay there no matter how intense the speech is made. These two kinds of data on the same people simply do not fit. Their ability to discriminate the sounds of speech is poor, and yet their ability to detect differences in the intensity of sounds is better than normal. Does this suggest that the ability to detect small differences in intensity is not particularly fundamental to the ability to understand speech? Here lies one of the most important paradoxical problems in contemporary clinical audiology.

DL for Frequency. Certain tests of frequency and intensity discrimination have been used to help predict the musical ability of children (Seashore). In addition to this general ability, specific ones have been attacked through the use of measures of the frequency DL. The sonar operator on a submarine must be able to recognize different pitches, and this fact has undoubtedly accelerated the work of Harris (1948a) on frequency discrimination at the U.S. Naval Submarine Base.

So far as a specifically clinical use of the frequency DL is concerned, we can cite only the phenomenon of diplacusis binauralis. If we present a tone of a constant frequency to one ear of an observer and then ask him to adjust the frequency of a tone presented to his other ear until the two tones sound equal (in pitch), he will ordinarily adjust the second to the frequency of the first plus or minus the associated DL for frequency. A listener with diplacusis will set the frequency of the second tone off by more than a DL. Another way of describing the phenomenon is to say that if we present two tones of the same frequency, one to one ear and the other to the other, a normal listener will hear the same pitch in both ears, while the diplacusic listener will hear two different pitches in his two ears (hence the name). Some individuals with normal audiograms show a certain amount of diplacusis, but larger deviations are associated with a pathologic audiogram in which the threshold increases very rapidly above a certain frequency. In short, a demonstration of the phenomenon of diplacusis in a listener with a hearing loss seems to confirm a diagnosis of the recruiting type of deafness. (See Davis *et al.*, 1950.)

Future Work. One always feels guilty when suggesting a new kind of test to be included in routine clinical audiometry. But in this case one would not know what particular test to suggest. We have not enough basic information on discriminatory behavior to suggest what pathologic conditions might influence the behavior for better or for worse. Certain relations are clear—for example, the relations between masking and the intensity DL. But others remain to be worked out. We can recognize different speech sounds on the basis of different spectra, but there is a distribution of different acoustic spectra that we identify as the same speech sound. Differential sensitivity for speech sounds is not finished but is really just starting, so far as the determination of the necessary physical conditions for recognition are concerned. The pilot and the mechanic get a large amount of information from the 'sound' of an engine, but the limits of man's discriminatory powers for the intensity, frequency, and spectra of different noises are far from being quantified.

In short, the ability of a listener to tell one sound from another is basic to his ability to use the acoustic events around him in everyday living. Certain data have already been gathered on some aspects of this very general ability. The fact that there remain inconsistencies between patients' audiograms and their ability to hear speech and otherwise adjust to their acoustic environments means that here is a field in which clinical research, related to basic psychophysical measurements, offers much future promise.

References for Further Study

Miller, G. A. (1947) Sensitivity to changes in white noise and its relation to masking and loudness. *J. Acoust. Soc. Amer.*, **19**, 609–619. In addition to presenting data from his experiment on white noise, the author writes coherently about the theoretical and experimental relationships of intensity discrimination, masking, and loudness.

Licklider, J. C. R. (1951) Basic correlates of the auditory stimulus. Chap. 25 in S. S. Stevens (Ed.), *Handbook of Experimental Psychology*. New York: Wiley. A section on Differential Thresholds summarizes recent data.

Stevens, S. S., and H. Davis. (1938) *Hearing.* New York: Wiley. Chapters 3 and 4 summarize the experimental work on differential sensitivity for frequency and intensity, respectively, up to 1938.

CHAPTER 8

LOUDNESS AND RECRUITMENT

EARLIER chapters have discussed the measurement of (1) the smallest acoustic energy that a listener can detect, either in the quiet or in the presence of another sound, and (2) the smallest change in acoustic energy that a listener can detect. These psychophysical thresholds provide valuable but limited information about the auditory system. For additional kinds of information we must turn to the psychological attributes of hearing.

The transition from the *threshold of intelligibility* to the *articulation score*, which was discussed in Chap. 5, is very similar to this transition from *psychophysical thresholds* to *psychological attributes*, which must be made if we are to be able to relate certain aspects of behavior to changes in the physical dimensions of sounds at intensities that are above the absolute threshold. For example, within a restricted range of intensities— the range of uncertainty—we know that the number of positive responses to a tone will increase as the intensity of the tone is increased. Thus we can say that, within a range of about 20 db around the absolute threshold, the *audibility* of a tone (*i.e.*, percentage of the time it evokes a response) is directly related to the intensity. As the intensity is increased beyond the point at which the listener reports that he hears the tone 100 per cent of the time, the audibility of the tone cannot be said to increase any further, since 100-per-cent response represents the maximum amount of audibility. Yet it is obvious that some aspect of the observer's experience continues to change: the tone becomes *louder*. And it is this psychological dimension of *loudness* and its relation to the physical dimension of *intensity* that we are about to discuss.

Suppose, for example, that we are waiting for a train. There comes a time when we begin to *just hear* the whistle of the train in the distance (*i.e.*, the intensity of the sound at our ears has now come up just to threshold). As the train approaches, the whistle becomes louder and more audible (the intensity at our ears increases), until we are sure that we hear the whistle all the time. Now, though the whistle cannot become more audible, it continues to become louder. And if one were to ask,

"How much louder is it now than it was one minute ago?" he would be asking for quantification of a psychological dimension (loudness), which could later be related to a physical dimension (intensity). Such are the relations to be discussed in this chapter.

PSYCHOLOGICAL AND PHYSICAL DIMENSIONS

In Chap. 1 we discussed a distinction between the physical dimensions of a sound and the attributes of the auditory sensation to which the sound gives rise. We noted that Fechner's work was prompted by a desire to relate the stimulus and the sensation (response) by a mathematical formula. The distinction between a physical and a psychological dimension is not always easy to make, because even physical measurements must be made, or at least recorded, by observing human beings. But the distinction between the physical and the psychological is essentially the distinction between the stimulus and the response. To be sure, the measurement of the stimulus requires that an observer read some instruments, but the readings on those instruments are independent of the observer, in the sense that the reading remains even if the observer goes away. (The falling tree does make a physical sound even if no listener hears it.) A response, on the other hand, cannot be measured or observed unless someone makes the response. These distinctions are at best superficial, and no high order of sophistication is pretended. In hearing we can measure the stimulus with microphones and voltmeters in terms of the physical dimensions of sound pressure, intensity, and voltage. Our responses and the psychological dimensions that are derived from them are produced by listeners.

Psychological Attributes of Sound

Loudness and Pitch.   We have already spoken of loudness as one of the ways by which we characterize sounds. Since the loudness of a particular tone increases as the intensity of the tone is increased, loudness and intensity have sometimes been thought to be about the same thing. But loudness is one of the psychological attributes of a sound, whereas intensity is a property of the physical stimulus. Loudness may change, even though intensity remains constant.

When we restrict our discussion to pure tones, we find that the two attributes that have been investigated most in the field of auditory psychophysics are *loudness* and *pitch*. The subjective scale of loudness runs from weak, or soft, to very strong, or very loud. Pitch, on the other hand, tells us about the *lowness* or *highness* of a tone. It is not surprising that these are the two most studied attributes in hearing, since they are commonly thought to be so uniquely tied up with the two basic physical properties of the pure tone, namely, intensity and frequency. Although it is true that loudness increases when intensity increases, it is also true that loudness may change when frequency is changed, while the intensity remains constant. Furthermore, although the pitch goes up when the frequency increases, pitch may also change when the intensity is changed, while the frequency remains constant.

Other Attributes. Loudness and pitch, of course, are not the only ways by which we describe even pure tones. As a matter of fact, a complete list of all the psychological attributes of pure tones would have to include

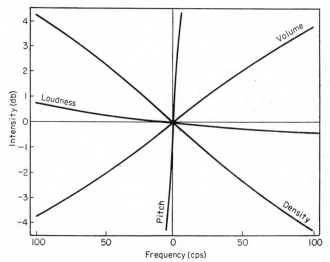

FIG. 8.1. Isophonic contours for four tonal attributes. Each contour connects all points that represent tones that sound equal to the reference tone (500 cps, 60 db) with respect to each of the attributes shown. (*From Stevens*, 1934.)

almost all the adjectives that people have used in describing the tones that they hear. Let us mention here, however, only those attributes that have yielded consistent results when they have been studied at one time or another in the laboratory. Experiments have been carried out on certain attributes of pure tones, such as volume, density, brightness, vocality, and annoyance. The *volume* of a tone has to do with its bigness or smallness, in a spatial sense. Roughly speaking, tones of low frequency sound 'bigger' or more voluminous than tones of high frequency. *Density* has to do with the compactness or hard-packed quality of a sound. Volume and density seem to be reciprocally related, except that both increase when intensity increases. The dependence of pitch, loudness, volume, and density upon frequency and intensity is shown in the isophonic contours of Fig. 8.1.

Brightness is perhaps a more abstract dimension that involves a comparison with brightness in other sense modalities. Tones have also been said to have *vocalic qualities*, certain tones seeming to give rise to characteristics that are best described by analogy to particular vowel sounds in speech. Observers have also reported different amounts of *annoyance*, or annoyingness, for different tones.

Other psychological attributes have been assigned to sounds that are more complex than the pure tone. Just as loudness and pitch have been thought to be closely related to the physical properties of intensity and frequency, so the quality, or *timbre*, of sounds has been associated with the number and amplitudes of the harmonics in a complex tone. It is probably on the basis of timbre that we characterize different sounds, judged to have the same fundamental pitch and loudness, played by each of several musical instruments. Sounds are thus clarinetlike, violinlike, pianolike, etc. Complex sounds, of course, can be characterized in many ways. We speak of them as irritating, noisy, sweet, mellow, harsh, tinny, rich, etc. But most of these attributes have so far been relatively difficult to quantify, and we shall pass them by.

The Measurement of Psychological Attributes

For a long time philosophers and psychologists have argued about the possibility of applying numbers to (*i.e.*, quantifying) aspects of experience. It is clear that psychological attributes preceded, historically, physical dimensions. We *heard* long before we had Fourier analysis. What people heard constituted the only auditory data before we had any techniques for specifying the physical dimensions. We should like to know whether certain relations might not exist between the psychological and physical dimensions. This interest is not new; it got psychophysics started. But in order to relate psychological and physical dimensions, we must be able to measure each.

We can get people to agree on and to distinguish among such concepts as pitch, loudness, volume, etc. But the next step is difficult—we must be able to scale the attribute in some way if we are to relate it empirically to a physical scale of the stimulus. A pitch may be described as high or low, and a loudness as loud or soft. These judgments, however, are relative to each other, and they boil down to a discriminatory response: is this tone louder or softer than another? Or, is this tone higher or lower in pitch than another? Such comparative judgments yield a scale with the property of rank order but nothing more. That is, we can know only that tone A has a higher (judged) pitch than tone B, but we cannot know how much higher, whether A is twice or three times as high as B. Nor can we know whether A is as much higher than B as is B than C. To obtain the answers to these questions, we must ask the observer directly, not only whether A is higher than B, but how much higher? Only then can we obtain a scale for our psychological attributes that has the same properties as the scales of our physical dimensions.

The application of numbers to these psychological attributes has evoked a long history of controversy, a major opponent to the idea being William James, who ridiculed the work of Fechner on the ground that a given sensory experience was not a sum of lesser sensory experiences. Said James, "Our feeling of pink is surely not a portion of our feeling of scarlet . . . ." (Boring, p. 44). In spite of such a "quantity objection," some psychological attributes have been scaled, and the variation of the attribute with a physical dimension has been plotted. An example is given in the following section.

LOUDNESS AND LOUDNESS LEVEL

A tone just above the absolute threshold sounds very soft. If the intensity of the tone is raised about 120 db, to just below the threshold of feeling, it will sound very loud. In between these two limits there are tones whose loudness will be judged to be somewhere between very soft and very loud. We may assume also that as the intensity is raised, between these limits, the loudness will increase. To obtain a suitable scale for the psychological attribute of loudness, we must make psychophysical measurements that will turn these semiquantitative comparative judgments into cardinal numbers.

We shall discuss only briefly the development of one scale of loudness merely to show that the job can be done. Fortunately for the patient, clinical use of loudness in certain tests does not depend upon a loudness scale, because we get along well enough with a physical scale of *Loudness Level* which tells us indirectly about the loudness of a given sound through a judgment of *equal loudness*. This is extremely convenient, because a judgment of equal loudness is undoubtedly easier for the naive listener than more complicated judgments like "twice as loud" or "half as loud" that are required for the loudness scale itself.

Loudness in Sones

Perhaps the simplest way to explain the method of developing a loudness scale is to go through some of the steps. The term *sone* was proposed as a unit of loudness by Stevens, who defines 1 sone arbitrarily as the loudness of a 1000-cps tone at an Intensity Level of 40 db. We ask a listener, or preferably several listeners, to adjust the level of a 1000-cps tone until it sounds *half as loud* as this standard of 40 db. Then we ask for an adjustment that yields a tone that sounds *twice as loud* as the standard.

These two loudnesses we will then label 0.5 and 2 sones, respectively. If we go further and ask for an adjustment that yields a loudness that is half that of the 0.5-sone tone, and another that sounds twice as loud as the 2-sone tone, we shall have added points on the loudness scale for tones of loudnesses 0.25 and 4 sones, respectively. This process can go on until the range of approximately 120 db is explored. Intermediate points

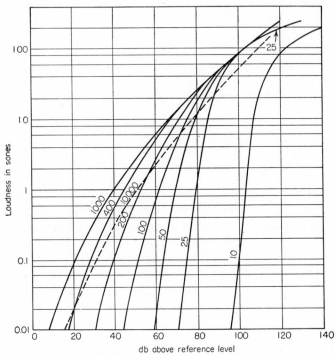

FIG. 8.2. Loudness as a function of Intensity Level. A loudness of 1 *sone* is defined as the loudness of a 1000-cycle tone at 40 db Intensity Level. All other points on the curves are related to this loudness by judgments of equal loudness, half loudness, twice loudness, etc. Note that the loudness for low-frequency tones grows much faster with Intensity Level than the loudness of the 1000-cycle tone. (*Reproduction by permission from Hearing: Its Psychology and Physiology by S. S. Stevens and H. Davis, published by John Wiley and Sons, Inc., 1938, p. 118.*)

are obtained by a method of bisection. For example, if we present tones of 2 and 4 sones loudness and ask the observer to adjust the intensity of a third tone until its loudness appears to be *halfway between* the loudnesses of the 2-sone and the 4-sone tones, the loudness of this third tone can be designated as 3 sones. We can now relate Intensity Level (in decibels) to loudness (in sones), as in Fig. 8.2. The loudness function for 1000 cps is shown as the leftmost line.

The loudness functions for the other frequencies shown are tied to the first curve at several points through an equal-loudness judgment between two tones of unequal frequency. The equality of loudness for tones of different frequencies is shown in Fig. 8.3. Each of these *equal-loudness contours* represents the Sound Pressure Level or the Intensity Level required at different frequencies in order that all tones on the contour

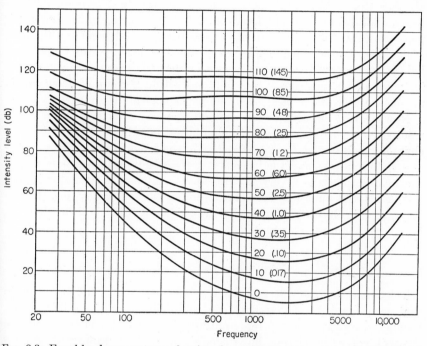

Fig. 8.3. Equal-loudness contours showing the relation between Intensity Level and frequency for tones at different Loudness Levels. The parameter is Loudness Level in decibels, or *phons,* defined as the Intensity Level of the 1000-cycle tone whose loudness is used as a standard for each contour. The 0-phon contour is the normal threshold curve (in a free field). The numbers in the parentheses show the loudness in *sones* associated with each contour. (*Reproduction by permission from Hearing: Its Psychology and Physiology by S. S. Stevens and H. Davis, published by John Wiley and Sons, Inc.,* 1938, *p.* 124.)

sound equally loud. The data from which the equal-loudness contours were drawn were obtained by Fletcher and Munson in a free field, while the threshold curve comes from the experiment (with earphones) of Sivian and White.

The fact that such a loudness scale can be constructed may not in itself be of such practical importance as the clarification that it introduces in our thinking about loudness and intensity in particular and about psychological and physical dimensions in general. When we asked the listener, for example, to adjust the intensity of a 1000-cps tone until it sounded twice as loud as a fixed tone at 1000 cps and 40 db IL (*i.e.*, 1 sone) he did not give us a result at twice the intensity, which would have been 43 db; nor did he adjust to twice the number of decibels, or 80 db; nor, furthermore, did he give us a result that was twice as far above the absolute threshold in jnd's as was the reference tone (Newman, 1933), a result that Fechner would have predicted. We have, rather, an independent scale of loudness in terms of quantitative judgments on the part of listeners. To the objector who asks, "But how can a person know what half a loudness is?" we can only answer that the results are acceptable in terms of the consistency that is found within a group of listeners. So much for the example of at least one psychological attribute.

Now we may proceed to less difficult operations for slightly different results. Note, before we leave the loudness scale, however, that we can characterize a *normal loudness function* in the following way: if we represent both loudness and the intensity of the sound on logarithmic scales, the loudness increases very rapidly at low intensities, while at higher intensities the function decelerates, indicating a smaller logarithmic increment in loudness for each successive logarithmic increment in intensity. We must refer to this fact when we consider certain pathologic cases.

Loudness Level

Telephone engineers have needed for a long time a subjective scale that corresponds to the strength of sound. They had the decibel, which became extremely useful in representing powers over the enormous range that is involved in hearing, but the effect of a certain number of decibels upon the average listener could not be told without further measurement. A loudness scale in sones might have been extremely useful to the engineer, but the job of translating from psychological to physical scales, along with the original problem of validating the loudness function through complicated observations with many observers, was probably more trouble than the results would have warranted. A compromise was reached in the concept of Loudness Level, which tells us, not how loud a tone is, but rather how intense a 1000-cps tone must be in order to sound equally loud. The only psychophysical measurement required is a judgment of equal loudness with respect to two tones of unequal frequency.

Consider the equal-loudness contours of Fig. 8.3. Each of these contours represents a set of tones of different frequency and intensity, all of which have the same (unspecified) loudness. Consider, for example, the contour marked "40." It should cross the 1000-cps ordinate at 40 db

IL.[1] The other points on this contour were obtained by presenting alternately to a single ear of the observer the 1000-cps 40-db tone and a tone of a different frequency, let us say 250 cps, the intensity of which was adjustable by the listener. He is asked to adjust the intensity of the 250-cps tone until it sounds equal in loudness to the 40-db 1000-cps tone. The Loudness Level of this 250-cps tone is then, by definition, 40 db or 40 *phons*.[2] In other words, *the Loudness Level of any tone is the Intensity Level of the 1000-cps tone to which it sounds equal in loudness.* Every tone represented on a single equal-loudness contour has the same Loudness Level, which is the Intensity Level of the 1000-cps tone on that contour, and each has the same loudness, although we do not know what the loudness (in sones) is. Such contours may be called also *equal-loudness-level contours.*

Since the Loudness Level of any tone can be obtained by the relatively simple judgment of equal loudness, the loudness of any tone can therefore be obtained mathematically or graphically from the loudness scale for 1000 cps alone. Consider, for example, the functions of Fig. 8.4. Here we see the Loudness Level for tones of different frequencies plotted as a function of the Intensity Level of the individual tones. These can be considered functions of loudness in a relative sense. That is to say, the Loudness Level is actually loudness relative to the loudness of a 1000-cps tone. By definition, of course, the Loudness Level of a 1000-cps tone plotted as a function of the Intensity Level of the 1000-cps tone is a straight line with a slope of 1, because these two quantities, for 1000 cps, are the same thing. If, now, we go through the necessary procedures for obtaining the loudness (in sones) of a 1000-cps tone, as is given in Fig. 8.2, we can put in the functions for all the other frequencies in Fig. 8.2 by subtracting according to Fig. 8.4. Thus the concept of Loudness Level is a unifying one that ties all frequencies, through judgments of equal loudness, to the loudness function that was obtained for 1000 cps.[3]

---

[1] It crosses actually at about 47 db, because the original contours were plotted relative to the Sensation Level of the 1000-cps tone. Since the threshold curve is assumed to represent a Loudness Level of 0 phons, this discrepancy of 6 to 10 db remains a problem (see Rudmose).

[2] The *phon* is a unit of Loudness Level and is exactly the same as the *decibel* for this scale only.

[3] It might be well to review the different 'levels' that we have mentioned so far: *Sound Pressure Level* is the level of a sound in decibels relative to the reference pressure of 0.0002 dyne/cm^2; *Intensity Level* is the level of a sound in decibels relative to the reference intensity of 10^{-16} watt/cm^2; *Sensation Level* (or Hearing Loss) is the level of a sound in decibels relative to the normal absolute threshold for that sound; *Loudness Level* of a sound is the IL or SPL of a 1000-cps tone that sounds equally loud. All four levels are *physical quantities!*

Among other things, we can see from the three preceding figures that loudness grows at different rates for tones of different frequency. A simple demonstration consists of the comparison between 100 and 1000 cps. The absolute threshold for 100 cps is about 45 db, IL, while for 1000 cps it is only about 10 db. Yet the IL's for these two frequencies at the 100-phon Loudness Level are almost the same, namely, 107 and 108 db,

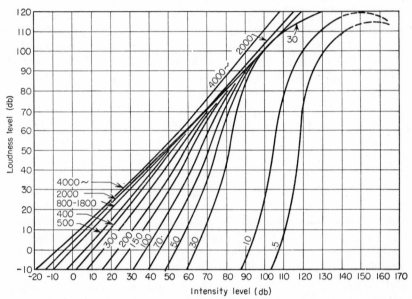

FIG. 8.4. Loudness Level as a function of Intensity Level. Since the Loudness Level for 1000 cps is defined as the Intensity Level of that tone, the curve for 1000 cps (800–1800 cps in the figure) appears as a straight line with a slope of 1. The Intensity Levels for all frequencies at any one Loudness Level constitute the equal-loudness contour for that level in Fig. 8.3. These functions permit the inclusion of frequencies other than 1000 cps in Fig. 8.2 without the necessity for establishing a loudness scale for each one. (*After Fletcher and Munson; and Békésy*, 1936b; *reproduction by permission from Hearing: Its Psychology and Physiology by S. S. Stevens and H. Davis, published by John Wiley and Sons, Inc.*, 1938, p. 126.)

respectively. In order to obtain the same range of loudness (*i.e.*, from threshold to 100 phons) the intensity of a 1000-cps tone must be increased 98 db, whereas that of a 100-cps tone must be increased only 62 db. The curves of Fig. 8.4 show such relations more generally. The loudness for tones of low frequency grows more rapidly with equal decibel increments of intensity than does the loudness for tones of higher frequencies. By way of introducing the next section, we may say that even in the case of normal hearing we have a phenomenon like *recruitment:* the loudness of low-frequency and very high-frequency tones increases more rapidly per decibel than does the loudness for tones of middle frequencies.

RECRUITMENT OF LOUDNESS

A Hearing Loss is usually measured in terms of the number of decibels a tone must be raised above the normal absolute threshold for a given person to hear the tone 50 per cent of the time. This Hearing Loss may remain constant as frequency is increased, or it may change with frequency. Although there are many exceptions, it is generally true that a more or less uniform Hearing Loss as a function of frequency is indicative of types of conductive deafness, while a Hearing Loss that increases with frequency is associated with inner-ear or nerve deafness. The shape of the audiogram is not, of course, the only means of distinguishing these two general types. Tuning-fork tests, bone-conduction measurements, and certain speech tests can help considerably. The phenomenon of recruitment constitutes another means, since it is now known to be associated with a pathologic condition that is more central than the middle ear.

Evidence for recruitment is obtained when it can be shown that the loudness of a given tone increases more rapidly than normal as the Sensation Level of the tone is increased in equal decibel steps. Suppose, for example, that a patient has a Hearing Loss (for 2000 cps) of 60 db in one ear only. If we introduce a 2000-cps tone into his normal ear at 100-db SPL (also 100 db above threshold for that ear), we shall find that the tone that sounds equally loud in his poor ear is also about 100 db SPL (40 db above his threshold for that ear). In spite of a deficiency at threshold, the ear with recruitment seems to 'catch up' with the normal ear in loudness. Although Fowler (1928) first used the term *recruitment* and suggested a method (see below) whereby it could be measured, Reger has pointed out that the first reference to the phenomenon was made by Pohlman and Kranz in 1924. Since that time recruitment has been investigated by many clinical workers, who have by now worked out many different ways of measuring the phenomenon.

Measurements of Recruitment

Before considering the various clinical procedures that are used to measure recruitment, let us devise a theoretical example in which we attempt to build a loudness scale (in sones) for patients with a Hearing Loss. In this way we will be able to discuss the basic kind of measurement that relates recruitment to loudness directly. The heavy curve in Fig. 8.5 shows the loudness function for 1000 cps (from Fig. 8.2) obtained with a listener with normal hearing. Now let us consider two other listeners with abnormal hearing, both of whom have a Hearing Loss of 40 db at

1000 cps. If we were to go through the same operations as were outlined
at the beginning of the section on Loudness and Loudness Level, we might
generate the two curves B and C in Fig. 8.5. Curve C shows that for any
given loudness in sones, the intensity required on the part of the hard-of-
hearing listener is always 40 db more than it is for the person with normal
hearing (curve A). Curve B, however, shows that although 40 db more
than normal is required at threshold, increasing amounts of loudness

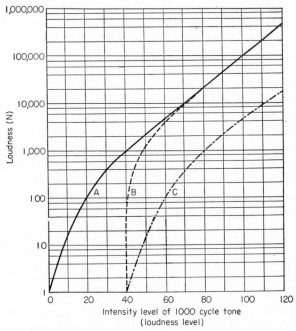

Fig. 8.5. Theoretical functions relating loudness to Intensity Level for three cases:
(*A*) normal hearing (see Fig. 8.2); (*B*) 40-db Hearing Loss of the variable type with
recruitment; and (*C*) 40-db Hearing Loss of the constant type with no recruitment.
(*From Steinberg and Gardner, 1947.*)

require progressively less than a 40-db increase over the normal. Eventually curve B 'catches up' with curve A, and we can see graphically
what we described above, namely, that the loudness for patients with
such a hearing loss increases more rapidly per decibel than it does for
either a normal person or a person with a conductive hearing loss.

   Since the Hearing Loss and loudness function represented by curve C
remain constantly separated from curve A by 40 db, Steinberg and
Gardner have called this the *constant-type hearing loss;* whereas curve B,
which shows a gradual reduction in the 'hearing loss' as the intensity is

increased above threshold, is called *variable-type hearing loss*.[1] Steinberg and Gardner's theoretical interpretation of the ideal recruitment function shown in Fig. 8.5 was as follows. The constant-type hearing loss is associated with a pathologic condition that removes a certain percentage of the sound energy and allows only a fixed percentage to get to the inner ear. Such a removal will then always result in a reduction of the effective stimulus by a certain number of decibels—the same at threshold as at higher intensities. The variable-type hearing loss is associated with a pathologic condition that involves, not a fixed reduction of the effective stimulus in decibels, but rather a fixed reduction in loudness, presumably contributed by a certain number of end organs on the basilar membrane.

Equal-loudness Matches for Tones of Different Frequency (Monaural). It has been pointed out that the equal-loudness contours of Fig. 8.3 (for normal ears) show a kind of recruitment in the growth of loudness of low-frequency tones relative to the growth of loudness for a 1000-cps tone. In a similar way we can measure clinical recruitment by comparing the rate of the growth of loudness for two tones of different frequency measured on the same ear. This method of measuring recruitment, so inextricably tied to the concept of Loudness Level, was introduced into the clinical literature in 1936 (Reger). By way of example, let us consider only the 0-, 40-, and 80-phon Loudness-level contours. These three contours, taken from Fig. 8.3, are shown again in Fig. 8.6. The broken line near the bottom of the figure shows the absolute threshold for pure tones for a listener who has a fairly sharp gap in his high-frequency hearing. His hearing, however, for 1000 cps and other frequencies outside of the 'hole' is quite normal. We present to his bad ear (the only one being considered here) alternately a 1000-cps tone at 40 db and a 6400-cps tone. The listener is asked to adjust the intensity of the 6400-cps tone until it sounds equal in loudness to the 1000-cps tone at 40 db. By definition, then, the intensity to which he adjusts the variable high-frequency tone corresponds to a Loudness Level of 40 phons for him. Other frequencies were measured and balanced in loudness in the same way against the 1000-cps tone at 40 db in order to generate enough points to show the curve that is labeled "40 phons." This procedure was repeated at a higher level to produce the 80-phon equal-loudness contour.

[1] Most English-speaking authors refer to the "variable type" with the term *recruitment*, which describes what happens to the loudness as the intensity is increased. DeBruine-Altes and other European writers have preferred the term *regression*, because it describes better what happens to the hearing loss, which regresses, or decreases, as the intensity is increased. We have introduced a general term, *hearing loss*, which refers to the number of decibels that a given listener requires above the normal quantity for a given response. The previously used term *Hearing Loss* (capitalized) refers to the response at absolute threshold.

Compare, in particular, the rate at which the loudness jumps from 0 to 40 to 80 phons at 6400 cps with the rate at which the same jumps were made at 1000 cps. The transition from 0 to 80 phons requires a change of about 80 db at 1000 cps but only about 10 db at 6400 cps. By virtue of the fact that the loudness for 6400 cps grows within an interval of only 10 db by the same amount as does the loudness for 1000 cps within an interval of 80 db, we can say that this ear shows recruitment at 6400 cps (and at neighboring frequencies between 4500 and 8000 cps).

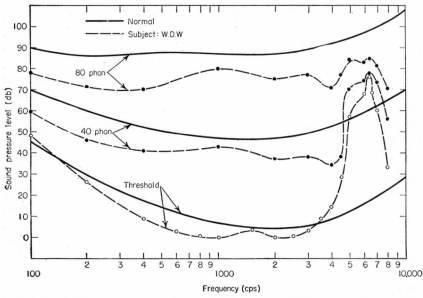

FIG. 8.6. Equal-loudness contours for normal hearing (solid lines) and for a patient with a high-frequency *dip*. The deviations between the threshold curves are much larger (in decibels) than the deviations between the 80-phon loudness contours Clinical data are given in SPL in a 6-cc coupler. (*From Hirsh, unpublished data.*)

To be sure, in clinical measurement it is doubtful that one would want to generate the complete equal-loudness contours for all frequencies and at several Loudness Levels. The easiest way to demonstrate recruitment using such a procedure is to show a difference in the rate of loudness growth for two tones of different frequencies. This can be shown only when the Hearing Loss for these two frequencies is different. Note in particular that the balance of loudness from one frequency to another is obtained for one ear only, and so this particular procedure for measuring recruitment may be applied to patients who have a Hearing Loss in both ears. A relatively easier procedure, which requires that one ear be normal or at least devoid of the *variable-type* deafness, follows.

Alternate Binaural Loudness Balance (One Frequency). The technique that Fowler originally described in 1928 requires only that the listener match in loudness two tones, both of the same frequency, presented alternately to the two ears.[1] Figure 8.7 shows an idealized representation of data that might be obtained with this procedure. Three curves are shown, corresponding to curves *A*, *B*, and *C* in Fig. 8.5. The ordinate

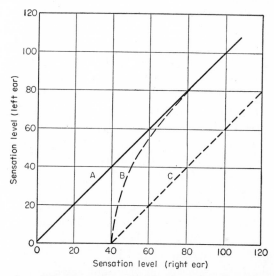

FIG. 8.7. Redrawing of the three theoretical loudness functions that were presented in Fig. 8.5 as they would appear as results of alternate binaural loudness matches. The three curves show the relation between Sensation Level on the left (normal) ear and Sensation Level on the right (pathologic) ear for equal loudness at several levels. All results are for one frequency and the three cases of hearing loss described in Fig. 8.5.

represents Sensation Level (decibels on the "Hearing Loss" dial) of the tone supplied to the left ear, while the abscissa represents the Sensation Level of the tone supplied to the right ear. The points on which the lines are based would be obtained by presenting a certain Sensation Level (Hearing-loss control on the audiometer) to one ear and asking the

---

[1] With a single audiometer and a single tone available, the test was carried out by having the patient switch the earphone from ear to ear. With the advent of binaural headsets associated with audiometers and, sometimes, with two oscillator circuits available, we may switch the tone from one ear to the other with different amounts of attenuation without having the observer remove the headphones.

listener to adjust the Sensation Level of the tone in the other ear until the two tones sound equal in loudness.[1] We assume that any two tones at threshold intensity have the same loudness, although this judgment has never been reported. Therefore one point goes at the intersection of 0 and 0 db of the two scales. Now we go up the vertical scale 20 db, indicating that we present to the left ear a tone at 20 db Sensation Level. If we ask a normal observer to adjust the intensity of a tone of the same frequency until it sounds equal in loudness, he should set the Sensation Level of the tone in his right ear at 20 db. This operation is repeated for as many points as we wish to obtain, and these points can be fitted by a straight line (curve A) with a slope of 1, indicating that equal loudness for the same frequency between two normal ears is given by equal Sensation Level.

Curve B represents the results that might be obtained from the ideal listener with recruitment (right ear) whose loudness function is shown as curve B of Fig. 8.5. Here we note that the first point of equal loudness at threshold is represented by 0 db Sensation Level on the left (normal) ear and 40 db Sensation Level on the right (pathologic) ear. This 'hearing loss' gradually decreases as loudness balances are made between the two ears for tones of the same frequency.

Curve C shows the result that would be obtained from the ideal listener with a conductive hearing loss (right ear) of 40 db. Here we note that points of equal loudness are represented by 40 db more intensity in the right ear than in the left for all levels.

As a matter of fact, the curves of Fig. 8.7 are actually the curves of Fig. 8.5, but the loudness scale for the right ear is now plotted relative to the normal loudness function of the left ear, whereas the ordinate for Fig. 8.5 was an absolute loudness scale. In Fig. 8.7 we have, by bending, made the normal curve A of Fig. 8.5 a straight line, and the others appear in Fig. 8.7 as bent by the same amount.

The judgment required in the alternate binaural loudness balance is easier than a monaural bifrequency balance (see above) for naive listeners, possibly by virtue of the fact that the tones to be balanced do not differ in frequency but only in respect of the ear to which the tone is delivered. This measure of recruitment is limited, however, by the fact that if two ears have the same hearing loss (of the same variable type) a straight line will show the relation between the loudnesses of the two ears. The devia-

---

[1] It is important that the presentation of the tones to the two ears be kept alternate, that is, that the two tones never be presented at the same time. The judgment of equal loudness between two tones presented simultaneously, one to each ear, is a very difficult one to make and is usually obtained by asking the patient to report when the sound appears to be in the middle of the head (see Chap. 9).

tion from a straight line, such as curve *B* of Fig. 8.7, can be shown only when the variable-type hearing losses in the two ears are different.

It is interesting to compare the results that are obtained with this method for one frequency with the results that are shown in Fig. 8.6. The frequency chosen is the one for which this listener had the most Hearing Loss. The left ear of this listener is normal. By using the alternate binaural loudness technique at a frequency of 6400 cps we obtain the curve shown in Fig. 8.8. The two ears are separated by about 50 db at

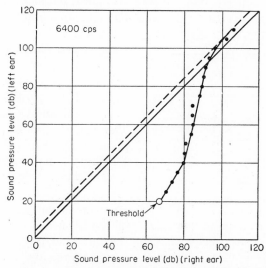

Fig. 8.8. Alternate binaural loudness balance for patient whose right threshold and equal-loudness contours were shown in Fig. 8.6. He adjusted the SPL of a tone presented to his right ear until it sounded equal in loudness to a tone in his left ear at different SPL's. The circle shows the thresholds for the two ears. Frequency of the tone in both ears was 6400 cps, the frequency at which his right ear shows maximum Hearing Loss. (*From Hirsh, unpublished data.*)

threshold. Relative to the growth of loudness in the left ear, the loudness in the right ear increases more rapidly per decibel. Note that the curve does not immediately rise from threshold at its maximum slope but rather acquires its maximum slope after accelerating to about 40 db SPL on the left ear.

Considerable significance has been attached to the points above the reference line. Four such points are seen in Fig. 8.8, corresponding to SPL's on the left ear of 95, 100, 105, and 110 db. We cannot conclude from these points that the right, pathologic ear becomes 'better' than the left ear as the intensity is raised above 90 db. Suppose, for example, that the left ear has a conductive Hearing Loss of only 5 db. Then the reference line would have to be shifted upward by 5 db to the position of the broken straight line that is shown. Then we should say only that recruitment is complete, but we should not have "hyperrecruitment." Such small Hearing Losses, which are difficult to measure, affect the results of such functions considerably.

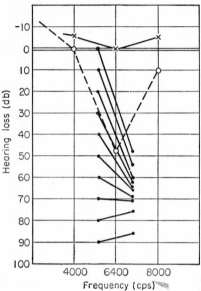

FIG. 8.9. The results from Fig. 8.8, plotted on an audiogram. The audiograms (absolute thresholds) are shown by the O and X for the right and left ears, respectively. Points of equal loudness are joined by straight lines that cross the vertical line of the frequency being tested. The Sensation Levels for the left ear are shown to the left of the frequency line and are increased at 10-db intervals. The Sensation Levels for the right ear are shown to the right of the line and are produced by the listener who adjusts the intensity of the tone in his right ear until it sounds equal in loudness to the tone in his left. (*From Hirsh, unpublished data.*)

It may be helpful to show these results on an audiogram, the type of record most frequently made in the clinic. Normally we let a circle (*O*) and an *X* represent the Hearing Loss for the right and left ears, respectively. We need to choose one frequency at which the Hearing Loss is different for the two ears to explore for recruitment with the alternate binaural loudness balance. The case represented in the audiogram of Fig. 8.9 is the same as in Fig. 8.8. We shall be concerned here with only half the points previously presented, those that represent 10-db increments of Sensation Level on the left ear. A tone 10 db above the threshold, presented to the left ear, is represented by a small dot at 10 db Hearing Loss placed just to the left (left ear) of the vertical line that represents the frequency being tested. The Sensation Level on the right ear, which the listener adjusts until it sounds equal in loudness to the 10-db tone on the left ear, is entered as a small dot just to the right of the same vertical line. These two points are joined by a straight line whose deviation from a horizontal line represents the difference in Sensation Level between the two ears for equal loudness. Successive pairs of such points may be joined for successively higher Sensation Levels. When recruitment is present these lines approach the horizontal as the Sensation Level of the test tone in the left ear is raised. In this case, at about 70 db the line is horizontal, indicating complete recruitment. The apparent "hyperrecruitment" is shown when the slope of the line reverses direction.

The two preceding methods are in common use in those clinics where recruitment is measured by asking the listener for judgments of equal loudness. In the first case, where different frequencies are equated in loudness on the same ear, the judgment is relatively difficult for a naive listener, but this method has the advantage that it can be used in almost all cases. The matching of the loudness of two tones at the same frequency that are presented alternately to the two ears is, although somewhat easier, less generally applicable, because it requires that there be a substantial difference between the two ears in the Hearing Loss for the frequency that is tested. We may call these two methods of measurement *direct*, since they measure recruitment through judgments of loudness, and we have defined recruitment in terms of loudness. The following section will describe certain other methods that have been proposed as indirect measures of recruitment, though they do not involve judgments of loudness directly.

Indirect Measurements of Recruitment

Ever since the phenomenon of recruitment has been examined in clinical situations, different workers have attempted to devise new, better, and easier methods for its measurement. Fowler's original technique, consisting of the alternate presentation of tones of the same frequency to the two ears, is limited to patients who have one normal ear for comparison. The interfrequency loudness matches, which were introduced in the experimental literature by Fletcher and Munson and were later applied by Reger to the clinical detection of recruitment, made the possibilities of loudness measurement more general, so that recruitment could be observed in patients who had defective hearing in both ears. The general feeling probably still remains among many clinicians that the judgment of loudness is a relatively difficult task for the patient who is inexperienced in the listening situation. In the last decade or so, therefore, we find several new methods which attempt to measure recruitment indirectly, that is, without actually getting judgments of loudness. Since the phenomenon of recruitment can be represented as a pathologic loudness function, it is not surprising that these indirect methods employ measurements of the difference limen, masking, and auditory fatigue, all three of which phenomena have been related to loudness both theoretically and experimentally in the literature on hearing (Stevens and Davis, Chap. 4).

Differential Sensitivity to Intensity. The rationale for using intensity discrimination as a basis for the measurement of recruitment is essentially the following: if the loudness is increasing more rapidly than normal as the stimulus intensity is increased, a smaller than normal amount of intensity change is necessary for a noticeable difference in the loudness. This argument does not depend at all upon the erroneous assumption that loudness is simply a cumulation of just noticeable differences above the absolute threshold.

In 1947 Békésy described a new audiometer (see Chap. 4) for measuring the absolute threshold as a continuous function of frequency. Not only

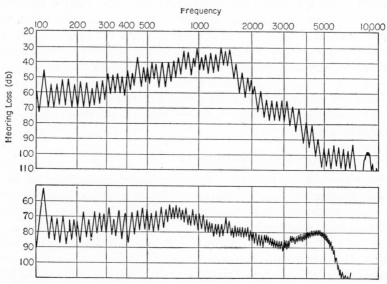

Fig. 8.10. Two audiograms obtained with the Békésy audiometer. The top audiogram shows a Hearing Loss that increases with frequency but the variability or *range of uncertainty* remains about the same for all frequencies, *i.e.*, no recruitment. The bottom audiogram shows a similar Hearing Loss, but the variability gets much smaller at high frequencies where the Hearing Loss is maximum, indicating recruitment. (*From Békésy, 1947.*)

does Békésy's audiometer permit an automatic recording of the threshold at all frequencies throughout the range of the instrument, but it also provides an estimate of the variability of the absolute threshold. This variability is shown by the length of the excursions above and below the average threshold that are produced in the interval between a just-heard tone and a just-not-heard tone. As a limiting case, this variability about the absolute threshold is a measure of the DL.

Two sample audiograms, taken from Békésy (1947), are shown in Fig. 8.10. The top one is the audiogram of a patient who shows no recruitment. The variations around the average threshold are of the order of 10 or 15 db from peak to peak and are roughly the same as the variations that would occur around the zero line of the audiogram for a normal listener. The bottom curve, however, shows the Hearing Loss with recruitment that gradually increases above 1000 cps. Note that the variability (DL) gets smaller at the higher frequencies.

Békésy's technique uses a measure of differential sensitivity at or near the absolute threshold. As we saw in Fig. 7.4, the intensitive DL is largest near the absolute threshold but then gradually diminishes to its constant (relative) value at a Sensation Level of 40 db. Lüscher and Zwislocki (1948, 1949) have proposed that the pathologic DL also be measured at 40 db Sensation Level (relative to the patient's threshold) because of its relative invariance with both frequency and intensity above that Sensation Level.

Their clinical technique is quite similar to the experimental procedure of Riesz (see Chap. 7) in that they use a continuous tone whose amplitude is gradually changed or *modulated*. The modulation voltage is mixed with the pure-tone voltage in such a way that the percentage of modulation, in voltage or pressure ($100\Delta P/P$), can be controlled by the experimenter. The patient reports when the continuous tone appears to fluctuate in loudness, and the DL, defining the percentage change that the listener can just detect, is compared with that of the normal listener for a comparable Sensation Level. Indeed the normal DL's, in terms of percentage, are entered on an audiogram blank at Sensation Levels of 20, 40, 60, and 80 db. One has, then, only to measure the patient's DL, in percentage, and to consult this normal audiogram to learn whether the patient's DL is normal or abnormally small.

On the assumption that in cases of recruitment loudness increases most rapidly at low Sensation Levels and less rapidly at higher ones, and on the further assumption that the DL is uniquely related to the growth of loudness, Denes and Naunton have pointed out that although the DL in recruitment will be abnormally small at low Sensation Levels, it will approach normality at higher Sensation Levels where the rate of growth of loudness becomes normal. The technique used by Denes and Naunton for measuring the DL involves the successive comparison of two tones whose frequency is the same and whose intensities are slightly different. The listener's DL is given by the point at which he can just detect the difference between the intensities of the two successive tones. A generalized result of their tests is given in Fig. 8.11. The heavy line indicates the size of the DL as a function of the Sensation Level of the reference tone. The two broken lines indicate two different amounts of recruitment.

In diagnostic work, Denes and Naunton conclude that if the DL (in decibels) decreases as a function of intensity, there is no recruitment present. But if the DL either remains constant or increases as a function of intensity, there is recruitment.

In view of the work that has been done relating differential sensitivity to recruitment, we cannot say that we have a single standard method for making the measurement. The three techniques discussed above differ with respect to the level at which the DL is measured and the method of setting up a difference between two tones. Békésy (1947) measures the DL indirectly at or near the absolute threshold. It would seem that this low level is particularly advantageous for demonstrating an abnormal DL, because the loudness is changing so rapidly near the absolute threshold. Such was the argument made by Huizing in a discussion of the Lüscher and Zwislocki (1949) paper (*q.v.*). Lüscher and Zwislocki prefer that the DL be measured about 40 db above the absolute threshold, because it is relatively invariant with both frequency and intensity above that level. A detailed examination of the relation between the DL for intensity and intensity, as reported in clinical studies and in the author's data (see Fig. 8.8), reveals that loudness in recruitment does not always increase at its maximum rate near the absolute threshold. A *standard* level for measuring the DL must wait upon more clinical observations.

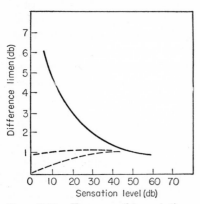

FIG. 8.11. Two possible relations between the DL and Sensation Level for persons with recruitment (broken lines) and the normal relation (solid line). The normal values are approximately doubled because the judgment used yielded the interval between just-noticeably *louder* and just-noticeably *softer*, not the interval between either one of those and *equal*. (*From Denes and Naunton.*)

Whereas Lüscher and Zwislocki ask an observer to listen for a change in a tone whose intensity is modulated, Denes and Naunton ask the observer to judge whether two successive tones are equal in loudness. Precedents for both procedures are to be found in the experimental literature. Again, we have no clinical evidence for deciding in favor of one or the other. More time is required for a complete function to be derived from the Denes and Naunton technique, but their own clinical experience has shown that useful information can be obtained when the DL is measured at only three, or even two, Sensation Levels (*e.g.*, 4, 24, and 44 db or 4 and 44 db).

Masking and Recruitment.   In view of the argument presented at the beginning of Chap. 7, that differential sensitivity for intensity is a special case of masking, it is not surprising that masking should find its way into these clinical measures of recruitment. The application of the measurement of masking to recruitment was suggested by Huizing at least as early as 1942. Using tones from two audiometers, Huizing measured the masking of one tone by another as a function of the intensity of the masking tone. His normal functions were related to those of Wegel and Lane. As a particular example, consider the masking of a 1000-cps tone by a 4000-cps tone. If a patient has a hearing loss and recruitment at 4000 cps, then the masking by the 4000-cps tone will increase as its Sensation Level is increased more rapidly than is the normal case in, for example, the data of Wegel and Lane. Such abnormally steep masking functions were shown by Huizing to be associated with hearing losses that exhibited recruitment by other criteria (*e.g.*, by loudness matches). This relation supports the hypothesis that a sound's ability to mask is directly related to its loudness.

There are many different combinations of low-frequency tones with high-frequency tones and vice versa that present a fairly complicated picture of what is to be expected. From earlier work, however, Langenbeck (1950*a*, *b*, *c*) has come up with a different measurement. We have already seen some equal-masking contours, obtained by measuring the masked threshold of pure tones at various frequencies in the presence of a white noise at several levels, in Fig. 6.3. Suppose we were to obtain sets of such equal-masking contours for patients with different kinds of hearing loss. Langenbeck has shown that the contours obtained from patients with either conductive or recruiting-type hearing loss are the same as those for normal listeners when plotted on an absolute intensity scale (like Fig. 6.3). Cases with nerve-type hearing loss without recruitment, however, typically show more masking than normal.   These results lead Langenbeck to claim the same diagnostic distinction as made by Dix, Hallpike, and Hood on the basis of recruitment measures (see p. 228).   In a sense, though, the results from masking are opposite to those of recruitment and the theoretical implications for the relation between loudness and masking are not at all clear.

The use of white noise in the measurement of the masked threshold for pure tones is probably the simplest of all the procedures, indirect or direct, that have been suggested for measuring recruitment. In addition to the relative simplicity of obtaining and graphing the results, measurements made in the presence of a random noise have proved to be remarkably stable and precise. But the results on a good-sized population are not available, and the interpretation of the results in the light of the concept of *critical bands* (see Chap. 6) offers some difficulties that remain to be worked out in the future. Furthermore, some clinicians object to the use of the masking procedure because they claim that many of their patients are disturbed by the presence of the masking noise. The amount of disturbance and the percentage of patients involved have not as yet been determined.

Auditory Fatigue and Recruitment. If we assume that auditory fatigue is a special case of masking, namely, the case in which the masked tone follows the masking tone instead of coexisting with it in time, the same reasoning that leads to the use of masking as a test for recruitment will also lead to the use of auditory fatigue. As was stated at the end of Chap. 6, it is difficult to specify a *normal* amount of fatigue unless all experimental parameters are fixed and stated. When they are so stated, however, a reasonable approximation to a normal fatigue can be made.

The reasoning put forth by Gardner (1947a), for example, is as follows: A given amount of auditory fatigue will be produced by a particular short-time exposure to a particular frequency, and this amount, found for normal listeners, is taken as normal. Now if a patient has a conductive hearing loss, the effective level of the sound reaching his inner ear is reduced by the amount of the conductive Hearing Loss. Thus we should expect the amount of fatigue for such an observer after exposure to the same sound to be less than normal; indeed, it will be equal to the fatigue that would have been produced in the normal observer by a tone that is less intense, less by the amount of the conductive Hearing Loss. A recruiting-type hearing loss will be fatigued by a normal amount or even more, because the effective stimulus arriving at the inner ear is not reduced. The fatigue produced by a given tone, then, is more directly related to its loudness than to its intensity.

Confirmations of this hypothesis appear not only in Gardner's (1947a) paper but also in the earlier work of de Maré (1939). It would be difficult to plot fatigue as a function of the intensity of the fatiguing tone over the ranges suggested by Gardner in routine clinical audiometry, but Huizing (1949) gives a specific test procedure that he has found useful in testing for recruitment. He states that a 2000-cps tone, presented 30 db above the patient's threshold, will normally produce a shift of up to 12 db. The range of amounts of fatigue extends from 5 to 12 db for patients with normal hearing, conductive hearing loss, or nerve-type hearing loss without recruitment. Patients with recruitment, however, when stimulated with the 2000-cycle tone for 3 min at 30 db above the *pathologic* threshold, give threshold shifts of between 19 and 22 db. Huizing concludes, as did Gardner, that the amount of fatigue produced by a tone depends upon its loudness.

Interpretations of Recruitment

What special significance does the phenomenon of recruitment have in clinical diagnosis and prognosis? It has been shown that recruitment is associated with a perceptive or nerve-type deafness as distinguished from a conductive deafness. We can think of the conductive loss as an attenuator placed in the auditory system that takes out of any sound that enters the auditory system a fixed number of decibels or a certain percentage of the energy. As an approximation only, it may be convenient to regard the perceptive loss with recruitment as a constant subtraction of a certain number of loudness units from the system, a notion that Steinberg and Gardner put forward in 1937. From some such general considerations as these, we should be able to predict the relation between a hearing loss with recruitment and the intelligibility of speech. That there is a relation is clear, particularly since, in her very careful summary, de Bruine-Altes gives the measurement of the *index vocalis* as one method for determining recruitment. This index is the ratio of required distance for whispered voice tests to the distance for spoken voice. It is to be expected that results from the whispered voice test, at low energy, will be more greatly affected by such a hearing loss than will be results from the spoken voice test, at higher energies where pathologic loudness functions have begun to catch up with the normal ones. Huizing (1948) discusses this relation more fully.

Recruitment and the Intelligibility of Speech. Rather than rely on a relation that is based upon the relatively uncontrolled spoken and whispered voice tests, we should like to inquire into the relation between recruitment and the threshold of intelligibility or the articulation score. In Chap. 5 we discussed two idealized audiograms (Fig. 5.15), one for conductive, the other for perceptive deafness. The first (*A*; conductive type) remained constant in frequency and completely predicted the threshold of intelligibility. This conductive type of hearing loss was associated with a very high articulation score when the intensity of difficult speech was made high enough. The second type of deafness (*B*; perceptive) showed Hearing Loss progressively increasing with frequency and recruitment. In this latter case we should expect at first glance that the rapid increase in loudness for those frequencies for which the patient has severe Hearing Loss would help his understanding of speech and would place him at an advantage relative to his fellow with a conductive hearing loss. The reverse, however, appears to be the case, since the low maximum articulation score is found for patients who show recruitment. The very patients who gain so rapidly in loudness for given frequency components and appear to have better than normal intensity discrimination are the ones whose articulation scores go up to 50 or 70 per cent and then level off, no matter how much the intensity is increased.

Harris and Myers have attacked one aspect of this problem experimentally in order to answer the question: Is there recruitment for speech? They find that there is recruitment for the loudness of speech; that is to say, if one performs an alternate binaural loudness balance using speech as the stimulus instead of a pure tone, one obtains results very similar to those for pure tones when the patient has a monaural hearing loss. In spite of this growth of loudness, however, the intelligibility is no better; in fact, it is usually worse than for an equivalent hearing loss without recruitment. The experiment of Harris and Myers offers quantitative validation of the statement heard so often from patients with a recruiting type of hearing loss: "Don't shout; you're talking plenty loud, but I don't know what you're saying!"

The measurement of recruitment can, therefore, be crucial in the establishment of a clinical prognosis, particularly with regard to hearing aids (Huizing, 1948). We shall discuss recruitment again in Chap. 11 when we bring together the kinds of auditory tests that may be used in the selection of hearing aids. By way of foreshadowing that discussion, we may mention the recent conclusions of Davis et al. (1947), that most of the patients in an experimental sample that included some hearing losses with recruitment preferred a flat frequency-response characteristic rather than one that was the mirror image, or approximately so, of the audiogram. This conclusion was reached on the basis of articulation tests, and the rationale was given in terms of the equal-loudness contours at the levels where speech would normally be heard. The hearing loss as a function of frequency is fairly constant if we consider the recruited equal-loudness contour at, for example, 80 db; whereas it varies widely as a function of frequency at the absolute threshold. This rationale (Huizing, 1948) is weakened by the lack of relation between the recruitment of loudness and the articulation score.

Recruitment and Diagnosis. This book has been oriented toward psychophysical relations. We have largely neglected the physiologic or pathologic implications of these relations. We cannot leave the subject of recruitment, however, without mentioning some recent extensions in the area of diagnosis. Until recently, the demonstration of recruitment in a patient was sufficient evidence for diagnosing a hearing loss as being of the nerve type. But there are many cases in which the bone-conduction threshold is exactly or nearly the same as the air-conduction threshold (another piece of evidence for nerve-type deafness) and in which recruitment does not appear. In 1948, Dix, Hallpike, and Hood advanced the hypothesis that recruitment is observed only in cases of pathologic conditions of the cochlea. When, however, the condition involves injury to the eighth nerve, as in acoustic neuroma, recruitment is absent. These workers used the alternate binaural loudness balance on a dichotomous population of patients, half of whom were diagnosed as cases of Ménière's disease (cochlear pathology) and the other half as having acoustic neuroma. The same differential diagnosis has been made by Langenbeck (1950*a*, *b*, *c*), who measures, instead of recruitment, masking by white noise. It is to be hoped that the results of these two studies can be validated on many more groups of patients at other clinics, so that this part of otologic diagnosis may become secure.

Another interesting measurement, which has *not* been made extensively on two such groups of patients, concerns the intelligibility of speech. If the factors that contribute to the recruitment of loudness are the same as those that contribute to a low maximum articulation score, persons with a hearing loss that is associated with a pathologic condition in the cochlea ought to have low maximum articulation scores, while patients with, for example, acoustic neuroma should have normal articulation-gain functions that reach the normal maximum, between 90 and 100 per cent, after a sufficient increase in intensity. This relation would be difficult to explain, however, because we already have data from the Bell Telephone Laboratories (see Fig. 5.13) that show that if a sufficiently wide band of high frequencies is cut off (for example, all frequencies above 2000 cps), the articulation score as a function of intensity will rise to a maximum of 60 or 70 per cent and then level off, going no higher as the intensity is increased further. This relation is very similar to that obtained in measuring the intelligibility of speech for patients whose audiograms cut off above a certain frequency—but the electrical filters that were used in the Bell studies to eliminate certain frequencies do not have any property that is analogous to recruitment.

References for Further Study

de Bruine-Altes, J. C. (1946) *The Symptom of Regression in Different Kinds of Deafness* (thesis). Groningen: J. B. Wolters. This thesis covers most of the history of the measurement of recruitment (regression) in clinical practice. The different methods for measuring are given, although rather sketchily, with the author's preference for her own method quite clearly stated. This is probably one of the best single sources on the subject of recruitment that is available.

Denes, P., and R. S. Naunton. (1950) The clinical detection of auditory recruitment. *J. Laryng.*, **64**, 375–398. This journal reference is given here because it reviews the several procedures that involve the measurement of differential sensitivity for evidence of recruitment. The methods of Békésy and of Lüscher and Zwislocki are discussed in relation to the method of the authors.

The relation between the DL and recruitment appeared in the literature after the publication of the summary work of de Bruine-Altes.

Stevens, S. S., and H. Davis. (1938) *Hearing*. New York: Wiley. Chapter 4 in this basic text is concerned with loudness. There one finds a discussion of the development of the loudness scale (sones) and the relations between loudness and intensity, loudness and Loudness Level, etc. Basic information on the DL and the relation between accumulated DL's and loudness is also included.

CHAPTER 9

BINAURAL HEARING AND BONE CONDUCTION

THE experimental procedures and results discussed in the preceding chapters are limited to those cases in which the stimulus is presented to one ear only. We have considered only monaural thresholds, monaural masking, and monaural fatigue. Except for certain complications at high intensities, such as cross-hearing, we can be reasonably sure that when we apply a sound pressure to the eardrum by means of an earphone and the intervening air of the ear canal, only one ear is stimulated. Listening with one ear, however, is not the way in which we ordinarily hear sounds in everyday life. Usually we have both ears open, and they are both stimulated simultaneously. We have said nothing about how this binaural hearing compares with monaural hearing, nor have we brought up the possible clinical value of testing binaural hearing relative to that of testing monaural hearing.

There are three ways in which binaural hearing can come about. First, both ears may be uncovered and the sound source may be situated in space external to the listener's head. Second, each ear may be stimulated by an earphone of a binaural headset. A third way, which may seem out of place in this chapter, is by means of bone conduction, in which we apply a vibrating force to the skull. The consequent reactions to such a vibrational force, as we shall see presently, involve both ears. Unfortunately, these three ways of stimulating both ears simultaneously do not give the same results for different experimental problems. But we can state some relations among them. With a slight bow to tradition, we shall group the first two types of binaural hearing by air conduction together and discuss them under the heading, Binaural Hearing; the process of bone conduction will be treated separately in the second section of this chapter.

BINAURAL HEARING

In diagnostic testing we are interested in only one ear at a time. A major reason for this one-sided interest is that most of the hearing tests that are used for diagnosis have been related only to more or less peripheral pathologic conditions. To find normal monaural hearing in each ear of a listener whose binaural hearing exhibited certain pathologic behavior would be to create a whole new set of problems in auditory pathology. But in addition to classic diagnostic procedures, certain kinds of tests with two ears reveal some interesting relations. The apparent location of the source of a sound is sometimes used in audiometric procedures as a clue to which ear is responding to a sound. In addition, we may draw certain conclusions from the following discussion concerning the use of hearing aids.

Binaural vs. Monaural Hearing

Are two ears better than one? What can we do with two ears that we cannot do with one? What can we do better with two ears than with only one? In order to answer these and similar questions we shall examine whatever experimental results pertain directly to a comparison of monaural and binaural hearing with respect to localization, absolute and differential thresholds, loudness, masking, and a special relation between localization and masking.

Localization. The most characteristically 'binaural' of all the auditory phenomena is localization, the process by which a listener reports the distance and direction of the apparent source of a sound. There is not very much information on the ability to judge the distance of a sound source, except that it seems to have something to do with the ratio of reflected sound to direct sound. If a sound source is very close to a listener, the sound coming directly from the source will be much greater than the sound reflected from any nearby walls. If, on the other hand, the sound source is quite far away from the listener, a good part of the sound heard may be due to reflections from walls, etc. But now let us concern ourselves with the direction of a sound source.

Although there is some evidence, experimental (Angell and Fite) and clinical, that persons with only one functioning ear can localize, or more precisely, directionalize, a sound source, most of the experiments that have been done on the phenomenon have assumed it to be a binaural affair. Suppose we place a small loud-speaker in the vicinity of a listener, both being located in an anechoic space, that is, one in which there are no reflecting surfaces to produce echoes. If the loud-speaker is directly in front of or behind the listener, the sounds at his right and left ear will be identical in respect of intensity and of time. By *time* is meant the time of arrival of short impulsive sounds like clicks, or time of arrival of the onset of a tone, or time of a given phase point in a sound wave. Now if the loud-speaker is off, let us say 30°, to the right, then the sound arriving at the right ear will be a little more intense than the one at the left, and it will arrive a little sooner (*i.e.*, the time of onset of the sound at the right ear will be earlier than at the left, or the right sine wave will lead the left by so many degrees). Both the time and intensity differences come about because of the difference between the distances from the left and right ears to the source. According to the inverse square law (see Chap. 2), the intensity should be greater at the right ear because it is not so far away from the source as the left. Also, since sound travels at less than infinite speed, it will take a little longer for a sound to have an effect on an ear a little farther away. Both the intensity and the time differences between the two ears play a significant role in localization.

In the case of pure tones, Stevens and Newman have shown that differences in intensity are more important at high frequencies, while differences in time of arrival (or phase, in the pure tone) are more important for low frequencies. This is entirely reasonable if we remember that the diameter of the average head (about 8 in) is approximately one-half the wavelength of 1500 cps. At 3000 cps, for example, a difference between the two ears of $\frac{1}{3000}$ sec would indicate a phase lag or lead of 360°, which is identical to 0°, and our corresponding judgment would be "center." In other words, phase information is retained for low frequencies in which the time differences between the two ears correspond to small phase changes, $i.e.$, less than 360° or even 180°. The relation between wavelength and the head's diameter also tells us that at low frequencies the effective difference between the distances from the sound source to the two ears is negligible when compared to the difference at high frequencies. Thus only the high frequencies provide circumstances in which differences in intensity between the ears are appreciable.

For very short sounds such as acoustic clicks, the difference in time of arrival seems to be the important factor for localization (Wallach, Newman, and Rosenzweig). These experimenters have also shown that a click generated in a reverberant room (with several echoes) will give rise to a single unitary perception localized toward the click source, in spite of the fact that physically there are many sets of clicks and reflected clicks arriving at the two ears with many different interaural time differences.

These statements in a sense summarize what we know about the physical factors that are important in the localization of actual sources of a sound situated in the external environment. Such external localization, although important for everyday listening, has relatively little to do with clinical auditory measurements, but we shall refer again to external localization later in this chapter in order to show certain relations to the use of hearing aids.

Another kind of localization is reported when sounds are delivered to the two ears through earphones. When one earphone alone stimulates one ear, we localize the sound at that ear. When both earphones of a binaural headset stimulate both ears at the same intensity and with the two earphones (and consequently the eardrums) in phase, the sound appears to be in the center of the head. Increasing the intensity or advancing the phase or time of arrival of the onset of a tone at one ear relative to the other makes the apparent source of sound move toward the ear of greater intensity or earlier time of arrival. Although this apparent source can be shifted by manipulating the difference between the ears in respect of either intensity or time, the localizations are usually reported within the head.

Such *intracranial* localization seems to be restricted to stimuli produced by earphones. In order to produce localizations that are reported to be

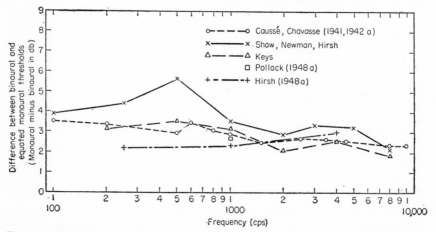

FIG. 9.1. Binaural summation at threshold as a function of frequency. The ordinate shows the amount by which the "equated" binaural absolute threshold is lower than the monaural. (*From Hirsh*, 1948c.)

outside the head, in the external environment, there must be, as a consequence of slight movements of the head, slight changes in the interaural differences (Wallach). Since the earphones ordinarily move with the head, with the result that no changes in the sound pattern are brought about, the localizations are referred to intracranial space. We shall return to the localization of sounds produced by earphones when we discuss the relation between monaural and binaural masking.

Absolute Thresholds. The normal absolute threshold, which was discussed in Chap. 4 (see Fig. 4.9), specifies the minimum sound pressure that is just audible to one normal ear. Is this minimum sound pressure the same when it is introduced into both ear canals simultaneously, or might a lesser amount suffice for both ears together to just hear the tone?

The search for an answer to this question has a long history (see Hirsh,

1948c), most of which was confused by the fact that investigators neglected to take into account the relative contributions of the two ears, each of which might have a slightly different threshold. If one takes this difference into account and stimulates the two ears, not at the same Sound Pressure Level, but instead at the same number of decibels relative to threshold for each ear, the binaural threshold, measured with the two ears thus 'equated,' is about 3 db lower than the monaural threshold for either ear alone (Shaw, Newman, and Hirsh; Caussé and Chavasse, 1941, 1942a; and Keys). The difference between the binaural and monaural absolute thresholds does not vary in any systematic way as a function of frequency, as is shown in Fig. 9.1. The 3-db difference between binaural thresholds holds also when the stimulus is white noise (Pollack,

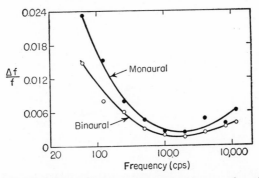

FIG. 9.2. Binaural and monaural frequency discrimination as a function of frequency. The relative DL ($\Delta f/f$) was measured at 40 db Sensation Level. (*After Shower and Biddulph; from Hirsh, 1950b.*)

1948a) and for the threshold of intelligibility (Shaw, Newman, and Hirsh). For detecting the minimum sound pressure in a quiet surround, two ears are clearly better than one—in fact, about twice as good (3 db = 10 $\log_{10} 2/1$). But this observation does not permit any conclusion about an energy-summating system that connects the two ears. It can be shown that it makes little difference whether the two ears belong to the same listener or each ear belongs to a different listener; the same summation would be predicted on a statistical basis (Smith and Licklider).

Differential Thresholds. A comparison of the monaural with the binaural ability to discriminate slight changes in the intensity or frequency of a pure tone is difficult to make, because the data are few, and what data there are must be extricated from experiments that were not designed primarily to make this comparison. Figure 9.2 shows the difference limen for frequency as a function of frequency for a Sensation Level of 40 db. The two curves show results from the experiment of

Shower and Biddulph for monaural and binaural listening. In Fig. 9.3 we see both monaural and binaural differential sensitivity for intensity at a frequency of 800 cps. These binaural and monaural minimum ΔI's as a function of Sensation Level were measured by Churcher, King, and Davies. In these two last figures we see again that the binaural threshold is lower than the monaural. Binaural differential sensitivity, as well as absolute sensitivity, is better than monaural.

Loudness. One of the underlying assumptions for the early construction of loudness scales (see Chap. 8) was that a given sound appears to be twice as loud when heard with two ears as it is when heard with only one. Another way of approaching the relation between binaural and monaural loudness is the following: What is the difference in intensity

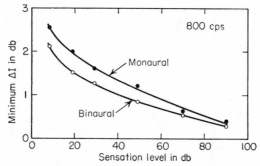

Fig. 9.3. Binaural and monaural intensity discrimination as a function of Sensation Level. The relative DL in decibels $\left(10 \log_{10} \dfrac{I + \Delta I}{I} \right)$ is shown for a frequency of 800 cps. (*After Churcher, King, and Davies; from Hirsh,* 1950*b.*)

between two sounds, one presented to one ear and the other presented to both ears, both of which sound equally loud? This difference at threshold (0-db Loudness Level) is 3 db. It increases to 6 db as the Sensation Level is increased to about 35 db and remains constant as the Sensation Level is increased further. This is shown in the results of an experiment by Caussé and Chavasse (1942*b*), plotted in Fig. 9.4. From a Sensation Level of 35 db upward, a sound must be increased by 6 db when presented to one ear in order that it sound as loud as it did when presented to both ears.

This figure is corroborated by the results of Hirsh and Pollack, who attempted to find the relation between interaural phase (see below) and binaural loudness. They found that interaural phase did not play any role in the apparent loudness of a tone presented binaurally unless the tone was heard against a background noise whose intensity approached that for masking. In the presence of such a noise, however, a comparison between binaural and monaural loudness showed results that depended upon the interaural phases of both the tone and the noise, in the same way as do masked thresholds (see below).

Masking. If the binaural threshold is 3 db lower than the monaural when measurements are made in the quiet, how does this difference change as the intensity of a masking noise is increased? Answers to this question are shown in Fig. 9.5, in which the ordinate shows the difference between monaural and binaural masked thresholds and the abscissa shows two scales of intensity of the noise. In the case of the 4000-cps tone, we see that the 3-db difference (binaural better than monaural) in the quiet

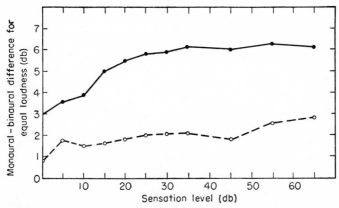

Fig. 9.4. Binaural summation of loudness as a function of Sensation Level. Ordinate shows difference in decibels between a tone presented to one ear and a tone presented to both ears, both tones judged to be equal in loudness. Data represent averages of results at 500, 1000, and 1500 cps. Broken line shows variance (σ^2) of the measurements. (*From Caussé and Chavasse, 1942b.*)

disappears as the over-all SPL of the noise approaches 100 db. For lower frequencies and for speech the difference not only goes to zero but even reverses in direction, denoting a condition in which monaural listening is superior to binaural listening. On further investigation it was found that the phase relations between the ears for both the signal and the masking noise are crucial for this peculiar *interaural inhibition* to appear instead of the more usual *binaural summation,* in which the binaural threshold is lower than the monaural. Thus it appears that there is more than one *binaural critical band* function (see Chap. 6), depending on phase relations between the ears.

We have already mentioned interaural phase in connection with the localization of pure tones, but now we should consider phase in more detail. The two ears or two earphones are said to be *in phase* when both eardrums or both earphone diaphragms move toward or away from the center of the head at the same time. They are *out of phase* when both are moving to the right or to the left at the same time.

These two interaural phase relations, namely, 0 and 180°, respectively, give rise to characteristic localizations of the sound source within the head. When a sound is in phase at one ear relative to the other, the sound appears to be in the center of the head, whereas when a sound is out of phase at the two ears, it appears to be situated out at the two ears. The

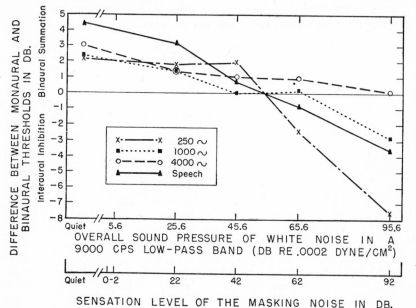

FIG. 9.5. Difference between monaural and binaural masked thresholds for pure tones and for speech in the presence of a white noise. Positive difference indicates that the binaural threshold is lower than the monaural (summation). As the intensity of the noise is raised, the difference goes to zero for high frequencies and reverses in direction for low frequencies and for speech. Both signal and noise were in phase at the two ears. (*From Hirsh*, 1948*a*.)

localizations associated with these two interaural phase relations are uniquely related to the binaural masked threshold. It has been found, for example, that interaural inhibition, in which the monaural masked threshold is lower than the binaural, occurs only when the interaural phase angles for *both* the signal and the noise are the same. In other words, the binaural masked threshold is higher (worse) than the monaural when both signal and noise appear to be in the same place in the head. If they are separated in intracranial space (as they are, for example, when the signal is in phase and the noise is out of phase), binaural summation is again observed, and now the binaural threshold is lower than the monaural by even more than 3 db.

These results (Hirsh, 1948b) are shown in Fig. 9.6, in which the ordinate represents the difference between binaural and monaural masked thresholds and the abscissa represents the frequency of the signal tone. The noise level was constant. Note that the large differences due to changes in the interaural phase relations appear most frequently at the low frequencies, where changes in phase are most important for localization (see above). Although these relations between the masked threshold and

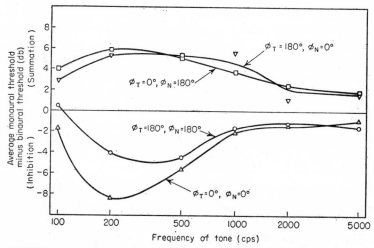

Fɪɢ. 9.6. Difference between monaural and binaural masked thresholds for pure tones in the presence of a white noise whose over-all SPL was about 95 db. The monaural thresholds for the several frequencies are used as the 0-db reference line for the binaural thresholds, which are shown relative to the monaural. Note that whether the binaural masked threshold is better or worse than the monaural depends upon the conditions of interaural phase. Normal operating conditions probably involve both the signal and the noise in phase at the ears. (*From Hirsh*, 1948b.)

interaural phase are complicated and difficult to understand without a fairly detailed discussion, they are of practical importance for the very common situation in which we use both ears to listen to tones or speech in noise. Licklider (1948) has shown that interaural phase plays a similar role in the intelligibility of speech that is masked by noise. We shall see presently how these relations hold when the apparent sources are not localized within the head but rather correspond to actual sources located in external space.

Localization and Intelligibility. When earphones are used, it is easier to detect a signal in a background of noise when the signal and the noise appear to be in different places in the head than when they both appear to be at the same place. This relation between the masking of one sound on another and the relative positions of the sounds in space can be generalized to space that is outside the head. It has been shown (Hirsh, 1950a) that the threshold of intelligibility for speech in the presence of noise is lower when the sources of speech and noise are separated spatially than when they are together. Between the least favorable (both sources together) and most favorable (speech on the side and noise in front) conditions, the masked thresholds of intelligibility differed by about 10 db. It was also shown that this difference, which was due to spatial arrangement of the sound sources, was not so large (if it existed at all) when the head was immobilized or when only one ear was used. In other words, cutting down on a normal listener's ability to localize, either by preventing head movement or by preventing binaural listening, reduced his ability to separate the sources of speech and noise in apparent space and consequently reduced his ability to understand the speech. This finding has broad implications for the patient with unilateral hearing loss or the patient who uses a hearing aid, which is a monaural listening system. We shall discuss these practical points in the next section.

Hearing Aids and Binaural Hearing

From our description of how a hearing aid works (Chap. 3) it should be apparent that the sole purpose of a hearing aid is amplification of any sound that impinges on its microphone. If a hearing loss is produced by some kind of attenuation in the auditory system, a hearing aid will compensate for the loss, because amplification and attenuation are precisely reverse processes. It is simple enough to so state the case for amplification, but we are disregarding certain shortcomings in the hearing aid outside of its amplifying characteristics.

Monaural Hearing Aids. If a hearing-aid user gets all his sound through the single earphone of his single hearing aid, then he is using only one ear. Not only that, but his ear is no longer on his head; that is, the thing that picks up the sound is now resting on his chest, or on an outside lapel in the case of recent hearing aids whose microphones are worn separated from the amplifier chassis. Such a hearing aid is, then, a monaural system and, in particular, is a monaural system in which the one ear is no longer in its usual place. As a consequence of this arrangement, persons who use hearing aids find especially difficult those situations in which they must listen to speech or music against a noisy background. On the basis of the discussion in the previous section we might have predicted this, because in a monaural system both signal and noise would appear to be in the same place even if their sources are actually separated, and hence we should measure a relatively high masked threshold of intelligibility for the speech.

Attempts have been made to correct this defect in the wearable hearing aid by supplying two earphones with a single hearing aid. But since there is only one microphone, this is still a monaural system in spite of the fact that both ears are receiving sound. The point is, of course, that they are both always receiving the same sound, namely, whatever sound was picked up by the single microphone and was amplified by the single amplifier. Indeed, there are certain possible arrangements of this double-earphone hearing aid that would permit interaural inhibition to operate—that is, certain arrangements in which the patient could hear more speech in a given amount of noise when he uses only one earphone (Hirsh, 1950b).

A Binaural Hearing Aid. If a person's ability to understand speech in noise can be improved by enabling him to localize the sources of speech and noise separately (see above), it is clear that a hearing-aid user would benefit from a gadget that would enable him to localize. Since localization seems to be dependent on at least two important factors, namely, head movement and two more or less independent ears that are separated in space by about 8 in, we must try to build these factors into a hearing aid. The outcome is not difficult to predict. Actually, we should have two independent hearing aids (though their amplifiers might be built on the same chassis or in the same case), and we should have each microphone mounted right next to its associated earphone, so that sound is picked up at the usual place (near the ear). Some preliminary observations have been made with such a hearing aid (Hirsh, 1950b), but the feasibility of production and usefulness in a large population has not yet been demonstrated.

Localization in Audiometry

In any audiometric test in which we apply a sound to one ear, we assume that the listener hears the sound at the ear being stimulated. Exceptions to this rule are to be found in cases of cross-hearing. Sometimes we may not have to go to the trouble of masking before we know about a *shadow curve* on an audiogram, because, as we introduce the sound into one ear, the patient reports that he hears it on the other side. Shifts in localization of this sort are generally brought about by differences in the loudness or the intensity of the sounds at the two ears. The role of phase in these observations is practically unknown.

A special case in which the clinician asks for a judgment of localization is the Weber test in bone conduction. This anticipates our discussion of bone conduction that follows, but we can note here that when a vibration is applied to the skull in a central position, the sound to which the vibration gives rise is normally localized in the center of the head. Certain pathologic conditions can render the vibration more effective than is normal in stimulating the end organs of hearing, and thus a unilateral condition of this sort will effectively produce a stronger sound on the defective side. The patient will then report that the sound seems to be on that side. The opposite occurs when the condition involves more central structures and does not enhance the sound produced by bone-conducted energy.

One other clinical procedure related to localization has already been mentioned in Chap. 8. When we ask a listener to compare the loudness of a sound in one ear with the same sound in the other ear, we should present these sounds one after the other. But when procedures for loudness balances are specified in some reports in the clinical literature (*e.g.*, Hood), it would seem that both sounds are introduced to the two ears simultaneously. In this situation it is difficult to compare the loudness of the sound on one side with the one on the other, because together these sounds have a unitary localization, usually (if they are in phase) in the center of the head. We can only conclude that some workers are substituting for a loudness balance a judgment of central localization. That is to say, we can either present the tone alternately to the two ears and ask the observer to adjust the intensity at one ear until it sounds equal in loudness to the tone in the other ear, or we can present it to both ears simultaneously and ask him to adjust the intensity at one ear until the sound seems to be in the middle of the head. We have no evidence that these two judgments produce the same results, because we do not know whether, granting that the sounds are in phase at the two ears, central localization requires equal intensity (physical) at the two ears or equal loudness (psychological) at the two ears.

BONE CONDUCTION

We have been discussing psychophysical measurements. We have emphasized that hearing can be measured when we know the physical dimensions of the auditory stimulus and can measure the response of a listener. This is what is known as a 'black-box' relation: we put in something known and measure what comes out; there is no need to discuss the anatomy and physiology of the system that intervenes between these two kinds of measurement. In applying the results and methods of auditory psychophysics to clinical audiometry, however, we must take into consideration certain clinical methods that are much less based on psychophysical experiments than have been most of the preceding topics. Such a topic is *bone conduction*, a process of hearing that has been extremely useful for some clinicians in making diagnoses.

But when this topic is introduced, we can no longer deal with the 'black box'; not that the input-output kind of analysis is no longer valid, but because we do not know how to specify the input. We must get inside and talk a little about some peripheral anatomy in order to distinguish between bone conduction and the more normal air conduction. As was stated in the Preface, it is assumed that the reader comes to this book on auditory measurement with at least some knowledge of the anatomy of the auditory system. On this assumption, the following discussion will introduce a few anatomical structures which are germane to the present issue, without either explaining them in detail or relating them to the other parts of the system.

The sounds of the external world that give rise to hearing normally do so through a path of *air conduction*. This path consists of the outer air and the air of the *external meatus*, through which sound waves are propagated to the *eardrum*. Alternating pressures against the eardrum are transformed into vibrations of the drum and the attached ossicular chain. The consequent vibration of the footplate of the *stapes* produces an alternating difference in pressure between the oval-window membrane and the round-window membrane; and any difference in pressure between these two is sufficient to produce a deformation of the *basilar membrane*. Let us agree that the deformation of this membrane is a necessary condition for hearing and that we can discuss, as a possible mechanism of conduction, any process that results in such a deformation.

Although the air-conduction path is most usual in everyday hearing, it is possible to by-pass this route and obtain hearing (*i.e.*, deformation of the basilar membrane) by applying vibrations to the skull. This latter method of conduction is used for certain hearing tests, but, as E. Bárány has shown, the over-all auditory system is designed to minimize the effects of bone conduction. Thus we do not hear very well the constant body noises of chewing, breathing, etc., and Békésy (1949) has shown that the auditory and speech systems are so designed that we do not hear our own voices so intolerably loud as we might. First let us see how bone-conduction hearing might come about, and then we shall apply certain of the principles to some clinical problems. The important basic papers from which the following discussion is almost entirely drawn are those of Bárány and Békésy (1932, 1948).

Mechanisms of Bone Conduction

A cursory examination of the clinical literature on bone conduction gives one the impression that the application of a tuning fork or other vibrator to the skull tests the sensitivity of the inner ear and the auditory nervous system. This test appears to be complementary to a test by air conduction, which measures the sensitivity both of the inner parts and of the conducting system in the external and middle ears. This is clearly not the case. There are as many factors entering into the 'conduction' process in bone conduction as in normal air conduction, if not more. Of course, if we adopt the view that the peripheral auditory neurons may be stimulated directly by mechanical vibration, the picture might be changed, but, as we shall see, bone-conducted vibration may simply produce deformations of the basilar membrane much as air-conducted vibrations do. Indeed both Békésy (1932) and Lowy have demonstrated that a tone introduced by bone conduction can be completely cancelled by proper adjustment of the phase and amplitude of a second tone introduced by air conduction.

According to Bárány and Békésy, we may distinguish at least two basic types of bone conduction: *compression bone conduction* and *inertia bone conduction*. Both probably operate in all cases of bone conduction, but one is more important than the other, depending on the frequency of vibration and the point of application of the vibrating force to the skull. It should be obvious why we discuss bone conduction as a special case of binaural hearing. With the mechanisms about to be outlined, it is almost inconceivable that we can stimulate one cochlea and not the other when a vibration is applied to the skull. The implication, which we shall develop in the clinical discussion, is that we cannot test one ear at a time by bone conduction unless the other ear is sufficiently masked. If both ears are stimulated almost equally, then we must keep one of them 'busy' with a masking sound while we test the other.

Inertia Bone Conduction. The mechanical properties of the human skull are responsible for the fact that the skull moves in quite different ways in response to different vibrating forces. Békésy (1948) has shown that at certain frequencies, primarily below 800 cps, the skull moves as a rigid body when a sinusoidal vibration is applied to it. This vibration pattern is shown in Fig. 9.7 for 200 cps. Now consider that the ossicles are suspended rather loosely in the middle ear cavity. If the skull moves in a particular direction, the ossicles will not follow that movement directly; they will demonstrate a resistance to acceleration, or an *inertia*, which will cause a lag between their movements and that of the skull. This means that there is movement of the skull relative to the ossicles whenever the skull is moved. Since the bone around the oval window is a rigid part of the moving skull, this bone will move relative to the stapes, and therefore the stapes will be displaced (relative to the bone) in much the same way as it is when sounds are introduced by air through the external meatus. One component of bone conduction, therefore, consists of the movement of the skull relative to the ossicles, which is the same thing as movement of the ossicles relative to the skull. This inertia bone conduction is most important at frequencies below 800 cps, but is always present to some extent. Attention must be called to the fact that inertia bone conduction will arise as a result of either translational or rotational movements of the skull as a whole. The relative importance of these two

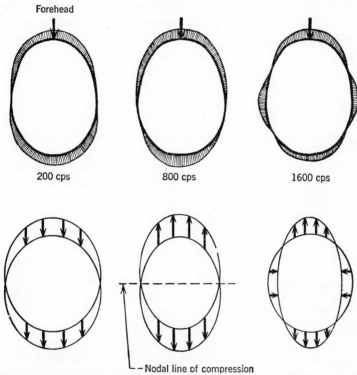

Forehead

200 cps   800 cps   1600 cps

— Nodal line of compression

FIG. 9.7. Vibration patterns of the skull when the vibration is applied to the forehead. At 200 cps, the skull exhibits the translational movements of a rigid body. Near 800 cps, the forehead and the back of the head move in opposite directions (single nodal line of compression). Above 1500 cps, the skull vibrates in sections separated by nodal lines of compression. (*After Békésy, 1932; reproduction by permission from Békésy, G. v., and W. A. Rosenblith, Chapter 27 in S. S. Stevens (Ed.), Handbook of Experimental Psychology, published by John Wiley and Sons, Inc., 1951, p. 1108.*)

components of skull movement is discussed by both Bárány and Békésy (1948).

Compression Bone Conduction. At above its resonant frequency (somewhere between 800 and 1600 cps) the skull no longer moves as a rigid body but rather shows deformations, two examples of which are shown in Fig. 9.7 for 800 and 1600 cps. At higher frequencies the skull may be alternately compressed and expanded in parts in response to an alternating

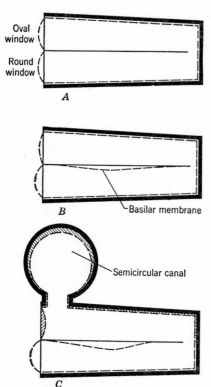

Fig. 9.8. Compression of the inner ear and the displacement of the basilar membrane. The broken lines indicate the position of the various membranes during compression. (*A*) shows a hypothetical case of equal yielding at both windows, symmetrical compression, and no movement of the basilar membrane. The round window actually yields more than the oval window (*B*), and the compression is nonsymmetrical, leading to a downward displacement of the basilar membrane. Since the semicircular canals are also compressed (*C*), more fluid is forced into the upper canal, and the basilar membrane is forced downward even more. (*After Békésy, 1932; reproduction by permission from Békésy, G. v., and W. A. Rosenblith, Chapter 27 in S. S. Stevens (Ed.), Handbook of Experimental Psychology, published by John Wiley and Sons, Inc., 1951, p. 1110.*)

vibration. This type of skull movement brings about a compression of the labyrinth and thus gives rise to a second type of bone conduction. Consider the two examples shown schematically in *A* and *B* of Fig. 9.8. The upper drawing illustrates what would happen in the cochlea as a result of compression if the stiffnesses of the membranes of the round window and of the oval window were equal. The labyrinth is squeezed as a result of an inward force, and since both membranes have the same 'give,' both will bulge by the same amount, and the basilar membrane will remain in the same position. Drawing *B* illustrates what is normally more nearly the case, namely, that the stiffness of the oval-window membrane is greater than that of the round-window membrane. As a result, an inward pressure on the labyrinth will produce a greater bulge at the round window than at the oval window. Since there is now a pressure difference between the two, the basilar membrane will be deformed, and we have another way in which hearing may be produced. Again, this compression bone conduction is probably effective throughout the whole frequency range, ʃbut it seems to be more important at frequencies above 1500 cps.

Bone Conduction by Air. The distinction between bone conduction and air conduction is not always easy to make. Sometimes the application of a vibrator to the skull produces reactions that give rise to pressure changes in the external ear canal that are transmitted in a normal way through the path of air conduction. Two examples will suffice. Both concern volume displacements of air in the external meatus that are brought about by movement of the cartilaginous wall. They are both effective when the ear canal is occluded.

In the first place, faulty placement of the stem of the tuning fork may result in vibrating the cartilage around the ear canal rather than the skull itself. When a patient is asked to move a vibrating source around until he finds a place that yields maximum loudness, he will often end up either on the ridge on the *mastoid process* that is formed by the insertion

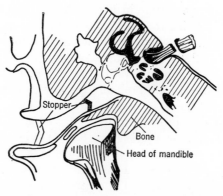

FIG. 9.9. Schematic longitudinal section through the external meatus and the temporal bone. The head of the mandible, being close to the canal, produces deformations in the walls of the canal. A stopper peripheral to the mandible will 'enhance' the bone conduction, whereas a stopper that is pushed into the bony portion of the canal will not. (*After Békésy, 1941; reproduction by permission from Békésy, G. v., and W. A. Rosenblith, Chapter 27 in S. S. Stevens (Ed.) Handbook of Experimental Psychology, published by John Wiley and Sons, Inc., 1951, p. 1109.*)

of the *sternocleidomastoid* muscle or down on the mastoid process near the cartilaginous portion of the *meatus*. Figure 9.9 illustrates how this latter position of a vibrator actually gives rise to pressure changes of considerable magnitude in the external canal. If the vibrations are transmitted directly to the cartilage of the meatus, there will be volume displacements in the canal. When the canal is open, of course, the effective volume is so large that the pressure changes will be negligibly small, but if the canal is closed by a finger or an earplug, these volume displacements will be very effective in producing hearing by air conduction.

Even when the skull itself is moving, however, volume displacements in the external ear canal may result from relative movement between the skull and the mandible, the condyle of which is embedded in the cartilaginous tissue below the meatus (Fig. 9.9). Again, these volume displacements are negligible if the canal is open but important if it is closed. And these displacements in the canal due to relative movement of the mandible and the skull will be most effective at those (lower) frequencies at which the skull vibrates as a rigid body. This agrees perfectly well with the observation of Kelley and Reger that the threshold for bone-conducted sounds (applied on either the mastoid or the forehead) when the ear canal is occluded is significantly lower than normal at frequencies 64, 128, 256, 512, and 1024 cps, but not at 2048, 4096, or 8192 cps.

On the basis of either of these two principles we can easily see why a given bone-conducted sound seems louder when the ear canals are blocked than when they are open. Note in Fig. 9.9 that if the earplug is pushed in so far that it is blocking the bony part of the meatus, bone conduction is not increased (neither sounds louder nor gives a lower threshold) relative to the open canal. This, of course, is owing to the fact that the volume displacements occur peripheral to the plug and in the open air.

We have sketched what are probably the most important mechanisms for various kinds of hearing in response to vibration of the skull. Nevertheless, we cannot now proceed to press the vibrator of an audiometer against the skull and know precisely with what type of bone conduction we are dealing. All three factors are operating. A pathologic condition that produces a conductive hearing loss will not facilitate bone conduction very much at low frequencies if it is central to the cartilaginous portion of the ear canal. We can suppose, however, that if the stapes is fixed, as it is in otosclerosis, bone conduction will be better than normal, but primarily for the high frequencies where compression bone conduction plays the major role. But in all these cases there are so many variables that affect the bone conduction besides the relatively minor effects of the particular conductive pathologic conditions that our diagnostic technique with bone-conducted sounds is far from precise.

Clinical Problems

On the basis of the preceding section, we can agree that tests of hearing by bone conduction are not necessarily and automatically tests of cochlear and neural function, independent of the transmitting system of the middle ear. We cannot assume that the application of a bone-conduction vibrator involves a by-passing of the conductive mechanism, because, as we have seen, the conductive mechanism plays an important role in results obtained from bone-conduction tests. But this is not to say that vibrating the skull is not a useful way to obtain certain diagnostic information. We do not have sufficient information on the basic processes involved to write a definite set of rules on the execution and interpretation of bone-conduction tests. Rather, the following paragraphs are written in a negative way, with the view to certain cautions that must be observed in testing and interpreting the results according to the more classic rules.

Absolute vs. Relative Bone Conduction. The absolute threshold for hearing by bone conduction is, or should be, measured in exactly the same way as the corresponding threshold for hearing by air conduction. For air conduction, the problem is to measure the energy, Intensity Level, or Sound Pressure Level for a given frequency at which a listener responds positively 50 per cent of the time. In the case of bone conduction the physical dimensions of the energy that is supplied through the vibrator are much more difficult to specify.

Although it is true that ear canals vary from person to person, there seems to be enough homogeneity with respect to acoustic impedance to permit the use of a representative physical model, a cavity of 6 cc with rigid walls. In representing the acoustic impedance of many skulls, the problem is made infinitely more difficult, not only by the greater variability among skulls of different individuals, but also by the fact that this impedance varies so widely on a single skull depending on the point of application of the vibrating force. Furthermore, we have not yet definitive grounds for stating the effective or important dimensions of the vibration —that is, whether we should measure displacement, velocity, pressure, energy, etc.

Now, of course, we can make relative physical measurements, as we did in the case of the earphone. We can measure the voltage across a particular vibrator that transduces electrical to mechanical energy. Then we can measure decibels of attenuation relative to a fixed voltage to obtain an estimate of the threshold on a reasonable sample of listeners. This is still an absolute threshold—the measurement is one of minimum energy, even though we do not know what the energy is.

Such is the status of the bone-conduction assemblies that are supplied with commercial audiometers. These vibrators are calibrated on a group of normal listeners, and the experimental variable is always voltage, or more precisely, attenuation relative to a fixed voltage. You cannot interchange the vibrators of different audiometers without expecting the scale for Hearing Loss by bone conduction to change. These changes are, however, probably no greater than the constant errors that clinicians seem to find in checking the *normal* values for bone conduction. In fact, many clinicians still prefer the classic bone-conduction tests with tuning forks. It is not the intent here to enter this professional controversy, but it is difficult to understand why many clinicians maintain that the tuning-fork results are more reliable than those of the audiometer. Let us examine the details.

The bone-conduction threshold, measured by the audiometer, is essentially the classic Schwabach test. According to the Schwabach test, one holds the stem of a vibrating tuning fork against the mastoid process and notes for how many seconds the patient still hears the tone. A normal Schwabach test is defined by a duration of time that is equal to the time that the clinician can hear (if his hearing is normal) the fork when he holds it against his own mastoid. Now clearly, such a time measure as such is not different from a measure of intensity. Rather this measure of time is simply a crude way of stating the intensity of the sound. We know that the amplitude of vibration of a tuning fork decays exponentially in time, and so a given *number of seconds* after the fork is struck (with a "standard blow") must mean a particular *intensity*. Thus when we say that a person stops hearing a tone after a number of seconds, we mean only that at that time the intensity of the sound had decreased to a level below the threshold of the listener.

With an audiometer, we make exactly the same measurement, but we control the intensity manually. If the intensity dial is left alone, intensity remains constant; it does not, like the tuning fork, decrease automatically. The dial setting for 0-db Hearing Loss corresponds to the intensity of the tuning fork at the clinician's ear after his normal hearing time has elapsed. Certainly the threshold measurements that can be made with present-day bone-conduction equipment in the commercial audiometers are far from perfect, but they can be at least as precise as the tuning-fork results, and probably more so. Many of the factors, to be discussed presently, that contribute to variability are not completely controlled, and perhaps clinicians will have to standardize a certain set of testing conditions along with their own *norms*.

When a clinical report states "absolute bone conduction increased," this must mean that the absolute threshold is lower than normal, that the Hearing Loss is negative on the audiogram for bone conduction, or that the Schwabach response is prolonged. It seems fair to say that most of the problems concerning the enhancement of bone conduction in conductive pathologic conditions refer *not* to such absolute increases but rather to improvement in *relative bone conduction*. By *relative* is meant either the bone conduction relative to the air conduction or the bone conduction 'heard' on one side relative to the bone conduction on the other side. Tests for these two kinds of relative bone conduction are the Rinne and the Weber,[1] respectively.

In the Rinne test we compare the time during which the tuning fork is heard by air conduction with the time during which it is heard by bone conduction. With an audiometer we may accomplish the essentials of

[1] The Weber test was discussed above under Localization.

the Rinne test by simply comparing the audiograms for air conduction and bone conduction. A negative Rinne test is shown by a bone audiogram that is above the air audiogram. That is to say, the patient's bone-conduction threshold is nearer to the normal bone-conduction threshold than is his air-conduction threshold to the normal air-conduction threshold. The time scale of the tuning fork is here converted to an intensity scale on the audiometer.

Of course, even for normal hearing, we must supply more energy to the skull in order to deform the basilar membrane than we do to the ear canal for air transmission. By placing the head in a sound field and measuring the thresholds by air and bone conduction, Békésy (1948) obtained a difference of approximately 60 db. Ordinarily, however, we do not vibrate the skull by moving the air around it. Instead, the audiometer manufacturer uses a more efficient device that applies vibratory forces directly to the skull. Therefore the 60-db difference between air- and bone-conduction thresholds does not show between the Hearing-loss scales for bone conduction and air conduction on the audiometer. Moreover, the electrical impedances of the earphone and vibrator are different and have, therefore, different effects on the characteristics of the amplifier. Furthermore, their transducing efficiencies are different because they are driving quite different mechanical impedances. The fact that these two sets of numbers (air and bone) on most audiometers are about 40 db apart has less to do with the actual difference between bone conduction and air conduction than with the electrical components of the audiometer.

Factors to Be Controlled in Bone-conduction Tests. In spite of some uncertainty about bone conduction and its practical application in clinical audiometry, we can set down certain precautions that, if observed, will tend to increase the reliability of our measurements. The more variables we leave uncontrolled, the less we learn about the important ones. We shall consider three factors outside the physical problems that are presently occupying a reasonable part of research activities of such laboratories as the Sound Section of the National Bureau of Standards.

First, the noise level in the testing room must be lower for bone-conduction tests than it need be for air-conduction tests, especially when we wish to measure the bone-conduction thresholds of persons with normal hearing. These measurements are made without any earphone and cushion over the ear to cut out some of the noise. If one were to recommend that the earphones remain on during the bone-conduction measurements, then, of course, the effects of the volume displacements produced in the ear canal by relative movements between the condyle of the mandible and the skull would play a role, and we should be confounding the bone-conduction measurement with the condition of the transmission system of the ear canal and middle ear. As a first approximation, we may say that an over-all noise level of not more than 30 db should be our goal. This is the level, roughly speaking, at which masking of the pure-tone threshold first begins. We needed to try for about 50 db in the case of earphones because we could count on 20-db attenuation by the earphones and their cushions.

Second, the type of vibrator used is very important. In addition to the tuning fork there are two principal types of electromechanical vibrators that are used with audiometers. The first is rather heavy and large and is ordinarily held in the patient's hand or by a strong headband. This is the type that is usually supplied with commercial audiometers. A second type that might be used is the small vibrator that is supplied with a bone-conduction type of hearing aid. Carhart and Hayes have shown that when this small hearing-aid type of vibrator is used, the clinical reliability of bone-conduction thresholds is easily as good as that of ordinary air-conduction thresholds. This undoubtedly comes primarily from the fact that one can put one of these small vibrators, with its headband, on the skull and leave it on in the same position and at a constant pressure for as long as the measurements may take. With a hand-held vibrator we have not only the possibility of its being moved after the measurements have begun, but also the rather high probability that the pressure with which it is held will vary. Of course, we cannot simply plug in the small vibrator and expect the audiometer's scale of Hearing Loss to remain valid. We must recalibrate the unit with a procedure like the one given in Carhart (1950, p. 800).

In this connection, we may mention a third important factor, namely, the point at which the vibrating force is applied to the skull. We persist in placing the vibrator on the mastoid process probably because of its proximity to the ipsilateral cochlea. That is, we probably feel that a vibrator on the right mastoid is having its maximum effect on the right cochlea. What we have already said should show that this notion is untenable and that both cochleas are subjected to similar effects no matter where on the skull the vibrating force is applied.

With this in mind, a better criterion for best placement might be: Where is the bone and other tissue most homogeneous over a reasonable area? Both Bárány and Békésy (1932) have shown such an area to be located on the forehead, and it seems that this might be the best place to apply vibrations for bone-conduction testing. The absolute threshold may be higher than it is when the vibrator is applied to the mastoid process, but the difference will not be very large, and, what is more important, the threshold will remain fairly constant even though the vibrator be moved about slightly. This is clearly an advantage over placement on the mastoid process, where the variability from place to place within a relatively small area is quite large.

Masking and Bone Conduction. If, as we have maintained, both right and left basilar membranes are deformed as a result of vibrations applied to the skull, we must have a method by which we can test one ear at a time. Particularly is this necessary when, as has been suggested above, the vibrating force is applied to the center of the forehead and is thus placed more or less symmetrically relative to the two labyrinths. The effect of a very small deformation of the basilar membrane (*e.g.*, at threshold) can be easily overcome by a masking sound in response to which the basilar membrane is deformed more and over a greater area.

We calculate the amount of masking needed here just as we calculated the amount needed to eliminate cross-hearing (see Chap. 6). The difference is, of course, that attenuation from one ear to the other for the test tone is no longer 50 db. It is small, of the order of 10 db, and may even be negative, *i.e.*, vibration applied on the right side may have more effect on the left cochlea than on the right.

The application of the masking sound is a problem. To use a binaural headset and introduce the masking sound through only one of the earphones amounts to partially occluding the masked ear. Of course, the possible enhancement of the bone-conducted sound in the ear being masked is negligible because of the masking, but the possible enhancement in the ear being tested detracts from the validity of the measurement. Since the volume under the earphone, however, is considerably larger than the volume in the ear canal under an occluding earplug or finger, it is doubtful that the effect will be very great. Whatever the effect, it may be decreased by inserting a layer of absorbent cotton or a gauze sponge under the earphone that is over the ear being tested. This effectively enlarges the volume without decreasing the attenuation. The experimental data on masking that are applicable here and were applicable to cross-hearing (see Chap. 6) pertain chiefly to white noise, and, as Carhart (1950) has pointed out, the noises that are provided in the commercial audiometers are not of this type. Either we must obtain precise masking data for the noises that are provided commercially in audiometers, or we shall have to persuade the manufacturers to use noise (*e.g.*, white noise) on which we already have considerable experimental data.

Summary

The testing of hearing by bone conduction is at a transition stage in its development. Many otologists still prefer tuning forks to the bone-conduction devices that are provided with audiometers. This preference is probably based on the fact that an experienced otologist who knows his forks can apply his fork at precisely the same point and with precisely the same pressure time after time. He does not have the same experience with the electromechanical vibrators. The pioneer studies of Bárány and Békésy (1932, 1948, 1949) show that a great deal is known about the physics of bone conduction, but there is so much more to be known that we can do no more than point to the many variables that must be controlled in this type of measurement. The bone-conduction equipment that is provided with audiometers is subject to variations from all these sources, and there is much work to be done, on both the physical and the psychophysical side. When certain precautions are observed and the reasons for them are understood, there is no reason why the absolute threshold for vibratory forces applied to the skull should not be measured with the same reliability as that for sounds that are conducted through the air and the bones of the middle ear.

References for Further Study

Bárány, E. (1938) A contribution to the physiology of bone conduction. *Acta oto-laryng., Stockh.*, Suppl. 26. This is a physically oriented monograph on the fundamental problem of bone conduction. Although there is not very much by way of practical suggestion for the clinician, a great step toward understanding the basic processes involved has been made.

Békésy, G. v., and W. A. Rosenblith. (1951) The mechanical properties of the ear. Chap. 27 in S. S. Stevens (Ed.), *Handbook of Experimental Psychology*. New York: Wiley. A section in this chapter entitled Hearing by Bone Conduction offers a brief clear statement of most of the experimental results on bone conduction by Békésy and others.

Licklider, J. C. R. (1951) Basic correlates of the auditory stimulus. Chap. 25 in S. S. Stevens (Ed.), *Handbook of Experimental Psychology*. New York: Wiley. The experimental results that have contributed to recent knowledge on localization and other binaural phenomena are summarized in this chapter in sections on Sound Localization and on Other Binaural Effects.

CHAPTER 10

CONDITIONING IN AUDIOMETRY

It HAS already been emphasized, particularly in Chaps. 1, 4, and 5, that any psychophysical measurement depends upon the kind of response that is observed. In measuring the absolute or masked thresholds for pure tones, we use responses like the pressing of a signal button or the raising of the finger. In measuring the intelligibility of speech, we observe the verbal responses of the listener. In differential sensitivity we observe either a verbal response, e.g., "same" or "different," or a motor response that has been made a substitute for the appropriate verbal response. The same kind of responses are involved in judgments of equal loudness. All these responses have one factor in common: they are motor responses involving contraction of skeletal striated muscles, and they are mediated by the *central nervous system*. In the development of this chapter, we shall see that other kinds of response can be observed in connection with auditory stimuli.

In addition to the *kind* of response that is used in psychophysical measurement, there is another, perhaps even more important factor, namely, the *means by which we get the observer to respond* to a given stimulus. In the preceding chapters we have made one important assumption about the occurrence of a response after a stimulus is presented. We have assumed that a listener would respond in a certain way by virtue of the fact that we have told him to do so. We have assumed that he would raise his finger after the presentation of a pure tone, that he would write down a word after it is spoken for him, that he would say "same" or "different" after a pair of stimuli has been presented, all because we have instructed him to respond in these specific ways. In usual clinical and experimental procedures, these instructions are verbal. We tell the listener to do something. We depend upon a history in which the listener has learned to use language. We assume that he follows our instructions to do something when he hears a tone, but we have no observable way of knowing this except for the temporal relations between the occurrence of the stimulus and that of the response.

There are many problems in clinical audiometry that seem to demand more 'objective' procedures than the classic ones. Clinicians sometimes complain that the traditional procedures are too 'subjective' and do not, therefore, tell us about a listener's *actual* ability to hear. It seems to the author that what are called 'subjective' procedures are those that involve verbal instructions; that the several 'objective' techniques that have been suggested in the clinical literature are different from the traditional techniques in that the instructions by which the listener is *taught* to respond are nonverbal, and the actual learning to respond goes on during the experimental period. To be sure, there may be other ways in which to differentiate these two types of procedure, but the dichotomy is a bad one anyway, as we shall see presently.

Let us first state the clinical problem. We tell a listener to raise his finger when he hears a tone; we turn on a tone; he does not raise his finger. Can he hear the tone or not? Does he really hear it but will not respond, either because he has misunderstood our instructions or does not wish to obey them? We shall not answer these questions satisfactorily in the paragraphs to follow, but it is hoped that the concepts that are about to be introduced will provide a framework in which we can think intelligently about the important problems raised.

In order to understand the role of instructions, we must first analyze the relation between stimulus and response. A most convenient framework for these training procedures is provided by conditioning, a process that has been of interest to psychologists and physiologists for more than half a century. We shall find that we can cast all our audiometric variables and parameters into their analogous roles in the conditioning experiment and in this way may find the relations among stimuli and responses easier to understand.

Conditioning seems to be a new term to clinical audiometry because it has been introduced only recently as a *method* in certain kinds of auditory tests. Conditioning and its attendant methods have been heralded in some clinical circles as a 'bag of tricks' for a definitive objective audiometry—heralded thus, not by the doers of the work, but rather by the talkers, well-meaning but misunderstanding enthusiasts. We shall show, in the following pages, that the principles of conditioning may be used equally as well to describe traditional audiometric procedures, in which we tell the listener what to do, as for such 'modern' tests as those that use the resistance of the skin or the dilation of the pupil in connection with nonverbal instructing stimuli. Instead of distinguishing between audiometric procedures that use conditioning and those that do not, we shall conclude that conditioning is used in all cases, and that we can distinguish the cases only on the basis of the specific conditioned (or instructing) stimuli that are used and of the dimensions of the response (number of responses or strength of a response) that are measured. Our first job will be to describe the general process of conditioning.

CONDITIONING

Most animals, including man, are born with a certain number of reflexes or responses that are normally elicited by particular stimuli. A few segments of such innately formed behavior exhibit a natural stimulus-response connection that may be demonstrated without instruction, training, learning, or other intermediate process. Innate stimulus-response connections, however, comprise a very small fraction of the total number of responses that make up the everyday behavior of adult human beings or even the behavior of a small child. We find responses and series of responses that occur in the presence of stimuli that certainly did not elicit these responses in the first place but rather have come to elicit them, or at least provide a situation in which they occur, after some training or experience in similar situations. Indeed, a behavioristic psychologist of the early twentieth century would have explained all these rather complicated pieces of behavior simply as additions or combinations of *conditioned responses*. Let us take a simple example. When we put food in our mouths, we salivate. This seems to be an innate response (no instruction needed) to the stimulus *food*. As we gain experience with mealtimes and consequent meals, we find ourselves salivating (our mouths 'water') when the dinner bell is sounded. A new stimulus, a sound, has come to evoke a conditioned response, which was previously evoked as an *unconditioned response* only by food.

It is not our purpose to go into the details of a subject that sometimes occupies whole chapters, indeed whole books, in psychology. Rather we shall attempt to describe just enough of the basic principles involved in conditioning to be able to demonstrate its role in the measurement of hearing.

Pavlovian Conditioning

The classic experiments on conditioning were performed by Pavlov at the end of the nineteenth century (see Hilgard and Marquis, Chap. 2). Pavlov started with an *unconditioned reflex*, namely, salivation (by a dog) in response to food. The unconditioned reflex can be any stimulus-response connection that is 'wired into' the organism, *i.e.*, one for which no demonstrable training is necessary. The aim of this conditioning experiment is to enable a second stimulus, which did not elicit salivation in the first place, to elicit salivation by being associated in time with the food. Of particular interest to us was Pavlov's use of an auditory stimulus, the sound of a bell, as the conditioned stimulus. The sound of the bell was presented to the dog immediately prior to each successive presentation of the food. After a sufficient number of such stimulus 'pairings,' the bell alone was sufficient to produce a flow of saliva. One speaks of the food as an *unconditioned stimulus* that is capable of eliciting an unconditioned response, the secretion of saliva. The sound of the bell, called the *conditioned stimulus*, comes to elicit a similar response that is called the *conditioned response*. The psychophysiological theory that Pavlov built on the basis of these experiments need not concern us here. Rather we have only to look at the experiments themselves and, in particular, certain developments that have occurred since Pavlov's time.

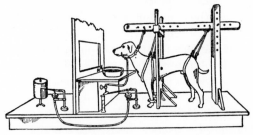

Fig. 10.1. Pavlov's method of establishing a conditioned salivary response. Just before each automatic presentation of food, a bell is sounded. After a sufficient number of stimulus pairings have occurred, salivation is elicited by the sound of the bell alone. A record of salivation is obtained by recording the movements of a lever on which drops of saliva fall from a tube that is connected to a fistula in the dog's cheek. (*After Yerkes and Morgulis; from Morgan and Stellar, p. 439.*)

Suppose that Pavlov, having conditioned a dog to salivate at the sound of a bell, had systematically decreased the intensity of the bell's sound until the dog no longer salivated when the bell was sounded. Would he not then have measured the auditory threshold of the dog for the sound of the bell? If we answer with an unqualified "yes," there will certainly arise the comment, "Well, he has measured the auditory threshold for an autonomic[1] conditioned response, but do we know what the dog's *real* threshold is?" Our reply must emphasize the principle that *there is no 'real' threshold, but rather there are as many different thresholds as there are different responses and stimuli in the measurement.*

When Pavlovian conditioning is used to study the relations between certain dimensions of a conditioned stimulus and a response, the measures

[1] Autonomic responses, mediated by sympathetic and parasympathetic divisions of the *autonomic nervous system*, involve the secretion of certain glands and the contraction of smooth muscle. They are distinguished from responses mediated by the *central nervous system*, which are usually contractions of striated muscle.

employed are somewhat different from those that were outlined in Chap. 4. For example, suppose we refine Pavlov's technique by using a loudspeaker that is fed by sinusoidal voltages so that pure tones are presented to the dog. The food itself will evoke a certain secretion of saliva, let us say 10 drops within a stated interval of time. After a suitable conditioning procedure, a tone of perhaps 60 db SPL will also come to elicit a response of the same magnitude. Note that we are measuring *the magnitude of the response*, in this case in number of drops of saliva. (In traditional audiometry we count *the number of responses* that are given to a certain number of stimuli. We do not ordinarily measure the amplitude of movement of the finger; we force an all-or-none character into the observed responses.) As we decrease the intensity of the tone, or as we change its frequency, the number of drops of saliva that will be secreted will decrease, and we have the problem of deciding arbitrarily what will be the magnitude of salivary response by which we shall define the *threshold*. Or we may, as in the traditional case, arbitrarily say that a response of, for example, five drops or more will be considered a true response, and that a secretion of any lesser amount will not be recorded. In this way we can count the number of responses (of five drops or more) that are elicited by a certain number of tonal stimuli. Then we can apply the 50-per-cent-response criterion for a threshold measure.

Something more should be said about the restricted nature of Pavlovian conditioning. The early experiments of Pavlov himself and those of his associates showed that the conditioned response was almost the same as the unconditioned response. This is to say that the salivation to the bell was the same as the salivation to the food, and furthermore, that the latency, or interval of time between the appearance of the stimulus and that of the unconditioned and conditioned response, was very nearly the same. When further experiments were done in the Pavlovian model, particularly by psychologists in the United States, it was found that the conditioned response differed somewhat both in amplitude and in latency from the unconditioned response (see Hilgard and Marquis, Chap. 2). These later experiments utilized skeletal motor responses (central nervous system). This general observation has led to the view that the Pavlovian type of conditioning is *strictly* applicable only to responses that are mediated by the autonomic nervous system (Skinner, 1950); for example, salivation, pupillary contraction or expansion, perspiration and the attendant change in skin resistance, etc. Some skeletal responses, under the control of the central nervous system, have been used in experiments on Pavlovian conditioning. But it appears that another kind of conditioning is more appropriate to such responses. We shall refer to this point again after we have discussed this other kind of conditioning.

Let us summarize by pointing out the essential characteristics that a procedure must have in order to exemplify Pavlovian conditioning. First, we must begin with a response (unconditioned)[1] that is normally reflexly elicited by a particular stimulus; and it is preferable, though not necessary, that the response be one that is mediated by the autonomic nervous system. Having demonstrated that each occurrence of the unconditioned stimulus produces a response, we shall cause a conditioned stimulus (tone, light, etc.) to precede the unconditioned stimulus by a fixed (short) interval of time. Conditioning is demonstrated when the conditioned stimulus alone can produce the response even when the unconditioned stimulus has been omitted. Applications of this procedure in audiometry will appear presently.

Instrumental Conditioning

At about the same time that Pavlov published his first results, Thorndike, in the United States, was conducting his experiments on the problem-solving behavior of chickens and cats. His experiments set the stage for a tremendous amount of work on animal and human learning that is still going on today. Thorndike's approach to the way in which stimuli interact to provide the proper circumstances for learning was different from that of Pavlov, and yet it has been formulated (Hilgard and Marquis, Chap. 3) as another type of conditioning. Let us cite an example from the experiments of Thorndike.

A cat is placed inside a box from which there is only one means of escape, namely, a door that is opened automatically when a small latchstring inside the box is pulled down. When the cat is first brought to this situation he exhibits several kinds of motor behavior, of which there is one (perhaps accidental) that includes the pulling of the latchstring. If the string is pulled, the door opens and the cat may walk out of the box and secure some food that has been placed just outside the box. The adjective *instrumental* is used to described such conditioning, because a response, the conditioned response, is instrumental in producing the reward, or the unconditioned stimulus. The string pulling is instrumental in bringing about an occasion on which the cat may secure food. In Pavlov's experiments the fact that the dog salivated had no bearing upon whether or not food would follow. In instrumental conditioning the occurrence of the conditioned response brings about a change in the environment of the responding organism that makes a reward or reinforcement more avail-

[1] Responses that have been conditioned in the Pavlovian manner include (1) autonomic: salivation, change in skin resistance, pupillary contraction, vasomotor reactions; and (2) skeletal: knee jerk, eye blink, change in respiration. (Hilgard and Marquis, p. 33.)

able. Upon further occasions of being placed in the box, more and more of the cat's random behavior is eliminated, and eventually (when the conditioning is 'complete') the cat immediately goes over and pulls the string whenever he is placed in the box. Systematic information on the growth of such responses in conditioning has been reported by Skinner (1938).

In terms that we introduced in connection with the Pavlovian conditioning, we may say that the conditioned stimulus is the box itself and any other stimuli that inform the cat that this is an occasion upon which he may secure food by performing a certain response. The instrumental or conditioned (in this case, more properly, *conditional*) response is the

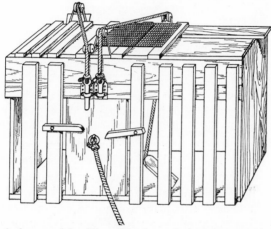

Fig. 10.2. Puzzle box used by Thorndike in early learning experiments with cats. When the cat is placed inside the box, he can escape and secure a food reward by pressing on the treadle, thus pulling on the door latch and allowing the door to fall open. (*After Thorndike; from Garrett, p. 43.*)

response that leads to the food. The unconditioned stimulus and response are, respectively, the food and the eating of it. The distinctive features of this instrumental type of conditioning are that a response is emitted by the organism (*i.e.*, occurs without being elicited by an observable stimulus) and that, if the circumstances following such a response are rewarding or reinforcing, the response tends to increase in frequency. Note that the occurrence of the unconditioned stimulus in this situation is dependent upon the occurrence of the conditioned response, while in Pavlovian conditioning the unconditioned stimulus is used to elicit the response in the first place.

It is unclear, so far, how instrumental conditioning can be used in a psychophysical measurement. We have shown only that it is possible to increase the frequency of occurrence of a particular response. Now we must set up a conditioned *discrimination*. In other words, we must teach the animal that his response will be rewarded only when certain stimuli are present and not when these stimuli are absent. Suppose, for example, that after the cat has learned to pull the latchstring in order to get food, we set out to have him pull the latchstring only when a tone is sounding. We should proceed by having the food outside the box only when the tone was sounding. Then pulling the latchstring would not lead to food during intervals of silence, and we should find the frequency of latchstring pulling high during times when there was a tone but relatively lower during the silent intervals.

RESPONSES TO SOUND

We shall now restrict our discussion of conditioning to those cases in which sounds are used as either conditioned or unconditioned stimuli. First we must ask, What are the innate unconditioned reflexes to sound that are observable in human beings? Suppose, for example, that we introduce a sound into the ear canal of a particular listener and then observe what happens—how or if he responds. We say and do nothing by way of instructing or suggesting what he should do when he hears the sound. We simply present a stimulus and observe the responses that follow. There are very few such unconditioned responses to sound that are built into the human organism, and so we must utilize conditioned responses in which the sound comes to be an adequate stimulus for the occurrence of a response only after a conditioning process. But with all these responses that may be shown to be dependent upon sounds, have we yet answered the question, "When does he hear?"

The aim of this discussion is to show that we must define *hearing* in terms of the specific conditions of measurement that are used. In traditional audiometry we tend to define *hearing* in terms of a raised finger or a pressed signal button after we have verbally instructed the listener to respond in that way. In more 'objective' procedures we may say that a man *hears* if his pupils contract, or if his skin resistance decreases, or if he presses a bar, or if he reaches for a ball, etc., after nonverbal instructions or conditioned stimuli. Or perhaps we have become used to saying that none of these 'objective' procedures tells us about when a man *really hears*. *Real hearing*, then, might mean responding in a certain way after *verbal* instructions; while just plain *hearing* may mean simply responding in any of several ways after any of several kinds of instruction or conditioning. To remain consistent with the discussion of measurement in Chap. 1, we must conclude that hearing is whatever a particular hearing test measures, just as intelligence is defined as that which the intelligence test measures. This may sound more circular than satisfying, but it is consistent with an empirical, operational approach.

Unconditioned Reflexes

Some responses are known to be evokable by particular stimuli without any conditioning or other training process. A blow to the patellar tendon will cause the leg to extend. A strong light in the eye will cause the pupil to contract. An electric shock will cause the resistance of the skin to decrease. But what about a sound? What responses will it elicit? We know, for example, that when its intensity is high enough a sound will produce contraction of the tensor tympani and the stapedius muscles of the middle ear. But these responses do not meet our criterion of observability except with special apparatus used under special conditions. There are also electrical responses in the auditory nervous system that have been observed in anesthetized animals, but again, these are not easily observable in the awake, intact human observer.

There are some unconditioned responses to sound that are more easily observed. Most of us are familiar with the *startle response* that follows almost any sudden intense stimulus. The adequate stimulus for a startle response may be a strong light, a strong electric shock, or an intense sound. There are a number of components of the startle response that may be identified and used in connection with stimulation by an intense sound. In examining the hearing of newborn infants, for example, Froeschels and Beebe tried to observe as many of these components as possible, and they found that the most frequent response to be observed was a sudden turning of the eyes. Other responses that have been used in clinical situations have been the Tullio reaction, the eye blink, and the contraction of the pupil (Unger). All these seem to be parts of the startle response and are, therefore, clearly elicited only after fairly intense sounds. A sound of low intensity, only a few decibels above the threshold (for finger raising), is not in itself an adequate stimulus for the elicitation of the startle response. Of course, we could define the auditory threshold for the startle response, but our prediction of an individual's ability to hear under everyday circumstances on the basis of such a threshold is extremely limited.

More quantitative information is available on the *galvanic skin response*. This response seems to be another part of the startle pattern when it is elicited (as an unconditioned response) by intense sounds or other sudden strong stimuli. We should speak of two kinds of skin response (Woodworth): the *Tarchanow effect* is a change in the electrical *potential* that exists between two points on the surface of the skin, while the *Feré effect* is a change in the electrical *resistance* between two such points, the measurement of which requires that an external voltage be applied. The latter *skin resistance response* may be elicited by intense sounds and has been shown to be correlated with the 'startle' that is experienced and reported by the observer (Coombs). The Tarchanow effect, or galvanic skin response, has also been shown to be elicited by both intense sounds and electric shocks, its magnitude being directly related to the intensity of the stimulus (Hovland and Riesen). The relations between these two types of skin response remain to be worked out completely.

Observable unconditioned reflexes to sound have one aspect in common: they are mostly elicited by sounds that are intense. This means, of course, that they cannot ordinarily be observed for sounds that are at or near *threshold* for some other response. We must, therefore, turn to responses that can be elicited by weak sounds by virtue of the fact that the weak sounds have become substitute or conditioned stimuli for previously nonauditory stimuli. This discussion will be clearer if we dichotomize, as we have done above, the two basic kinds of conditioning, the classic, or Pavlovian, and the instrumental.

Pavlovian Conditioned Responses

The first experiments that employed Pavlovian conditioning in connection with auditory stimuli were those of Pavlov himself. For our purposes, however, these experiments do not warrant a detailed discussion, because Pavlov was not interested in the relation between the responses measured and the dimensions of the auditory stimulus. At least it is not clear that he systematically varied the physical dimensions of intensity or frequency in the bells and buzzers that he used. We must suppose that he used sounds that were well above his threshold and therefore were assumed to be above the threshold of the dog.

The most highly developed clinical application of Pavlovian conditioning is to be found in the work of Bordley, Hardy, and Richter.[1] These workers began with an unconditioned stimulus-response connection: the lowering of the skin resistance (Feré effect) in response to an electric shock. Throughout the conditioning period the electric shock is preceded by a tone. After conditioning, tests are made with tones of various frequencies and intensities in order to determine the limits, in respect of both these dimensions, within which the conditioned skin-resistance response is observed.

A typical arrangement of equipment for carrying out such a conditioning procedure in conjunction with the conventional audiometer is shown

[1] Details of the procedure are given more fully in the later papers of Bordley and Hardy and of Hardy and Bordley.

in Fig. 10.3.[1] The electrodes that are used for measuring the resistance of the skin are placed either on the back and palm of the hand or on the top and sole of the foot. The skin surface becomes, through the connecting wires, one arm in an electrical Wheatstone bridge circuit, and the resistance is measured by the amount of current that flows through the bridge when a small external voltage is applied. This current is amplified so that a signal is produced that is suitable for automatic recording in ink on a piece of moving paper. An electric shock, delivered to the arm or leg,

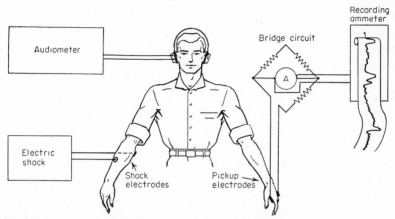

FIG. 10.3. Apparatus used for measuring changes in skin resistance in response to electric shock and conditioned auditory stimuli. The shock alone is adequate to elicit a decrease in skin resistance which is measured by the imbalance in the Wheatstone bridge. Current changes noted on the ammeter in the bridge circuit may be amplified and fed to a recorder, which traces out changes in skin resistance as a function of time. If a pure tone precedes the shock each time the shock is delivered, eventually the tone alone can elicit similar changes in the skin resistance.

produces a deflection of the pen that indicates a decrease in skin resistance. This apparatus can be calibrated with a resistance box in place of the hand or foot, so that not only the initial level of skin resistance is known but also the amount of resistance change in ohms.

The first tones are presented at relatively high intensity, and each tone is followed after 4 or 5 sec by the shock. Adaptation of the skin-resistance response (Coombs) is compensated for in the clinical procedure by increasing the intensity of the shock when needed. The time interval between the tone and the shock is long enough so that separate responses can be shown, one to the tone and the second to the shock. The intensity

[1] Circuits of the apparatus used by Bordley and Hardy are given in Richter and Whelan; similar apparatus, used by the author, is described by Haggard and Gerbrands.

of the tone is gradually reduced until a point is reached where no response is given to the tone alone. Repetitions, involving both ascending and descending intensities, provide a distribution from which the threshold for the conditioned skin-resistance response to a tone can be calculated.

It is unfortunate that so far we have relatively few quantitative data on the use of this technique in clinical audiometry, because there are certain experimental difficulties that have to do with interpretation of the results. It has been shown that the conditioned response that is mediated by a tone of a particular frequency and a particular intensity may also be elicited by tones of other frequencies and intensities. This observation is an example of what has been called *stimulus generalization*. We find, for example, the following statement in a clinical report: "It has been found that a patient conditioned to one tone is thereafter conditioned to all tones audible to that individual." (Bordley and Hardy, p. 6.)

The difficulty here, of course, has to do with the use of the word "conditioned." Different degrees of conditioning may be shown by relating either the amplitude of the response (*e.g.*, the number of ohms of resistance change) or the frequency of response (*e.g.*, the number of times the response exceeds a certain criterion amplitude) to the frequency or intensity of the conditioned stimulus. Measurements of such relations have been published by Hovland (1937*a*, *b*), who showed that generalization, *i.e.*, response to a tone that is different from the tone that was used during conditioning, is high immediately after the initial presentation of the second tone but is reduced after continuous presentation of this tone. The strength of conditioning, therefore, cannot be said to be maintained at the same high level throughout the testing procedure when tones of different frequency or intensity are used. Standard procedures must employ reinforcement for all frequencies to be tested. But how much and how often?

The use of the skin-resistance response in conjunction with auditory stimuli is undoubtedly a fruitful way of exploring relations between an autonomic response and the dimensions of the auditory stimuli used. The wide acceptance of this procedure in clinical audiometry, however, should be preceded by more information on the role of several variables.

The galvanic skin response (Tarchanow effect) has been employed in similar situations by Doerfler and by Michels and Randt. Both Doerfler and Michels and Randt used sound as an unconditioned stimulus for the galvanic skin response. Doerfler attempted to reduce the intensity of the sound to approximately threshold intensities by using a light as a signal, or preceding unconditioned stimulus. (Here is a case in which conditioning was attempted by using as an unconditioned stimulus a light, that had not been shown to be adequate for eliciting the response in the first place.) Michels and Randt mostly used intense sounds to test for *deafness*, rather than to measure *Hearing Loss*. Knapp and Gold used the sounds of speech as stimuli, taking advantage of the general emotional character of particular kinds of words and of the relations between the skin-resistance response (Feré effect) and emotionality. Their work was directed specifically at diagnosing certain forms of psychogenic deafness (Martin).

Instrumental Conditioned Responses

The use of instrumental conditioning is seen in the early studies on the hearing of dogs (Johnson; Finch and Culler). Finch and Culler trained a dog to lift his paw whenever a tone was sounded. If he did not lift his paw after the tone was sounded, an electric shock was delivered to his leg. Although it is difficult to speak of a shock as a reward, it is relatively easy to see that the absence of a shock or escape from a shock can reinforce paw lifting in response to any type of conditioned stimulus that we may wish to use. With this procedure these authors were able to show certain types of hearing loss in these dogs following exposure to very loud sounds.

How can instrumental conditioning be adapted for use in measuring the hearing of humans? You remember that the essential features of instrumental conditioning are (1) the response must be emitted, perhaps fortuitously; (2) immediately following the occurrence of such a response a reinforcing or rewarding stimulus must be presented; (3) the frequency with which the response is thereafter emitted will increase as a function of the reinforcement. In the clinical literature on audiometry we find such instrumental conditioning exemplified in the test of Dix and Hallpike. A sketch of their "peep show" is shown in Fig. 10.4.

Let us review the steps of their procedure in order to show how it fits our paradigm of instrumental conditioning. There are essentially two parts: an audiometer and a series of gadgets designed to introduce reinforcement into the situation. Just in front of the door of a kind of doll's house there is a small push button. When this push button switch is closed, the interior of the doll's house lights up and a very pleasant picture is illuminated. The switch will light the doll's house only when a tone is on. The tone is introduced, either through a loud-speaker or through earphones, by the operator's closing a tone switch. Only the coincident closing of these two switches, the operator's and the child's, will produce the illuminated pictures, which at least for some children constitute a considerable reward.

The frequency with which the child presses on the push button, particularly in the presence of tones, will increase as a function of the reinforcement provided by the illuminated pictures. Eventually the child will be conditioned to a point where no attempt will be made to push on the button during periods of silence, and the button will be pushed as rapidly as the child pleases during periods when the tone is on. Although

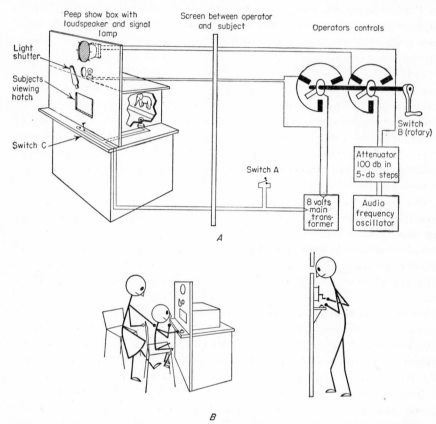

Fɪɢ. 10.4. Apparatus for the "peep-show" technique for measuring auditory thresholds in young children. In (A) we see a schematic diagram of the essential components. The ganged rotary switch is used by the operator to introduce a tone and is also a necessary condition for the illumination of the picture inside the box. If the patient closes switch C while switch A is closed, the picture will be illuminated. The second light, shown below the loudspeaker, may be used as a visual conditioned stimulus in place of or in conjunction with the auditory conditioned stimulus. A sketch of the apparatus in use is shown in (B). (*From Dix and Hallpike.*)

it is perhaps possible to improve on some of the details, providing for an easier response in the case of young children and also providing other types of reward than pictures for very young children, the basic procedure is completely in line with the formulation of instrumental conditioning that has come down through the last fifty years in the experimental psychology of learning.

With reference to this one example, we can point out several essential differences between the adaptation of instrumental conditioning and that of Pavlovian conditioning to audiometry. Note, first of all, that instrumental conditioning, exemplified in the peep show (Dix and Hallpike), uses a skeletal response that is mediated by the central nervous system. Pavlovian conditioning, as exemplified in the shock–skin-resistance test (Bordley and Hardy), uses a response that is mediated by the autonomic nervous system. As in most instrumental conditioning, the measure of response in the "peep show" is one of frequency, that is, the number of times that a particular response is made in a given time or after a number of stimuli have been presented (or, a special case of the same, whether or not a particular response occurs at all). Pavlovian conditioning, being usually confined to response of the autonomic nervous system, employs a measure of response in terms of amplitude.

One can impose a measure of the frequency of response in Pavlovian conditioning by selecting a particular criterion amplitude and counting up only those responses that exceed that amplitude. For example, after initial conditioning we might observe that each time a tone is presented the skin resistance decreases. But by how much? We may show, perhaps, that the more intense the tone the greater the change will be in skin resistance. We may for convenience choose a criterion amplitude, let us say a decrease in skin resistance of 200 ohms, and say that we shall simply count the number of responses that are made to tones of different intensity when such responses exceed this basic amplitude of 200 ohms. Of course, these measures of amplitude and frequency are inseparable, since the frequency of responses greater than 200 ohms will increase as the individual responses become larger. At least it is clear that, in the Pavlovian case, the amplitude and frequency measures of response are almost interchangeable.

In the case of instrumental responses this is not so clear, since the amplitude factor is imposed on the responding organism by the experimenter. For example, in the peep show the child is reinforced for making responses that exceed a certain amplitude, in the sense that he must overcome whatever force there is in the spring of the switch in order that the switch be closed. If we analyzed the response in terms of individual muscle twitches and eventually in terms of electrical responses of individual muscle fibers, we should eventually find an all-or-none kind of response; but at the molar level of observation there is undoubtedly a factor of response amplitude that could be measured if we were sufficiently interested. It is not clear in the case of instrumental responses that the frequency and amplitude or strength of response vary in the same direction. As a matter of fact there is some evidence (Skinner, 1950) that as the frequency of an instrumental response increases, its amplitude or strength decreases. The child may begin by banging very hard on the push button, but he will find out in time that he need press it only slightly in order to produce the desired reinforcement. There is no necessary relation between the frequency and amplitude of an instrumental response, because the amplitude may be manipulated by selective reinforcement.

Before leaving the instrumental-conditioning paradigm we must note that most of the special procedures that have been suggested in the clinical literature for measuring the hearing of young children (Utley) have exemplified, at least crudely, the application of instrumental, or operant, conditioning. Froeschels, for example, has described a chute that leads from a control room into a small playroom. A ball is rolled down this chute immediately after a tone is sounded, and the child reaches for the ball as soon as it comes out of the chute into his playroom. Eventually it can be demonstrated that if the child hears the tone he will show a reaching response even when the ball (the unconditioned stimulus) is absent. Bloomer presents pictures of objects that are associated with tones of different frequencies. The child may cause a tone to cease sounding by placing his finger over the correct picture. In this case, the very fact that a response is instrumental in bringing about a change in the stimulus situation seems to be rewarding enough to warrant a high frequency of discriminating (among different tones) responses. The techniques described by the Ewings, which are used by many teachers, also exemplify this type of conditioning. Many ingenious variations on this basic theme have been and can be arranged by varying the response to be used, the kind of reward that is used, etc., and we must know that the relation between the frequency of response and the intensity of the stimulus is the same for all these variations before we can say that the techniques are interchangeable as psychophysical tests.

The Clinical Problem

A simple way of demonstrating the relations among the audiometric applications of conditioning is to present an example of a single response to be made after the presentation of a tone, under different conditions of training. Suppose that we decide arbitrarily that the patient must raise his index finger whenever a tone is presented. We shall define the perception of a tone in terms of this finger-raising response. Let us now construct some *hypothetical* situations based upon the principles that have been discussed above.

First, can we use the finger raising as an unconditioned response to sound? It is clear that if we simply present tones to an observer without giving him any instructions, verbal or otherwise, his index finger will not automatically be raised in response to the sound.

But now let us further suppose that our observer has no language at his disposal, that he is perhaps a two-year-old child who has not learned to speak or to understand the speech of others. How are we to instruct him to raise his index finger when he hears a tone? Let us first apply the principles of *Pavlovian conditioning*. What stimulus will produce the finger raising as an unconditioned response? We might guess that the administration of an electric shock to the tip of the index finger that is resting over an electrode upon the table will cause the finger to be withdrawn, and if we limit the movement of the hand by strapping it to the table, the withdrawal will be made in one direction, producing the response of raising the finger. Each time we present such a shock, the finger will be raised. Now we must employ the tone as a conditioned stimulus, allowing the tone to precede the shock by some interval of time. For this particular response the optimum interval of time has been found to be about $\frac{1}{4}$ sec (Wolfle). Note that if we adhere strictly to the Pavlovian paradigm we must strap the small electrode to the end of the index finger, so that if the preceding tone successfully evokes a conditioned response and causes the finger to be raised, there is still opportunity for shock to be delivered at the appropriate interval.

The same basic procedure may be used to establish an *instrumental conditioned response* of finger raising. Instead of waiting for the raising of the finger to be emitted spontaneously by the subject (as we should in instrumental conditioning), we can force the response by administering a shock immediately after the presentation of the tone. Hereafter, however, the shocking electrode will remain on the table, so that if a person raises his finger immediately after the presentation of a tone, he will avoid being shocked. This latter situation, with the electrode on the table, allows us to bring in the contingency after which instrumental conditioning is named; if the conditioned response is made to the presentation of the conditioned stimulus (the tone), the unconditioned stimulus or reward is presented, namely, the *absence* of the shock.

Either of these conditioning procedures might be used in order to produce a finger-raising response after the occurrence of an auditory stimulus, but the frequency of response will undoubtedly increase faster if the instrumental procedure is used. To put this in everyday language, the subject does not achieve anything by raising his finger when he hears a tone if the electrode remains strapped to his finger; he will be shocked anyway. On the other hand, if he can successfully avoid a shock by raising his finger after hearing the tone, the frequency with which this finger raising will follow the presentation of a tone will increase very rapidly.

Now let us return to what we might call the traditional audiometric procedure. The response to be emitted on the occasion of a tone is the same: the finger is to be raised. We avoid these relatively cumbersome conditioning procedures by saying to the patient, "Please raise your finger whenever you hear a tone." If, then, the patient raises his finger when we present a tone, may we not say that he has been completely conditioned? He has learned that carrying out verbal instructions usually leads to certain kinds of reward. The verbal instructions of the clinician are a conditioned stimulus that tell the patient that this is an occasion on which finger raising, after a tone, will be rewarded in certain ways.

In terms of the preceding discussion, it seems that a distinction between 'subjective' and 'objective' responses is much less meaningful, if we must make such a distinction at all, than a distinction between *subjective* and *objective sets*. In the above paragraph we have discussed ways of establishing such a *set to respond* by conditioning. We have also discussed certain types of response in which the set to respond was 'wired in' at birth or at least at some level of development. And now we have a case in which the set is established by verbal instruction. For everyday use, therefore, the distinction between subjective and objective procedures may be based upon the fact that what have been called "subjective procedures" have involved the establishing of a set to respond by the use of verbal instructions, whereas those procedures that have been called "objective" are characterized by the use of nonverbal instructions or stimuli.

INTERPRETATION OF TESTS

The reader who has been seeking *the method* or a conglomeration of gadgets to provide sure-fire auditory tests for all kinds of patients must be, by now, utterly disappointed. We have been saying that different ways of testing hearing are different, and that we can describe these differences in terms of certain concepts that have been developed in psychology in the field of conditioning. It is very interesting to talk about our different procedures in a new way and perhaps display a little more erudition, but are we not ignoring certain clinical problems? Have we not suggested that there is almost no possibility of comparable audiometric data, owing to differences in procedure that must be maintained because there are differences among people and therefore different ways must be used to approach them?

Certainly we can have standard procedures (including standard verbal instructions) that will be used on a majority of patients. Then procedural variations that are necessitated by young children and other special cases may be brought into line in one of two ways: either a relation may be established between the threshold that is obtained with a novel technique and the threshold for the traditional procedure, or a new *normal threshold* must be set up for each technique. But these questions about standards and norms may be more academic than useful if we do not go a little further and hazard some reasonable guesses about the diagnostic implications of the results of different procedures.

To be very unscientific, we might say that the 'highest' form of hearing or auditory perception is exemplified by the person who follows verbal instructions and 'voluntarily' responds in a predetermined way to the oncoming of a sound. This is the kind of hearing that we test in what we have called the traditional audiometric procedures. But of course, the audiogram gives information about more than the auditory system. If it is normal, we know not only that the auditory system is intact but also that the person tested has command of at least enough language to follow verbal instructions that are given and furthermore has the ability to make whatever response we have demanded, namely, finger raising, button pressing, or saying "yes." Furthermore, if we can specify a *Hearing Loss* of, let us say, 30 db, we know that if a given sound is made 30 db more intense than one that a person with normal hearing would hear, all other features of the measurement are 'normal.' In other words, given a stimulus at 30 db Sensation Level, our patient can understand verbal instructions and make the appropriate response in a normal way.

Now suppose that we cannot get a patient to raise his finger when a tone is presented. Is he deaf? Before answering, we might find out whether or not he can raise his finger when a tone is presented if each presentation of the tone has been followed by an electric shock that causes his finger to go up. If we can observe such a response to a tone alone after a certain amount of instrumental conditioning, we cannot say simply that he is deaf. Perhaps he is 'malingering' and therefore will not follow our verbal instructions. His motives for malingering, however, may become secondary when he finds that he can escape from a shock by raising his finger at the appropriate time (as in instrumental conditioning). But malingering is not our only choice of interpretation; it is, after all, only one kind of psychological disorder for which we are more likely to 'blame' a patient than we are for more serious psychological problems. Even aside from such psychological disorders, however, we have also the possibility that the patient has a kind of receptive aphasia, which means simply that he does not understand spoken language. A decision among these latter alternatives is, in the clinical situation, probably beyond the person who is responsible for measuring the hearing. Conditioning comes into audiometric procedures, not so much as a tool for finding out what is wrong with the patient, but rather to determine whether the auditory system itself is intact.

Now where does the auditory system end? There is a question whose answer will be entirely arbitrary. One arbitrary answer might suggest that the auditory system extends from the pinna through the peripheral auditory system, through the midbrain structures, and up to the temporal cortex (and probably other cortical regions). Such anatomical considerations can be best applied to the use of Pavlovian conditioning in audiometry as exemplified by the skin-resistance test. Suppose that the patient whom we have discussed above shows a change in skin resistance, after an appropriate period of conditioning, when a tone at 0 db Sensation Level is presented. Is his hearing normal? We can say only that those parts of the auditory system and of the autonomic nervous system that are necessary for the mediation of this response are intact. There is enough anatomical evidence to guess at least that a connection between these two systems might be at a relatively low level in the nervous system. In other words, it might not be necessary for the auditory cortex to be intact in order to show a normal response, by the autonomic nervous system, to a conditioned auditory stimulus. The interpretation of a positive result from the skin-resistance data is, therefore, a very difficult one. A negative response, on the other hand—that is, a lack of response to the conditioned acoustic stimulus—tells us that something is wrong either with a more or less peripheral part of the auditory system or with the autonomic system. And this latter alternative can be eliminated as a possibility if it can be shown, for example, that a light used as a conditioned stimulus can elicit the response.

Our knowledge about the relations between certain psychophysical measurements and various conditioning procedures is so limited that we cannot be conclusive or specifically definitive in this discussion. Our basic observations are that different procedures may be used in measuring hearing in order to get at some observable response of persons whose response repertoire is limited in some way. We cannot yet tie these procedures together because we have an insufficient number of published observations by which to compare the results. No one can doubt that we can measure more responses by using nonverbal conditioned stimuli in the testing situation than by using traditional procedures in which verbal instructions presuppose learning that is not under the control of the tester. This application of conditioning is relatively new in audiometry, although we can cite examples of such applications in rudimentary form in older work. That we can cast both old and new procedures into the conceptual framework of conditioning means that these procedures can be meaningfully related on a common behavioral basis.

References for Further Study

Ewing, I. R., and A. W. G. Ewing. (1946) *The Handicap of Deafness*. New York: Longmans. Chapters 6 and 7 contain examples of clinical applications of instrumental conditioning to the testing of hearing in the preschool child.

Hilgard, E. R., and D. G. Marquis. (1940) *Conditioning and Learning*. New York: Appleton-Century-Crofts. Chapters 2 and 3 differentiate, with examples, Pavlovian and instrumental conditioning. The whole book serves as an excellent summary of the experimental work in conditioning.

Watson, L. A., and T. Tolan. (1949) *Hearing Tests and Hearing Instruments*. Baltimore: Williams & Wilkins. Chapter 9 reviews most of the important clinical 'techniques' for the detection of malingering, including the recent speech-masking test for malingering by Doerfler and Stewart.

CHAPTER 11

CLINICAL AUDIOMETRY

THE theory and practice of clinical audiometry is an important part of the training of persons who work on problems of hearing and hearing loss. From a very practical point of view, we can say that this part of the training should at least provide the trainee with a knowledge of how to carry out those auditory tests that are particularly useful in otologic and audiologic practice. It would be foolish to entertain the proposition that every clinical audiometrist should be able to carry out all the clinical and experimental procedures that have been discussed in the preceding 10 chapters. Rather we must distill out of this complex array those procedures that have been shown to be applicable in the clinic.

Some of the problems that arise in clinical work stem from the lack of standardization or general agreement about specific audiometric procedures. Indeed, it was the desire for such standardization on the part of different professional and administrative groups that first prompted the writing of this book. As various clinical areas were studied and their experimental bases examined, however, it became obvious why such standardization is difficult to obtain.

Standardization in any field comes about either when there are enough experimental data to suggest the standard unequivocally or, lacking these, when there is agreement among reputable specialists on what the standard should be. Results from experiments on hearing have not yet yielded enough information about the role of all the variables that remain uncontrolled in the typical clinical procedure. Nor has there been any general agreement among clinical specialists on what standard procedures should be used. Without an accepted standard procedure, then, audiometrists usually acquire their training according to individual experience and the preference of their particular instructors.

In the preceding chapters, we have attempted to review the experimental findings that pertain to most of the audiometric procedures that have been or might be used in clinical practice. In examining these experimental results, we have become aware of the limitations of many of our 'traditional' procedures. But these 10 chapters fall far short of the original hope of setting down some rules for various kinds of audiometry—rules that could be shown to be based on experimental facts. Rather it seems that the writing of a *definitive* clinical manual or rulebook for the measurement of hearing would be premature at the present time.

Despite this lack of bases for standardization, clinical audiometry is carried out every day in many hearing clinics and otologists' offices. We should not, therefore, conclude a work on auditory measurement without attempting to summarize some clinical procedures and to suggest certain disadvantages and limitations of techniques that are used routinely. Many of the suggestions will be supported by references to the appropriate material in earlier chapters. Other suggestions may be implied only by less directly related experimental results. Still others represent only the considered opinion of the author or of more experienced clinical workers who have shared their experiences through the periodical literature.

This chapter is not intended, therefore, to be a rulebook by which any student of audiometry can learn his trade. Rather it is meant to be a limited survey of present audiometric technique, considered in the light of such information as has been presented in the first 10 chapters. In part it is a repetition, under different organization, of the clinical material in Chaps. 4 and 5.

AIMS OF CLINICAL AUDIOMETRY

Before discussing the audiometric procedures themselves, let us consider the reasons for doing audiometric tests in the first place. For the present, we shall divide these reasons among three main categories: *screening, diagnosis,* and *therapeutic evaluation.* The three corresponding clinical questions to be answered are (1) Does a person hear as well as a person of normal or standard hearing? (2) How much can a person actually hear, or how much and what kind of a hearing loss does he have? (3) How has a certain kind of therapy affected his hearing?

Screening

Screening tests of hearing are designed to separate two groups of persons: one that can hear as well as or better than a particular standard or criterion, and the other that cannot hear so well. They are designed to accomplish this aim as rapidly and for as many people as possible. Applications of such tests are to be found in public schools, where we want to separate out or 'screen' those children whose hearing may need individual attention from those whose hearing is as good as or better than a standard that is usually set by health officials. In industry and military service, screening is particularly useful when related to a standard that is established either with respect to requirements of hearing for a particular job or in the interest of protecting the hearing.

Diagnosis

Now assume that we have found some individuals whose hearing appears to be below standard. Then, individual audiometry is necessary to find out *how much Hearing Loss* is present and what is *its kind*. Furthermore, we may wish to administer tests of hearing to predict the kind of therapy that will be most beneficial to the patient. In short, we are now interested in doing *diagnostic audiometry;* that is, making measurements of hearing that will help the otologist and audiologist in prescribing the best course for the patient to follow. The very nature of the problems indicates that diagnostic audiometry involves more elaborate and varied measurements than those employed in the screening tests.

Therapeutic Evaluation

Now assume further that we have performed various audiometric tests and that the results of these, together with the results of otologic and other examinations, permit us to know the type of hearing loss involved and what kinds of therapy to recommend. Indications for a fenestration operation or a hearing aid, for example, may be good, and we should like to know how much benefit the patient has received from one or several of these different kinds of therapy. More of the same and other tests permit us to evaluate the therapy or to tell how much improvement has been brought about by surgery, a hearing aid, or certain types of training. Such types of audiometry will be treated under a third division, *therapeutic evaluation.*

Keeping in mind the several functions that screening tests, diagnostic audiometry, and therapeutic evaluation may have in clinical practice, we are now ready to review the various tests that are employed in clinical audiometry.

SCREENING TESTS

The concept of Hearing Loss is basic to both screening tests and diagnostic audiometry. In screening, however, we do not measure *how much* Hearing Loss a person has; rather we find out only whether he has *more* or *less* than a certain *standard* Hearing Loss. In screening, we are interested in obtaining this information on as many people in as short a time as possible. In individual diagnostic work we must take more time to measure the actual amount of Hearing Loss.

The foundation of any generally used screening test for hearing is the standard or criterion relative to which the screening is done. Standards vary from state to state, from school to school, from industry to industry and, unfortunately, from one military service to another. The standard may be stated as a Hearing Loss (in decibels) for certain pure tones, or it may be stated as a Hearing Loss for Speech. In spite of differences among large users of screening tests, we may, for our present purpose, consider as a dividing line Hearing Losses of 15 or 20 db either for pure tones in the middle range of frequencies or for speech.

Screening with Pure Tones

Most of the standards used in public-school programs for the conservation of hearing, as well as in military application, are stated in terms of Hearing Loss for pure tones. This is undoubtedly due to the wide use that the pure-tone audiometer now enjoys compared to the more limited use of devices employed for measuring hearing for speech. A genuine attempt has been made, however, by the makers of screening tests to restrict the pure-tone measurements to those that have been shown to be important for the hearing of speech. Thus the three middle frequencies (500, 1000, and 2000 cps) are used most in screening.

Individual Sweep Check. The earliest form of screening with pure tones was a particular kind of technique of individual pure-tone audiometry, which has come to be called the "sweep check." In making a diagnostic kind of audiogram, we usually select one frequency at a time and at each frequency vary the Hearing-loss or intensity control until we obtain a level at which the patient can just barely hear (see next main section). This requires that we spend some time at each frequency, and we cannot test a large group in this way in any reasonable period of time. But in screening we do not wish to make an audiogram; that is, we do not wish to know *how much* Hearing Loss a listener has at each frequency. We wish only to know whether or not he can hear at a certain level.

Let us assume that we use, as a criterion, 15-db Hearing Loss (Sensation Level). We can then set the Hearing-loss control of an ordinary commercial audiometer at 15 and vary the frequency, either stepwise or continuously, depending on the particular audiometer and our own wishes. Relative to the tests that are ordinarily used in making an audiogram, the test question has now been turned around, and we ask: What frequencies can he hear and what frequencies can he not hear, if the Hearing-loss control for all frequencies is set at 15 db? The time required for each test and for a large group of tests is, of course, much less, and one can screen large groups of listeners in this way much more rapidly.

The sweep-check technique has been adapted by Johnston, in the Massachusetts Hearing Test, for testing groups of children. The children record on a paper form either a "yes" or a "no" each time the tester indicates a test period. It is much simpler than the group tests to be discussed in the next paragraph but provides the tester with more limited information.

Pulse-tone Technique. The method of introducing a pure tone into the ear of a listener in short bursts or pulses, as used by Gardner (1947b) and by Reger and Newby, is particularly well adapted to screening. Although it takes a little longer to measure a single individual's hearing by having him count pulses than by the individual sweep technique outlined in the above paragraph, the pulse-tone technique may be used successfully with groups of listeners all listening at the same time. Since a listener can respond by reporting the number of pulses heard, he can just as well write down that number as speak it aloud.

Special equipment, in addition to the usual commercial type of audiometer, is required for the pulse-tone technique, and some manufacturers have made such equipment available in conjunction with their pure-tone audiometers. One of the simplest kinds of additional equipment, described by Reger and Newby, uses a mechanical pulsing system that can be manipulated very easily by the audiometrist.

The screening level is set at, for example, 15 db. Then during test periods, which are announced by a signal light, groups of different numbers of tones are presented. The groups may differ not only in the number of tones but also in the frequency of the tones. If the listener reports or writes down the correct number of tones for a given group, his hearing is assumed to be as good as or better than the criterion or screening level. Those individuals whose hearing is deficient (*i.e.*, more than 15-db Hearing Loss) are easily detected by their incorrect responses at one or several frequencies.

When the pulse-tone technique is used to make an individual audiogram (see below), that is, to find out *how much* Hearing Loss is present at different frequencies, the testing procedure becomes more complicated. One must *program* such a test by predetermining the number of pulses that will be presented at each level and each frequency. For example, a shortened version of such a program might involve presenting 4, 2, 3, 1, 3, and 2 pulses of 1000 cps at Hearing-loss settings of 50, 40, 30, 20, 10, and 0 db, respectively. Again the listener's task is to report correctly the number of pulses that were presented at each level. In this descending series, we should say that his threshold lies somewhere below the last level at which he reported the number of pulses correctly and above the first level at which he reports incorrectly. When such a technique is used for individual listeners (see Gardner, 1947b), the number of pulses heard is reported orally by the listener, whereas when the test is administered to a group of individuals, each person writes down the number of pulses he hears.

The relation between thresholds measured by this technique and those obtained by more traditional techniques has not yet been establisbed, except for a small group of listeners (Gardner, 1947*b*).

Screening with Speech

The first systematic attempt to set up a screening program in the public schools made use of the Western Electric 4-A audiometer (see Appendix A and Chap. 5). This audiometer (now 4-C) consists of a phonograph whose output is delivered to almost any desired number of earphones, mounted in spring headbands. The records contain lists of two-digit groups recorded at gradually decreasing intensities. The listeners simply write down the numbers that they hear, and the threshold for this material is defined as the lowest level at which about half of the correct numbers are written down. The fact that the digits used differ from each other in their main vowel sounds and that the monitoring of the speech does not always yield decreasing intensities with time has made these records useful only in a very rough way. (The 4-A audiometer was recommended for screening in public schools in the syllabus of Newhart and Reger.)

Although it has not been suggested in the clinical literature, it seems that we might construct a screening test using the spondee words that are used for measuring the threshold of intelligibility or Hearing Loss for Speech (see Chap. 5 and below) in a way that is completely analogous to the pure-tone screening at a particular level. Let us say, for example, that we wish to screen out of a given population all listeners whose Hearing Loss for Speech is greater than 15 db. We should use spondee words spoken or recorded at a constant level and set the level 15 db higher than the normal threshold of intelligibility for those words, *e.g.* at about 35 db SPL. Then we could administer the test to a group of individuals, who would write down the words that they hear, and we should reject or refer for further examination all those who did not write down more than 50 per cent of the words correctly at that level. The nature of such speech material, in addition to the standardization that has been achieved from its use, makes such an application of recorded spondees to screening quite feasible. Obviously, the use of such a test would be restricted to groups of listeners who are familiar with the vocabulary.

DIAGNOSTIC AUDIOMETRY

The purpose of any diagnostic test of hearing is to determine how much hearing loss the patient has, to describe the kind of hearing loss, and to predict the site of the pathologic condition. The essential difference between diagnostic tests and screening tests is not one of kind but of degree. In other words, the basic principles are the same, but more care and precision are desired in diagnostic tests. Although it is true that time is an important consideration in routine clinical practice, it is also true that it is of secondary importance when compared to its status in a screening program

Pure-tone Audiometry

The history of clinical audiometry has shown a long interest on the part of the otologist in the absolute sensitivity to pure tones, that is, the minimum amount of sound energy required at each of several different frequencies in order that the system respond at all. This absolute threshold for pure tones has been tested with tuning forks, vibrating strings, whistles, and, more recently, vacuum-tube audiometers. We shall consider next the three main methods for measuring the absolute threshold for pure tones. And since this is a clinical summary, we shall be concerned only with the relative threshold or Hearing Loss.

Tuning-fork Tests.   It would be beyond the scope of this book to treat thoroughly auditory tests that are done with tuning forks. This subject is already well covered in several books (*e.g.*, Bunch; Fowler, 1947). We shall sketch them here, however, in order to relate them to their more precise successors.

The three most important tuning-fork tests are the Weber, the Rinne, and the Schwabach tests. The otologist who has had experience with these tests, administered with a particular set of tuning forks, makes extremely accurate diagnostic judgments. It seems fair to say, however, that these tuning-fork tests are limited in that they are mostly designed to tell the clinician whether his patient has a hearing loss of the conductive type or of the more central perceptive, or nerve, type.

The *Weber test* concerns the apparent localization of a sound that is heard when the stem of a vibrating tuning fork is placed somewhere along the mid-line of the skull. A person who has normal hearing in both ears usually localizes the sound either in the center of the head or 'nowhere.' A patient with a unilateral conductive loss will usually report that the sound is heard on the side of the affected ear. A person with a unilateral perceptive-type loss will report that the sound appears to be on the side of the healthy ear. There are many variations of these judgments, depending on combinations of these different types of hearing loss and various amounts in the two ears. Also, the effect of a conductive lesion on the Weber test differs according to the frequency of vibration of the fork (see Chap. 9).

The *Rinne test* compares a patient's ability to hear the vibrations of the tines of a tuning fork by air conduction with his ability to hear the vibrations of the stem of a tuning fork by bone conduction. The durations of vibration that would describe normal hearing by air or bone conduction depend upon the individual tuning fork and its frequency of vibration. (In general, the longer the tines or the lower the frequency, the less rapidly the vibration will decay.) One compares the length of time a patient hears a fork by air conduction with the length of time he hears the same fork by bone conduction. Of course, there is no a priori reason for assuming that a person with normal hearing will be able to hear the same fork just as long by air as by bone, and, as a matter of fact, this rarely occurs, since a normal or positive Rinne response is defined as a longer time for hearing by air conduction than by bone conduction. This positive result holds so long as the conducting apparatus of the external and middle ear remain intact, that is, for normal hearing and for perceptive hearing loss. If, however, a pathologic condition exists in the peripheral conducting system, the Rinne test shows the time for bone conduction either the same as or longer than the time for air conduction.

The *Schwabach test* is essentially a crude test of absolute threshold by bone conduction. Time, rather than intensity, is used as a dependent variable. The clinician tries to strike the fork in such a way that the initial amplitude is always the same; and, since the decay of the fork may be assumed to exhibit the same characteristics on successive trials, the clinician may use time as a measure (because he usually has a watch for measuring it). But such a time measure is really derived from the patient's threshold intensity. The duration that the clinician measures is the time taken by the fork to decay from its initial amplitude to whatever amplitude corresponds to the patient's threshold.

In clinical practice it is not usual to make this an absolute measure; rather, the clinician has either decided upon or accepted a standard duration as normal, and the patient is said to have a *shortened* or *prolonged* Schwabach response according as he can hear the sound a shorter or longer time than the normal duration.

In the hands of a precise, experienced clinician it appears that the tuning fork is a more useful diagnostic instrument than is the more precise pure-tone audiometer in the hands of an inexperienced, careless tester.

The Audiogram (Air Conduction). Although there seems to be no official name for a test for hearing by air conduction in which the clinician holds the vibrating tines of a tuning fork just outside the ear canal of a patient and counts seconds, it is certainly possible that such an "air-conduction Schwabach" test can yield useful results. It is difficult to do, however, because of various physical factors involved in the vibration of the tuning fork that remain uncontrolled.

The pure-tone audiometer is a more precise instrument for carrying out the same measurement. An audiogram, which results from measurements made with a pure-tone audiometer, is a chart that shows the difference (in decibels) between the sound energy required by a particular patient to just hear a tone and the sound energy required by a normal listener, for several different frequencies. The most general method for making an audiogram includes the use of one of the audiometers that is commercially available and has been accepted by the Council on Physical Medicine and Rehabilitation of the American Medical Association (see Appendix A).

We have reviewed the basic parts of a typical audiometer in Chap. 3. Now we are concerned with manipulating the controls by which we turn a tone on, change its frequency, and change its intensity. These controls are usually labeled "interrupter key," "frequency," and "hearing loss."[1] There is no standard method for manipulating these three controls in making an audiogram. The effects of varying different aspects of the procedure have been reviewed in Chap. 4. In suggesting a procedure to be used in making an audiogram, the author is drawing on several clinical sources, including Bunch and the 'almost standard' audiometric procedure that is given in the syllabus of Newhart and Reger (pp. 17 to 18).

Before beginning the test, the audiometrist should acquaint the patient with the purpose and nature of the audiometric test. He may suggest that the test is designed to find out how "soft" a tone the listener can hear. He can suggest further that the tones will be different in quality or pitch, some sounding like high whistles and others like foghorns. The patient should be instructed to raise his finger whenever he hears a sound come on and to withdraw his finger as soon as the sound disappears. The withdrawal is almost as important as the raising for the tester who would distinguish between the responses to tones that are actually presented and those that may be produced by head noises and imagined tones. For the experienced tester the rate at which the patient moves his finger may also be diagnostically significant (see Chap. 8, Indirect Measurements of Recruitment). The signal light that is provided with audiometers has been found by at least some clinicians to be more trouble than it is worth, and they prefer the extending of the finger as the response.

After noting that the patient is seated comfortably, the audiometrist should help him to adjust the earphones so that they are centered over

---

[1] Since these controls are different in the many available audiometers, it is suggested that the reader supplement this discussion with the detailed instructions that are contained in the instruction booklet provided with his audiometer.

the ears. There should be enough tension in the headband spring so that the earphones remain at the same place throughout the test.

The first actual testing step usually consists of presenting a 1000-cps tone at about 30 or 40 db ("Hearing Loss" dial). If the patient does not signal that he hears this, the intensity may be increased until the patient gives a sure response. (The intensity should not be changed while the tone is on; rather the tone should be interrupted during the times that the "Hearing Loss" dial is moved.) When the tester is sure that the patient hears a tone (*i.e.*, that the intensity is well above threshold), he may decrease the intensity in 10-db steps until the patient no longer responds to the onset of the tone. Then the intensity may be increased again, in 5-db steps, until a sure response is observed.

The threshold should be crossed several times (*e.g.*, more than two) before one puts a mark on the audiogram card that indicates a level above which the patient responds almost always and below which he responds rarely or never. The criterion of responding to 50 per cent of the tones presented, which is usually adopted in psychophysical experiments, is slightly academic in the clinical situation, because we do not ordinarily present enough tones at each level to adopt any particular percentage of response. If we agree that it should be less than 100 per cent and greater than 0, the error involved will not be large relative to the steps of 5 db that are provided in most audiometers. (The use of the term "consistent response" in the syllabus of Newhart and Reger implies nearly 100-percent response.)

The above procedure may then be repeated at each of the other frequencies to be tested. The order does not seem to be too important, except that many clinicians begin at 1000 cps and then go either upward or downward.

Having measured the Hearing Loss for one ear at each of the frequencies to be tested, the audiometrist can then proceed to measure the Hearing Loss on the other ear. If the audiograms for both ears show that there is a large difference between the Hearing Losses of the two ears, the hearing of the worse ear must be retested while the better ear is masked (see Chap. 6).

Some of the techniques that have been introduced for special purposes (*e.g.*, pulse-tone technique for screening) may also be used for individual audiometry (Gardner, 1947*b*). There is little evidence in either the experimental or the clinical literature to suggest that one technique is any more valid than others for measuring an individual's Hearing Loss, but this is not to say that the results for all techniques will be the same (see Chap. 4).

One special procedure which seems to be potentially useful for clinical audiometry is the one employed in Békésy's audiometer (1947), in which the intensity is under the control of the patient. The special advantage of measuring the DL around the absolute threshold has been discussed in Chap. 7. Not only is this DL important for the detection of recruitment, but also its magnitude gives the clinician a rather precise estimate of how surely or how vaguely the patient is responding to liminal stimuli.

Testing Children. The application of the traditional procedures to measuring the Hearing Loss for pure tones in children is accompanied by many complications. The clinical literature suggests that these traditional procedures may be used with children who are more than six or eight years old. Below this age, however, there are two quite distinct sets of problems. First, the attention span of even a child who has enough hearing so as to have acquired language is limited, and he will insist on some kind of play before all frequencies on both ears are tested. In such cases, therefore, it is well to plan on several testing sessions before a complete audiogram is obtained.

The more serious set of problems has to do with testing the hearing of young children who have not acquired language. As we have pointed out in Chap. 10, the very nature of most of the traditional audiometric techniques lies in the verbal instructions, and, since the child who has no language cannot respond to such instructions, we must devise other means for telling him what to do when a tone is heard. In general, two types of conditioning have been applied to the solution of this problem, and they are best typified, in clinical audiometry, by the skin-resistance technique of Bordley and Hardy on the one hand and by a "peep show" of Dix and Hallpike on the other. Since these are rather special procedures, they will not be discussed here, and it is suggested that the reader review them in Chap. 10 and in the original sources.

The Audiogram (Bone Conduction). Bone-conduction audiometry represents a more precise way of arriving at the results of tuning-fork tests. The psychophysical technique used in measuring the Hearing Loss for pure tones by bone conduction is essentially the same as that used in tests by air conduction. The main difference between the two types of audiometry is the method by which sound energy is made to perform displacements of the basilar membrane within the cochlea. In the case of air conduction, changes in pressure in the ear canal produce displacement of the eardrum and the ossicles and thus produce differences between the pressures at the oval and round windows. The principal ways by which this difference in pressure is set up when the skull is set into vibration have been outlined in Chap. 9. Now we are concerned with the clinical technique for obtaining a threshold for this bone-conducted sound.

The Hearing Loss or the intensity relative to normal for bone-conducted sounds is usually given by a second scale of the Hearing-loss control of an audiometer. The vibrator that is used in place of the earphone which was used for air conduction is not nearly so simple to apply as the earphone. Many of the vibrators that are supplied with commercial audiometers are suspended in a spring headband so that they need not be held in the hand of the patient. Even so, the clinician must explore the mastoid process in order to find the point that gives maximum hearing. This point on the mastoid process is mentioned here for traditional reasons only (see Chap. 9). The mastoid region gives rise to considerable variability, and at least the experimental literature suggests that the forehead might be a more reliable site for such testing (even though the threshold might be higher than that for the mastoid). But it has been used very little in actual clinical practice.

Using the bone-conduction scale of Hearing Loss and the indications of frequency, the procedure for measuring Hearing Loss at each of several frequencies is the same as that given above for air conduction. The one major complication here is that no matter where we apply the vibrator on the skull, both ears are stimulated, and we cannot, no matter how carefully we place the vibrator, test either ear alone. Both must be assumed to be responding almost equally well to energy (especially at low frequencies) that is moving the entire skull. The only way of testing the threshold for a single ear by bone conduction is to mask the opposite ear (see Chaps. 6 and 9). Masking should be considered a routine part of audiometry by bone conduction.

Recruitment Tests. So long as the only diagnostic information desired is a distinction between a hearing loss that is produced by lesions in the conducting apparatus and one that is produced by pathologic conditions in the cochlea or in the central nervous system, the audiograms for air conduction and for bone conduction are probably sufficient if they are obtained properly. But, particularly among European otologists, recruitment (see Chap. 8) is also considered an important clinical datum. It is probably useful, however, as a phenomenon having more to do with decisions concerning the use of a hearing aid, etc., than for otologic diagnosis alone. On the other hand, the recent work of Dix, Hallpike, and Hood and of Langenbeck (1950*a*, *b*, *c*) indicates that the presence of recruitment may be useful in distinguishing lesions of the end organs in the cochlea from those in the more central part of the auditory nervous system.

Clinical procedures for detecting the presence of recruitment have already been presented in some detail in Chap. 8. Strictly speaking, recruitment, defined in terms of the growth of loudness with increasing intensity, can be tested only by the alternate binaural loudness balance or the monaural interfrequency loudness balance (see Chap. 8, Measurements of Recruitment). Measures of differential sensitivity (Békésy, 1947; Lüscher and Zwislocki, 1948, 1949a), of masking (Huizing, 1942; Langenbeck, 1950a, b, c), and of fatigue (Gardner, 1947a) have been suggested as substitutes for the loudness-balancing techniques. But, although these indirect measures produce results that are highly correlated with measurements of recruitment by loudness balance, it is not clear that these tests may actually be used as substitutes. There is the further possibility that a severe Discrimination Loss (see Chap. 5 and next section) may also be distinctly related to the presence of recruitment.

It is clear at least that the presence of recruitment indicates a nonconductive hearing loss and also one that will be very difficult to help with a hearing aid. Besides these general relations, the phenomenon of recruitment appears to be only an extremely interesting clinical phenomenon that has very interesting implications for a physiological theory of hearing.

Speech Audiometry

The analysis of a patient's Hearing Loss for pure tones at different frequencies probably gives us the most detailed information possible, so far as otologic diagnosis is concerned. But there is a seeming lack of validity in hearing for pure tones, especially since most humans use their auditory systems tô hear speech and other more complicated stimuli. Although many attempts have been made to calculate or estimate the ability to hear speech (see Chap. 5) on the basis of the ability to hear pure tones, the most promising measure seems to be that of the hearing of speech itself.

The notion of measuring the patient's ability to hear speech is quite old, and we find in otologic practice a very widespread use of the voice and whisper tests, both in a room and through a speaking tube. More recently, however, the measurement of the ability to hear speech has been made more precise by introducing the kinds of control that are afforded by vacuum-tube equipment and the phonograph. Let us turn now to three basic measures of the ability to hear speech that are used in clinical practice.

Uncontrolled Speech Tests. Perhaps the adjective *uncontrolled* is too strong to describe the speech tests about to be reviewed, but in comparison with the more precise speech tests, to be described in the following section, it seems justified.

Most trained otologists have learned to speak numbers, words or sentences at a fairly fixed intensity in an open room. This somewhat nebulous constant level seems to be adequate to evoke repetition of the words spoken by a person with normal hearing standing about 20 ft away from the tester. When the same items are spoken in a whisper, a person with normal hearing can repeat them if he stands about 15 ft away.

Distance fractions have been used to express results from such tests of a patient's ability to hear speech. If, for example, a given patient cannot hear the spoken voice at 20 ft, but rather has to come to within 10 ft of the tester, his hearing for the spoken voice is said to be 10/20. His hearing for the whisper would be 6/15 if the tester must come to within 6 ft of the listener, instead of 15, when he is whispering.

The pitfalls of these crude tests have been mentioned briefly in Chap. 5. If one must use them, it is well that the room in which the test is done be free of flat reflecting surfaces. Rugs on the floor, drapes on the windows and walls, and absorbing material on the ceiling will help. Even if the reflecting surfaces have been eliminated, there remains the problem of the control of the intensity of the tester's voice or whisper. His variability can be overcome to some extent if he uses a monitoring meter in conjunction with a microphone, so that he has a visual indication of the intensity of his voice or whisper.

It should be remembered that, just as time is really an indirect measure of intensity in the tuning-fork test, so in these speech tests, distance is an indirect measure of intensity. If one tests in a 'perfect' room, for example, and finds that a patient requires a 10-ft distance instead of a 20-ft distance, he has actually found that the patient requires 4 times the energy (6 db more) required by a normal listener to hear the same items (see *inverse square law*, Chap. 2).

Many otologists find that the use of the speaking tube is extremely helpful in diagnostic work. The speaking tube has a definite advantage over the usual spoken-voice or whispered-voice test in that the acoustic properties of the room do not play a role. The problem of variability in the intensity of the voice or whisper is more severe, however, because the clinician attempts to vary this intensity either by controlling his breath or by varying the distance between his lips and the mouthpiece.

The acoustic-transmission characteristics of the speaking tubes that the author has examined are not at all constant for all frequencies. Rather these tubes show a peaked response at about 1000 cps. Thus the speaking tube appears to have a frequency-response characteristic that is similar to that of a poor hearing aid whose response shows a single high peak in the middle frequencies.

In connection with both the speaking-tube tests and tests that are conducted in an open room, it must also be pointed out that the frequencies that are *required for* the *intelligibility* of voiced speech are roughly the same as those required for whispered speech. The notion that the whisper tests high-frequency hearing while the voice tests low-frequency hearing is not tenable. One can say only that there is present more low-frequency energy in voiced speech than in whispered speech.

Hearing Loss for Speech. We must review next the methods for measuring the difference (in decibels) between the intensity of speech that is required by a patient in order to hear a certain percentage of the words and the intensity required by a normal listener to hear the same percentage (see also Chap. 5). In other words, we want a measure of the ability to hear speech that is comparable to the audiogram, a measure of the ability to hear pure tones. In both cases we are measuring a quantity called Hearing Loss, which we have defined as a difference (in decibels) between the intensity that a patient requires for a certain response and the intensity required by a normal listener for the same response. If we assume that the intensity at a listener's ear, 20 ft away from a speaker, is the normal intensity or threshold for the items of speech used, then the distance fraction, converted appropriately to intensity ratios and decibels, is a kind of measure of Hearing Loss for Speech.

We can measure this quantity more precisely, however, if the intensity of the speech can be controlled accurately and conveniently in steps of some multiple of the decibel. Equipment for doing just that is provided in the speech audiometer, which is described in Chap. 3 and specified in Appendix A.

The normal threshold of intelligibility is defined as the intensity at which a normal listener can repeat 50 per cent of the words spoken. Now we are interested in a test that will yield this 50-per-cent level quickly and reliably. Two groups of test items have been found particularly useful in this respect: two-syllable words with a spondaic stress pattern, and sentences. Examples of spondee words will be found in Appendix B.

The procedure for measuring the Hearing Loss for Speech may employ, as a source of speech, either the live voice of the tester or speech that has been recorded on a phonograph disc or magnetic tape. If live voice is used, precautions must be taken to provide the speaker with a visual indication of the intensity of his voice so that he may, with practice, monitor his voice and so keep his intensity constant. The control of the intensity of speech arriving at the listener's ear should be accomplished with attenuators in the equipment, not by varying the intensity of the speaker's voice. Fairly detailed procedures for carrying out the measurement of the Hearing Loss for Speech (with Auditory Tests No. 9 and

No. 12 of the Psycho-Acoustic Laboratory) are given by Hudgins *et al.* and by Hirsh (1947). Procedures are also detailed in manuals that are usually provided with the purchase of a recorded speech test (see Appendix B) or a speech audiometer. We shall outline only one procedure here.

For practical reasons, which have to do with the repeatibility of the results both from day to day and from place to place, it is recommended that where possible the Hearing Loss for Speech be measured with phonographically recorded speech. The author is most familiar with Auditory Tests No. 9, 12, and 14 of the Psycho-Acoustic Laboratory, Harvard University, and the more recent Auditory Tests No. W-1 and No. W-2 of the Central Institute for the Deaf. These latter tests have been prepared especially for distribution to clinical users and are intended, within this clinical frame of reference, to supplant Auditory Tests No. 9 and No. 14, which have been used widely in clinics up to the present time. Actually, tests W-1 and W-2 have been adapted from Auditory Tests No. 14 and No. 9, respectively. There will undoubtedly be other sources for similar recordings in the near future, when the newly written specifications for speech audiometers have their effect on the demand and supply of instruments and test material.

Some kind of meter must be used to indicate the intensity of the recorded speech that is delivered by the tester, in order that the intensity may be controlled. If one uses a record on which all words are recorded at the same level, one should begin by delivering the speech at an intensity that is high enough to permit the listener to repeat correctly almost all the words. The tester may then decrease the intensity (or increase the attenuation) until the patient repeats correctly approximately 50 per cent of the words. The difference between this level and the average level at which a group of normal listeners repeats 50 per cent of the words correctly is the Hearing Loss for Speech in decibels. When the speech material to be used for the measure has become standardized, it is hoped that the normal threshold of intelligibility will be incorporated as a O-db reference in the clinical speech audiometer, in much the same way as the different levels for different frequencies correspond to O-db Hearing Loss in the pure-tone audiometer.

Auditory Tests No. 9 (PAL) and No. W-2 (CID) both contain groups of spondee words that are recorded at successively lower levels. This is done to expedite the measurement of Hearing Loss—the tester need not decrease the intensity manually. He has only to set up an initial level that is high enough so that the patient repeats correctly all the words in the first group, and then an estimate of the threshold may be made on the basis of the total number of words that he hears throughout a period of decreasing intensity. Specific instructions for making this calculation are usually supplied with the test records. For Auditory Test No. 9 (PAL), complete instructions are given in Hudgins *et al.* In CID Auditory Test No. W-2, each successive three-word group is reduced in intensity by 3 db, so that each successive word represents a decrease of 1 db, on the average.

Discrimination Tests. The absolute threshold, either for pure tones or for speech, tells us how small a sound energy we may supply to a listener and still have him respond in a certain way. The diagnostic tests that we have discussed so far in this second main section tell us only about the absolute sensitivity to small energies in pure tones or in speech.

From this threshold information we can know how much Hearing Loss there is. And from the relation between the Hearing Loss for Speech and the Hearing Loss for pure tones at 500, 1000, and 2000 cps, we can know something of the consistency of the patient's response for two different kinds of stimuli. Furthermore, from the shape of the audiogram and the difference between the audiograms for air conduction and bone conduction, we can know whether the hearing loss has been caused by lesion in the conducting apparatus, peripheral to the oval window, or is due to a lesion in the cochlea or auditory nervous system. On the basis of this information alone, the otologist can make important diagnostic decisions.

But additional information is required before we can predict whether a patient will receive benefit from certain types of surgery, from a hearing aid, or from training. We want to know how a patient interprets sounds that are well above his threshold. Sometimes we may wish to know what loudness or pitch he might associate with a pure tone. And, in the case of speech, we wish to know how fine a discrimination he can make among speech sounds when the intensity in the speech sounds is no longer an important factor.

The ability to distinguish among the sounds of speech has been tested clinically by using lists of short, one-syllable words. Such lists were made up in connection with tests of communications equipment, during World War II, by members of the Psycho-Acoustic Laboratory of Harvard University. They have been called *phonetically balanced* lists, or more simply, PB lists (Egan). In general, each of these lists of 50 one-syllable words contains a distribution of consonant and vowel sounds that approximates the distribution of their relative occurrence in conversational American English.

These words are more difficult to repeat correctly than the spondees. For example, almost all listeners will, if the intensity is high enough eventually repeat 100 per cent of a list of spondees. But only some listeners will achieve an articulation score of 100 per cent on a PB list, even when the intensity is so high that a further increase in intensity will not increase the score. It is this maximum articulation score, or *discrimination score*, that is used as the clinical measure of discrimination. In other words, so far as present clinical usage is concerned, the PB lists are always presented at a high level, well above the threshold, and the measure that is obtained is one of the percentage of words repeated correctly. *Discrimination Loss* is not measured in decibels but rather is the difference between the percentage of words heard correctly by a patient and 100 per cent, a presumed maximum score for normal listeners.

The procedure for obtaining a measure of Discrimination Loss is extremely simple. A list, or preferably two, is presented at 100 db SPL (or sometimes 40 db above the threshold of intelligibility). If a patient gets 90 per cent or more correct, we may assume that his discrimination is normal; *i.e.*, a Discrimination Loss of 10 per cent or less is insignificant. When, however, a patient's articulation score at a high intensity is significantly less than 90, the Discrimination Loss becomes an important clinical datum.

Although some patients may not have reached the *ceiling* at 100 db SPL and may require the lists to be presented at 110 or 120 db before a true maximum is reached, we realize that such therapeutic measures as fenestration or a hearing aid cannot decrease this type of loss. These two kinds of therapy in particular serve only to make more intense the effective sound energy that produces displacement of the basilar membrane. And since we have already shown, in our maximum discrimination score, that an increase in intensity will not improve discrimination, we must conclude that these two kinds of therapy will not improve discrimination.

The diagnostic significance of Discrimination Loss remains to be worked out. It is apparent that a significant Discrimination Loss is associated with cases that also demonstrate recruitment, but there is not enough evidence to permit us to use a discrimination test as a means for indirectly detecting recruitment.

Over-all Estimate of a Person's Hearing

There are many practical situations in which it would be desirable for the clinician who measures hearing to be able to give a single number that would represent the total hearing ability of an individual. It was such a desire that prompted the formulation of a method for calculating the *percentage hearing loss for speech* from the audiogram, which was sponsored by the American Medical Association in 1942 and revised in 1947. Although this method has been used widely in recent years, its nature has been misunderstood by some who have used it.

In the first place, the percentage that is obtained from the audiogram by the AMA method has nothing to do with the percentage of words that a person would understand. Rather it represents the percentage of an individual's total hearing capacity that has been lost. There was no objective measure of this capacity presented at that time or since. Rather the estimates that went into the computation represent practical considered opinions of a group of experts with much clinical experience.

At the present time there seems to be nothing better to suggest for use in courts of law, industrial medicine, compensation boards, etc. where hearing has been lost in connection with a man's job and the responsibility* for this loss is thought to lie with the employer. Because of the fact that this AMA method is at the time of writing of this chapter under consideration for revision, it will not be presented in detail here.

It must be remembered that any estimate of hearing ability that is calculated from the audiogram cannot show differences in the ability to discriminate (see above), because there seems to be no easy relation between the discrimination of difficult words and the absolute threshold for pure tones.

The Social Adequacy Index for hearing, which was discussed in Chap. 5, represents a more recent attempt to assess a man's ability to hear with respect to everyday communication. The SAI is also a percentage, but this percentage is not intended to be related to a unidimensional total capacity to hear. Rather this percentage refers to the average percentage of words that will be repeated correctly by a listener at three levels, which correspond to weak, moderate, and loud conversation. Although a scale relating the SAI to a total capacity to hear might be set up arbitrarily, the SAI itself cannot be used directly for deciding such practical issues as how much a man should be paid for a certain amount or type of hearing loss.

Theoretically it is almost impossible to set up a scale in one dimension that will describe a man's ability to hear. This is because the ability to hear has several dimensions, among which are absolute sensitivity, the ability to discriminate different frequencies and different intensities of pure tones, the ability to discriminate among speech sounds, and the ability to detect signals in the presence of noise. If all these abilities were simply related and if each could be predicted from a knowledge of the other, a simple, single estimate of hearing might be used—and research on hearing would be simple indeed.

THERAPEUTIC EVALUATION

Having obtained as much diagnostic information as we can from such tests as have been described in the previous section and from the otologist's examination, we should be in a position to recommend to the patient what course of action he should follow in order to either overcome or compensate for his hearing loss. In general our recommendations for therapy are of three kinds: medical and surgical, prosthetic, and educational. Of course, it will be the medical or otologic member of the clinic who will make the final decision about medical treatment, including surgery, but he may wish to have the participation of a more diversely oriented clinician in making recommendations about a hearing aid or various kinds of training. It would be quite beyond the scope of this book to enumerate the different specific steps that are used in the therapy of hearing loss. Instead, let us take one example from each of the three kinds of therapy already mentioned and show how we might apply certain audiometric procedures in order to find out what benefit the therapy has produced.

Surgical Treatment

For many years, surgery has been the principal way in which otologists have treated deafness or hearing loss. Tonsillectomy, adenoidectomy, mastoidectomy, and other types of surgery having to do with infections of the respiratory system have been shown to alleviate certain types of hearing loss. The evaluation of the benefit to hearing that is brought about by any one of these surgical procedures may be exemplified by considering a more recent type of surgery, the fenestration operation.

When the hearing loss is fairly constant as a function of frequency, when the bone-conduction audiogram is near normal, and when additional clinical evidence establishes that a patient has otosclerosis, the patient may be advised to have the fenestration operation. The surgeon should be anxious to show what improvement the operation has brought about. We shall assume that before the operation we have obtained the following data: Hearing Loss (by both air and bone conduction) for pure tones at frequencies from 250 to 8000 cps, Hearing Loss for Speech, Discrimination Loss, and, perhaps, a negative result on any of the tests for recruitment.

After the operation, and preferably at several intervals of time up to several years, the same measurements can be made. A successful result is shown by a decrease in the Hearing Loss for pure tones and for speech of about 20 to 30 db. There is also some evidence that the threshold by bone conduction may change, but this change seems to be due rather to the change in the transmission characteristics of the skull than to a beneficial effect on the end organs or the nervous system.

It would be unusual indeed if the Discrimination Loss should change, but it may be that after a time, with his new lower threshold, the patient, having been exposed to more sounds, may learn better discrimination among speech sounds, and this may be evidenced by a decrease in the Discrimination Loss.

Detrimental changes in the cochlear structures may be evidenced by an increase in the Hearing Loss for high frequencies for both air and bone conduction, the appearance of more recruitment than was present before operation, or a further increase in the Discrimination Loss at a high intensity. As we shall see in the next paragraph, it is easier in some respects to evaluate the effects of a fenestration operation than to evaluate the benefit afforded by a hearing aid, because, in the case of a surgically treated ear, we may still deliver the sounds through earphones.

Selection of a Hearing Aid

The most common form of prosthetic therapy is the vacuum-tube hearing aid, which was described in Chap. 3. As in the case of the fenestration operation, this kind of therapy is designed to do only one thing: to bring more sound energy to the inner ear.

When we place a wearable hearing aid upon a patient, we have moved his ear from the side of his head to his chest or the lapel of a coat. We can no longer test his aided ear by placing an earphone over his ear—there is already an earphone there, which belongs to the hearing aid. In order to evaluate the hearing of a person who is wearing a hearing aid, we must produce our sounds in a room by means of a loud-speaker. This means, of course, that in order to compare this evaluation of aided hearing with that of the hearing before the hearing aid was put on, we must also have tested the hearing with the loud-speaker previously.

Although the use of a loud-speaker is necessary when conducting tests that measure the benefit provided by a hearing aid, its use is beset with many pitfalls. In general, the loud-speaker should be set up in a room that is quiet or free from outside noise and is also nonreflecting within its walls. Unless special construction can be obtained, the use of rugs, drapes, and other absorbing material is mandatory. The problems are similar to those that attend the use of the traditional spoken-voice and whisper tests. Even more caution, however, must be used in the case of a loud-speaker, because the clinician assumes more precision with electronic gear than with a single nonmonitored talker.

The effect of reflecting walls and other deficiencies in the acoustic properties of the testing room may be compensated for to a certain extent by placing the listener as close to the loud-speaker as possible. In this way the ratio of direct to reflected sound is kept high. The advantages to be enjoyed by having several yards between the listener and the loud-speaker can be sought only where the room is quite free from reflection.

Several test procedures may be used with a loud-speaker. The most difficult stimuli to handle are pure tones, because slight movements of the head or of the hearing aid may have profound effects on the results. It is not recommended, therefore, that the pure-tone threshold with and without the hearing aid should be measured in a sound field. Measurements of the hearing of speech, however, can be made more reliably, and these latter measurements are more important practically because the patient is going to use his hearing aid mostly to help him understand the speech of others.

Hearing Loss for Speech. Without a hearing aid, a patient should show the same Hearing Loss for Speech in the sound field as he did when the measurement was made with earphones. It must be remembered that a speech audiometer can be calibrated (*i.e.*, known to produce speech at a certain SPL in the ear canal) when earphones are used because the distance between the earphone and the ear canal does not vary appreciably. If a loud-speaker is substituted for the earphone, however, calibration must be made in the particular clinical situation, with the position of the loud-speaker and the listener held constant. If there is no sound-level meter available, one can make a relative calibration for a speech audiometer coupled to the loud-speaker.

It must also be remembered that the loud-speaker may have a different electrical impedance from that of the earphone, and also that the loud-speaker requires more electrical power than does the earphone. A loud-speaker cannot, therefore, simply be plugged into a receptacle that was designed to receive an earphone. Either an auxiliary circuit for the loud-speaker must have been provided by the manufacturer, or else additional elements must be provided. The relative calibration can be made by testing a group of listeners known to have normal hearing, one at a time, in the same position relative to the loud-speaker. Although the SPL at the ears of each of these listeners is not known, the reference voltage on a meter preceding the loud-speaker together with a certain number of decibels on the attenuators may be used as a clinical normal value.

The binaural Hearing Loss for Speech of a patient seated in the same position is then simply the difference between the decibels of attenuation at which he repeats correctly 50 per cent of the test items and the decibels of attenuation that were noted for the normal listeners. The voltage relative to which these attenuations are made must be kept constant.

Now, if we place a hearing aid on the patient and have him seated in the same position, we can measure a new Hearing Loss for Speech, which should be less than the unaided Hearing Loss by approximately the amount of amplification provided by the hearing aid.

One criterion on the basis of which a hearing aid is evaluated or is selected from a number of possible hearing aids is the reduction in the Hearing Loss for Speech measured in a sound field. There is one very serious complication in the use of this criterion for the selection of a hearing aid: the gain control of a hearing aid cannot be adjusted precisely in any easy manner. One suggestion that has been made is that the patient adjust the gain control of each hearing aid before the test in such a way that continuous discourse at 50 or 60 db SPL measured at the microphone of the hearing aid sounds "comfortably loud." Although this sounds like a very sensible way out of the problem, it is clear that the range of intensities that would be judged to be comfortably loud may be considerable. Another possibility that has been suggested for fixing the gain control of a hearing aid is to set it at some fraction of the total range of gain. For example, the gain control may be set at "full," "half," "three-quarters," or "one-quarter" volume and the test be run at one or several of these settings. This problem of how to adjust the gain control is probably the most troublesome part of the clinical evaluation of a hearing aid. Fortunately, however, it is a serious problem only for the measurement of the threshold of intelligibility or the Hearing Loss for Speech.

Discrimination Loss. Since the change of Hearing Loss for Speech that is brought about by the use of a hearing aid can be predicted fairly well from the knowledge of the over-all amplification provided by the hearing aid, it is less interesting, from the clinical point of view, than a measure of the change in discrimination that is provided by a hearing aid. It should be remembered from our discussion of the two dimensions of hearing for speech, which were discussed in Chap. 5 and illustrated in Fig. 5.16, that the hearing aid should affect only the intensity or Hearing Loss dimension. If all hearing aids amplified all frequencies equally well, this would actually be the case, and a change in discrimination should never be expected.

Most wearable hearing aids, however, do not amplify all frequencies equally well. Their frequency-response characteristics reveal unfortunate peaks at certain frequencies and practically no amplification for certain other frequencies. As we have already emphasized in Chap. 5, whenever a speech audiometer is used, the patient is actually trying out a hearing aid that has a better frequency-response characteristic than any wearable aid that he will ever encounter. In speech audiometry, for example, when we say that a man has a 40-db Hearing Loss for Speech, we really mean that if speech is brought to him at a level that is 40 db higher than normal he will respond as if his hearing were normal. When we test his discrimination with a speech audiometer for speech at 100 db SPL, we are quite sure that all the frequencies necessary for the intelligibility of speech are present. Since most wearable hearing aids transmit a narrower band of frequencies than that transmitted by most speech audiometers, we must find out which hearing aid reduces his discrimination least, or, in other words, which hearing aid brings him difficult speech at a sufficiently high level with the largest portion of his normal discrimination still remaining.

The procedure for comparing the unaided with the aided Discrimination Loss in a sound field is relatively easy to carry out, particularly because slight changes in intensity are not important. Before a hearing aid is tried, the patient is seated in the same standard position and listens to PB lists that are transmitted by the loud-speaker so as to produce approximately 100 db SPL at the ears of the listener. Then the patient may try several hearing aids, while seated in the same position, having adjusted the gain control so that the words are not intolerably loud.

If the intensity of the speech coming from the loud-speaker remains the same as it was before the patient put the hearing aid on, the amplified speech sounds in his ear canal may be of the order of 120 to 130 db. In order to keep the patient from turning the gain control of his hearing aid down to an unusably low level, the original speech may be attenuated by 30 or 40 db.

It will be found that the Discrimination Loss may be much lower than before, even at high intensities, particularly when we use a hearing aid that has a sharply peaked response. It is unusual to find that the Discrimination Loss for speech through a hearing aid is significantly less than the Discrimination Loss without a hearing aid, unless the unaided discrimination was measured at an intensity that lay below the patient's ceiling.

Educational Therapy

A major portion of the therapeutic part of clinical audiology is devoted to training. The training program has the over-all aim of allowing the patient to receive as much information from his fellows as his hearing and other senses will permit. For pedagogical reasons, the training is usually divided in three parts: speech reading (formerly lip reading), auditory training, and speech training. These three parts have to do, respectively, with receiving information through the visual system, receiving information through the auditory system, and transmitting information through the speech mechanism. The application of auditory measurement to such therapy is made most easily when we use auditory training as an example.

Before the auditory training is begun, we know the patient's Hearing Loss for Speech and his Discrimination Loss, both with and without a hearing aid. After several months of auditory training, we may wish to know how his hearing, and in particular his hearing for speech, has changed as a result of the auditory training.

Just as it is unusual for a hearing aid to change Discrimination Loss, so it is unusual for auditory training to change Hearing Loss for Speech. Most teachers of auditory training do not have the lowering of any thresholds as an aim. They do not propose to change the characteristics of the auditory system as such. Rather they hope only to increase the use that the patient makes of the auditory capacities that he already has. We have noted in previous discussions (especially Chap. 5) that there are no known surgical or prosthetic means of improving the discrimination score at a high intensity. It appears that the only way to improve this discrimination score is through auditory training. We cannot speculate on the mechanism of this change, but we have reports of some successfully trained patients who have shown reduction in Discrimination Loss after auditory training.

To evaluate this change clinically is really a part of the auditory training program. When the patient entered the clinic we measured the Discrimination Loss at 100 db SPL (or at a higher level if we had reason to believe that more intensity would improve the score). As training proceeds we may measure this same score over and over again at this same level. If the Discrimination Loss decreases significantly, the effect of the auditory training is considered to be favorable.

Discrimination Loss is only one particular clinical measure, having to do with the intelligibility of one-syllable words, which has been found useful in diagnostic audiometry. It is not, however, the only measurement that would be useful for the teacher of auditory training, because many more aspects of hearing may be and should be evaluated at the same time.

SUMMARY

We have attempted to describe the kinds of auditory measurement that are used in clinical practice. We have organized these procedures according to their function. Although there may be other important aspects of practice which we have neglected, the three testing functions that we have considered—namely, screening, diagnosis, and therapeutic evaluation—are basic.

The basic procedures have been developed within diagnostic audiometry. Screening tests and therapeutic evaluation have arisen as applications of several diagnostic procedures.

The reader who is interested in routine pure-tone audiometry may use this chapter and the last sections of Chap. 4 as a basis for reading more detailed instructions, such as are provided by the manufacturer of the audiometer. As we have repeated several times, all the problems are not solved, and the audiometrist who is interested in finding all the answers will be disappointed, no matter what rulebook he consults.

It seems fair to say that speech audiometry is just beginning to be used generally in clinical practice, in spite of the fact that much of the spadework has been going on at least since the late 1920's. In order to set up a useful program of speech audiometry, one may use the pertinent facts of this chapter and the practical sections of Chap. 5 as a basis for more detailed study.

It is to be hoped that the organization of the present material is such that the reader finds a unified approach to the over-all measurement of the auditory capacities of patients. Each type of measure that we have discussed in this and previous chapters must be somehow related to all the others. The future may reveal what some of these relations are, and this information will contribute immeasurably to our understanding of hearing and to our clinical proficiency.

SPECIFICATIONS FOR AUDIOMETERS

In order to acquaint the reader with the characteristics of an acceptable commercial audiometer, and also to permit him to know what features are considered essential by two responsible organizations, this Appendix will include specifications for audiometers as stated by the Council on Physical Medicine and Rehabilitation of the American Medical Association (AMA) and by the American Standards Association (ASA).

Three types of audiometers will be specified. The most general is the pure-tone audiometer that is used for diagnostic purposes. More recently, specifications have also been drawn up for a pure-tone screening audiometer and for a speech audiometer.

The AMA specifications tell the prospective purchaser of an audiometer what characteristics that audiometer must have in order to be accepted by the AMA Council. The names of those audiometers that were found acceptable as of June 1, 1951, are included after the specifications.

The second part of this Appendix represents specifications for the diagnostic pure-tone audiometer as stated by the American Standards Association. In principle, there is no difference between the specifications of the ASA and those of the AMA, but the ASA specifications give more detailed information. (At the time of this writing, the ASA Standards for speech audiometers and for screening audiometers were in the final stages of being adopted.)

The *normal threshold of audibility*, which is left undefined in the Glossary, will be found in these specifications for particular earphones.

PART I. SPECIFICATIONS OF THE COUNCIL ON PHYSICAL MEDICINE AND REHABILITATION OF THE AMERICAN MEDICAL ASSOCIATION

Minimum Requirements for Acceptable Pure Tone Audiometers for Diagnostic Purposes*

An audiometer is a device used to measure sensitivity of hearing. The particular type of audiometer with which this specification is concerned is the pure tone audiometer designed for general diagnostic use with individual subjects. This specification has been prepared with the objective that the measurements obtained on any audiometer shall truly represent a comparison of a person's auditory threshold at prescribed frequencies with the corresponding normal thresholds. A hearing test of a given person on all audiometers designed in accordance with the standards should yield substantially the same results when performed under similar conditions of ambient noise.

The normal threshold of hearing at a given frequency is the modal value of the minimum sound pressure, at the entrance to the external auditory canal, which at that frequency produces a sensation of pitch in a large number of normal ears of persons in the age group from 18 to 30 years, inclusive. The threshold of hearing is measured by presenting tones of successively greater or less intensity to a listener.

1. GENERAL REQUIREMENTS

(*a*) The audiometer shall be an electroacoustic generator, with associated earphone and bone conduction receiver, which provides pure tones of selected frequencies covering a considerable portion of the auditory range. The frequency and intensity shall be controllable. A device for interrupting the tone shall be provided.

(*b*) The audiometer shall operate by electrical power from one or more of the following sources: battery power supply, direct current at line voltage of 117 volts and alternating current at 60 cycles per second and 117 volts, or such supply as regional requirements demand. Tests for compliance with the requirements of Section 2 shall be made at line voltages of 105 and 125 volts or at the extremes of the usable range of battery voltages recommended by the manufacturer or at the voltage required by regional demands. Tests for compliance with the requirement of Sections 3, 4, 5, 6 and 7 shall be made at a line voltage of 117 volts or at the battery voltage recommended as operating voltage by the manufacturer.

(*c*) In a battery-operated instrument some means of determining when the loaded limiting battery voltage has been reached must be provided.

(*d*) The audiometer shall have a nameplate giving the manufacturer's name, the serial number, the voltage and frequency (or frequencies) of the power supply, and the power consumed by the audiometer.

(*e*) A spring headband shall be provided to hold the earphone or earphones firmly against the ear. Cushions and/or other coverings for the earphone and the

* Reprinted with permission from *J. Am. Med. Assoc.*, **146**(3), 255–257, May 19, 1951.

spring tension shall be designed with due consideration of (1) acoustic seal, (2) comfort, (3) ease of rapid and accurate placement and removal, (4) ease of cleaning and (5) maintenance of the proper size of cavity for which the earphone is calibrated. If only one earphone is provided, a dummy earphone with proper cushion or covering to cover and close the opposite ear shall be provided and suitably marked. The headband shall be easily and rapidly adjustable to fit the heads of adults or children.

2. FREQUENCIES

(a) The audiometer shall produce at least the following definitely identified frequencies: 125, 250, 500, 1,000, 2,000 and 4,000 cycles per second for both air and bone conduction measurements, and also 8,000 cycles per second for air conduction measurements. Dials shall be marked so that frequencies in cycles per second can be easily read.

(b) Each frequency generated by the audiometer shall have a value within ±5.0 per cent of the corresponding frequency reading.

3. INTENSITY INTERVAL AND INTENSITY RANGES FOR AIR CONDUCTION

(a) The readings of the intensity dial or scale shall be hearing loss readings; i.e., when the intensity dial is set at zero the intensity of the tone produced shall be at the normal threshold of hearing for that frequency as defined in Section 4a, and other readings shall indicate the ratio, expressed in decibels, of the intensity of the test tone to the corresponding normal threshold of hearing. Values of hearing loss for air and for bone conduction shall be clearly differentiated.

(b) Hearing loss readings shall extend from 10 decibels below threshold by intervals of 5 decibels or less up to at least the values given in Table 1.

TABLE 1. VALUE FOR HEARING LOSS READINGS

Frequency, cps	Hearing loss readings in decibels above normal threshold
125	65
250	80
500	85
1,000	95
2,000	95
4,000	90
8,000	75

(c) At each of the foregoing frequencies the measured difference (in decibels) of the intensity levels corresponding to any two graduations of the intensity dial shall agree with the indicated difference in hearing loss readings within 1.5 decibels. Thus for a 5 decibel interval on the intensity dial, the measured difference in intensity levels shall not be less than 3.5 decibels or more than 6.5 decibels. The difference in the intensity levels shall be determined by measurement of the voltage levels at the input of the earphone with the earphone coupled to the National Bureau of Standards Coupler 9-A or its acoustic equivalent.*

4. SOUND-PRESSURE OUTPUT OF THE EARPHONE

(a) The sound-pressure produced by the earphone at each hearing loss reading shall not differ from the indicated value, as referred to normal threshold, by more than 4.0 decibels at the indicated frequencies of 125, 250, 500, 1,000 and 2,000 or by more than 5.0 decibels at 4,000 and 8,000 cycles per second. Measurements of sound-pressure output shall be made with the earphone coupled to the National Bureau of Standards Coupler 9-A or its acoustic equivalent. The sound pressures in Coupler 9-A corresponding to normal threshold have been determined by the National Bureau of Standards for several types of earphones. For other types the methods of comparison advised by the National Bureau of Standards or specified by the American Standards Association, Inc., shall be employed. When an audiometer is submitted for acceptance the manufacturer shall inform the Council what type of earphone is employed. For Western Electric Type 705-A earphone the threshold pressures, determined by loudness balancing with the earphones used in the National Health Survey Hearing Study, are given in Table 2.

(b) The normal thresholds for any indicated frequencies other than those listed in Table 2 shall be obtained by graphic interpolation on a smooth curve drawn through the normal threshold values determined by the National Bureau of Standards for the appropriate type of earphone. If the National Bureau of Standards performs such an interpolation, the values which it derives shall be employed. If additional frequencies between 125 and 8,000 cycles per second are indicated as test frequencies, the standard of accuracy established in the first sentence of this section shall be maintained, i.e., ±4.0 decibels relative to the values given by the National Bureau of Standards for frequencies of 2,000 cycles per second or less and ±5.0 decibels for frequencies above 2,000 cycles per second. The manufacturer shall indicate clearly on the instrument that hearing loss readings for frequencies above 8,000 cycles per second are only rough approximations.

* The National Bureau of Standards Coupler 9-A has been used by audiometer manufacturers and the National Bureau of Standards as a standard coupler for many years. Its volume is approximately 6 cc. Recently the American Standards Association, Inc., has issued American Standard Z24.9-1949, in which a coupler designated American Standards Association Type 1 is recommended. Adaptation of the American Standards Association Type 1 Coupler, or of any other coupler, to the different earphones supplied by audiometer manufacturers involves research, and consequently the issuance of this standard would be delayed by one or more years, if any coupler other than No. 9-A were to be incorporated into the standard. The American Standards Association, Inc., plans to rewrite American Standard Z24.9-1949 as soon as the basic research has been completed. The industry and the requirements of the Council on Physical Medicine and Rehabilitation will then change gradually from the National Bureau of Standards Coupler 9-A to a standard coupler approved by the American Standards Association. The phrase "or its acoustical equivalent" in the present requirements is intended to include any standard coupler approved by the American Standards Association as a substitute for or replacement of the National Bureau of Standards Coupler 9-A.

(*c*) The sound-pressure produced by the receiver at each specified frequency when the instrument is set to the 60 decibels hearing loss readings shall not vary by more than ±1 decibel as the line voltage is varied through the range from 105 to 125 volts.

(*d*) The sound-pressure output of an audiometer shall be measured directly at the hearing loss settings of 60 decibels. It shall be measured with the receiver coupled to the National Bureau of Standards Coupler 9-A or its acoustic equivalent. If appropriate apparatus is available for measuring acoustic pressure down to 40 decibels or less above 0.0002 dyne per square centimeter, the direct measurement of acoustic pressure is the preferred method for obtaining the sound-pressure output at other hearing loss settings. An alternative method is to combine the pressures measured at 60 decibels with the results of the measurements of hearing loss intervals.

TABLE 2. THRESHOLD PRESSURES FOR WESTERN ELECTRIC TYPE 705-A RECEIVER

Frequency, cps	Root-mean-square sound pressure in decibels above 1 dyne/cm²
125	−19.5
250	−34.4
500	−49.2
1,000	−57.3
2,000	−57.0
4,000	−58.9
8,000	−53.1

(*e*) If two or more earphones, substantially similar in appearance and interchangeable in their connections, are furnished with a pure tone audiometer, each earphone must meet the "minimum requirements" even when connected to either output, if two outputs are provided. If a clear color code or else a connector that will not allow connection of an earphone to the wrong circuit is provided, the output of each earphone need meet the specifications of Section 4 only when the earphone is connected to its intended circuit.

5. PURITY OF TEST TONES OF THE EARPHONE

The sound pressure of the fundamental signal shall be at least 25 decibels above that of any harmonic when measured with the earphone coupled to the National Bureau of Standards Coupler 9-A or its acoustic equivalent. The harmonics shall be measured at the frequencies and hearing loss settings listed in Section 3*b*, even though the manufacturer may provide a maximum intensity higher than is specified in that section.

6. NOISE

(*a*) The root-mean-square weighted sound pressure due to all frequencies except the signal frequency and its harmonics shall be either less than 1.0 by 10^{-3} dyne per square centimeter or at least 60 decibels below the sound pressure due to the signal frequency and its harmonics at all specifically designated frequencies and hearing loss dial settings. This measurement shall be performed with the interrupter switch in the "off" position. The other conditions of this measurement and the relative weights employed in the calculation shall be those specified by the American Standards Association, Inc., for this purpose (American Standard Z24.9-1949 and American Standard for Audiometers for General Diagnostic Purposes, if and when adopted).

(b) If an audiometer is provided with two or more earphones the signal in any earphone for which the switch is set to "off" should be at least 10 decibels below the normal threshold for a signal of that frequency. This test should be applied, by a listener (or listeners) with appropriately acute hearing, with the audiometer set for 60 decibels hearing loss and at all of the frequencies specified in Section 2.

(c) Neither the bone conduction receiver nor any other part of the audiometer shall radiate sound to such an extent that the sound reaching the tympanum through the auditory meatus might influence the validity of the bone conduction measurement. As judged by an observer with normal hearing, the sound received at the ear by air radiation from the audiometer shall have a sensation level at least 5 decibels below the level which the receiver generates by bone conduction when in contact with the head.

This test of sound radiation from the bone conduction receiver shall be performed by determining the bone conduction threshold in the usual way, and then, with the bone conduction receiver held in approximately the same position as in the threshold measurement, but with the driver element or contact area of the receiver resting on the soft flesh at the end of the operator's finger and with coverage comparable to that provided by contact with the mastoid, the threshold at which any auditory sensation is perceived shall be noted. Care must be taken that no direct contact be made between the finger and skull. The threshold of auditory sensation shall be at least 5 decibels above the direct bone conduction threshold. A jury of at least six persons with hearing losses for air-borne sound not greater than 10 decibels at the frequencies employed shall perform the test and the mean of their results taken. The above test is not required at frequencies above 2,000 cycles per second.

7. TONE INTERRUPTER

An audiometer shall be equipped with a device for turning the tone on and off without introducing an objectionable click (i.e., transient extraneous frequencies, audible to a normal ear) in the receiver.

8. AUDIOGRAM BLANKS

If the manufacturer supplies with his instrument blanks for plotting measured hearing losses, these blanks shall comply with the following specifications: The blank shall be ruled with rectangular coordinates, with frequencies in cycles per second on a logarithmic scale as the abscissas and hearing loss in decibels on a linear scale as the ordinates. Frequencies shall be shown by vertical lines equally spaced at octave intervals. (For an instrument that produces test tones at intermediate frequencies, vertical lines to correspond to these frequencies should appear at the proper fractional parts of the octave intervals.)

Normal hearing for both air-borne and bone-conducted sounds shall be indicated by a single horizontal line marked 0 (zero), near the top of the blank. "Hearing loss in decibels" shall be indicated by horizontal lines, equally spaced at 10 decibel intervals and numbered downward from the 0 line. One octave on the frequency scale shall be the same distance as 20 decibels on the hearing loss scale.

9. SHOCK HAZARD

Audiometers shall be free from electric shock hazard. A shock hazard shall be considered to exist at an exposed live part if the open circuit potential is more than 25 volts and the current with a 1,500 ohm load is more than 5 milliamperes.

10. GUARANTIES

The manufacturer shall make to the purchasers the following guaranties:

(a) Any defect other than those due to accident or damage from improper use that may appear within a period of one year from date of purchase will be corrected and the instrument recalibrated at no cost to the purchaser except for transportation charges; replaceable parts which may deteriorate with use, such as vacuum tubes, shall, by agreement, be supplied at reasonable cost.

(b) The maker will provide adequate instructions for the proper care and upkeep of his products and will encourage the purchaser to send his audiometer at reasonable intervals to the factory or to a qualified distributor for check as to performance and needed servicing at a reasonable cost.

11. MARKETING AND ADVERTISING

Rules of the Council on Physical Medicine and Rehabilitation shall be adhered to by manufacturers of acceptable audiometers.

RECOMMENDATIONS FOR PURE TONE AUDIOMETERS FOR DIAGNOSTIC PURPOSES

The following features are not required, but they are recommended for the guidance of manufacturers.

1. GENERAL

(a) Two earphones should be provided, and a switch on the operating panel that allows the operator to transfer the test tone from one ear to the other. Each of the two earphones should meet the requirements for accuracy of sound-pressure output.

(b) A battery-operated instrument should be provided with a device that will insure that the batteries are turned off when the instrument is closed or covered for transportation.

2. FREQUENCIES

If test tones in addition to the series 125, 250, 500, 1,000, 2,000, 4,000 and 8,000 are provided, the preferred frequencies are 1,500, 3,000, 6,000 and 12,000.

3. TONE INTERRUPTER

(*a*) The interrupter should operate either as normally "on" or normally "off" at the choice of the operator.

(*b*) The acoustic output should reach a level within 1 decibel of its final level not sooner than 0.01 second and not later than 0.5 second after the interrupter switch is operated for "on." The output should not overshoot its final level by more than 1 decibel. The test tone should decay at least 20 decibels and preferably more within 0.5 second after the interrupter switch is operated for "off."

4. BONE CONDUCTION THRESHOLDS

(*a*) A spring headband or other device for regulating the force of application of the bone conduction receiver to the mastoid is highly desirable.

(*b*) A recommended procedure for establishing the normal threshold of hearing for bone-conducted sound as measured by a particular audiometer is as follows: Determine at each frequency the intensity level, as measured by the hearing loss setting of the audiometer, which can just be heard when the bone conduction receiver is pressed firmly against the mastoid just back of the ear of each of 6 subjects with hearing losses at the frequencies employed of not more than 10 decibels by air conduction. The ear canal shall not be occluded during these measurements. The mean of the six measurements at any frequency is taken as the normal threshold for bone-conducted sound of that frequency. All measurements specified in this section are to be made in a room free from extraneous sound of sufficient intensity to vitiate the measurements. Acceptance tests on this requirement may follow the same procedure.

5. MASKING NOISE

Provision for masking noise is highly desirable. The noise should have a wide acoustic spectrum, at least from the lowest to the highest frequencies indicated for measurement of hearing loss by bone conduction. The noise should be delivered to the ear through an earphone and the intensity should be calibrated over a range of effective masking of at least 40 decibels. The loudest level should be about 60 decibels above the level that in a normal ear will just mask a tone of threshold intensity at 1,000 cycles per second (Table 2). An intensity scale showing relative levels at 5 decibel intervals should be provided.

Audiometers for Diagnostic Purposes Accepted as of June 1, 1951

Maico Audiometer, Model D-5. *J. Am. Med. Assoc.* **114,** 139, Jan. 13, 1940.
Maico Audiometer, Model D-8. *J. Am. Med. Assoc.* **120,** 205, Sept. 19, 1942.
Maico Audiometer, Model D-9. *J. Am. Med. Assoc.* **138,** 428, Oct. 9, 1948.
Maico Audiometer, Model D-10. *J. Am. Med. Assoc.* **144,** 315, Sept. 23, 1950.
Maico Audiometer, Model H-1. Report not yet published.
Maico F-1 Portable Audiometer, Model 36-M. Report not yet published.
Mfr: The Maico Company, Inc.
    21 N. 3rd St.
    Minneapolis 1

Microtone ADC Audiometer, Model 53-C1. *J. Am. Med. Assoc.* **144**, 1375, Dec. 16, 1950.
Mfr: The Microtone Company
    Ford Parkway on the Mississippi
    St. Paul 1
Sonotone Audiometer, Model 20. *J. Am. Med. Assoc.* **124**, 94, Jan. 8, 1944.
Sonotone Audiometer, Model 21. *J. Am. Med. Assoc.* **139**, 1079, April 16, 1949.
Mfr: Sonotone Corporation
    Elmsford, N.Y.
Western Electric Audiometer, Model 6BP. *J. Am. Med. Assoc.* **114**, 1634, April 27, 1940.
Mfr: Audivox, Inc. Successor to
    Western Electric Hearing
    Aid Division
    259 W. 14th St.
    New York 11

Minimal Requirements for Acceptable Pure Tone Audiometers for Screening Purposes*

An audiometer is a device used to measure the response of the hearing mechanism (human) to sounds of different measured intensities. These requirements and recommendations are concerned with the pure tone audiometer used for screening purposes. "Screening" is the detection of hearing losses greater than some minimum amount. It is not intended that medical diagnosis should be based on screening measurements, but merely that persons should be assigned to groups according to auditory sensitivity.

1. GENERAL REQUIREMENTS

(*a*) Except as otherwise specified, an audiometer for screening purposes must meet all of the minimal requirements for acceptable pure tone audiometers for diagnostic purposes.

(*b*) An audiometer for screening purposes must carry on its operating panel an easily legible label clearly designating the instrument as "screening audiometer" or "for screening purposes only."

(*c*) A spring head band shall be provided to hold the earphone or earphones firmly enough against the ear to insure an acoustic seal. Cushions and/or other coverings for the earphone and the spring tension shall be designed with due consideration of (1) acoustic seal, (2) comfort, (3) ease of rapid and accurate placement and removal, (4) ease of cleaning and (5) maintenance of the proper size of cavity for which the earphone is calibrated. If only one earphone is provided, a dummy earphone with proper cushion or covering to cover and close the opposite ear shall be provided and suitably marked. The head band shall be easily and rapidly adjustable to fit the heads of adults or children.

* Reprinted with permission from *J. Am. Med. Assoc.*, **144**(6), 465, Oct. 7, 1950.

2. FREQUENCIES

The audiometer shall produce at least the four following definitely identified frequencies: 500, 1,000, 2,000 and 4,000 cycles per second.

3. INTENSITY RANGE

Hearing loss readings shall extend from zero (at normal threshold) to 60 decibels by intervals of 5 decibels.

4. SOUND PRESSURE OUTPUT

The sound pressure produced by the receiver at each hearing loss reading shall not differ from the indicated value, as referred to normal threshold, by more than 4.0 decibels at the indicated frequencies of 500, 1,000 and 2,000 or by more than 5.0 decibels at 4,000 cycles per second. Measurements shall be made as specified in the Minimum Requirements for Acceptable Pure Tone Audiometers, *The Journal*, July 30, 1949, p. 1095 (revision in press). The sound pressures corresponding to normal thresholds as specified for acceptable pure tone audiometers for diagnostic purposes shall be employed.

5. STABILITY OF OUTPUT

(*a*) The acoustic output of the instrument shall not vary through a total range of more than 2 decibels with variations in line voltage over the ranges specified for audiometers for diagnostic purposes or as the voltage of the batteries of a battery-operated instrument varies within the limits recommended by the manufacturers. Measurements for this requirement shall be made at the 60 decibel hearing loss setting and the 1,000 cycles per second frequency setting by the method specified for audiometers for diagnostic purposes.

(*b*) In a battery-operated instrument there must be some means of determining when the loaded limiting battery voltage has been reached.

6. PURITY OF TEST TONES

The purity of the test tones shall be measured at the 60 decibel hearing-loss setting at the four indicated frequencies specified in Section 2.

7. BONE CONDUCTION

A bone conduction receiver is not required.

8. AUDIOGRAM BLANKS

Audiogram blanks are not required.

RECOMMENDATIONS FOR PURE TONE AUDIOMETERS FOR SCREENING PURPOSES

The following features are not required, but they are recommended for the guidance of manufacturers.

1. GENERAL

(*a*) Two earphones should be provided, with a switch on the operating panel that allows the operator to transfer the test tone from one ear to the other. Each of the two earphones should meet the requirements for accuracy of sound-pressure output.

(*b*) A battery-operated instrument should be provided with a device that will insure that the batteries are turned off when the instrument is closed or covered for transportation.

2. FREQUENCIES

If test tones in addition to the series 500, 1,000, 2,000 and 4,000 cycles per second are provided, the frequencies recommended are 250 and 6,000 cycles per second.

If additional test tones beyond the four specified as the minimum are provided, the requirements for accuracy of sound pressure output need not be met at the additional frequencies, but it is expected that manufacturers will make every reasonable effort to maintain the same standard of accuracy at all indicated frequencies.

3. NOISE

If an audiometer is provided with two or more earphones the signal in any earphone for which the switch is set to "off" should be at least 10 decibels below the normal threshold for a signal of that frequency. This test should be applied, by an observer (or observers) with appropriately acute hearing, with the audiometer set for 60 decibel hearing loss and at all of the specified frequencies.

4. TONE INTERRUPTER

The interrupter should operate either as normally on or normally off at the choice of the operator. The objective of the interrupter is to establish and to eliminate the test tone as rapidly and promptly as possible without producing an audible click or a transient.

Audiometers for Screening Purposes Accepted as of June 1, 1951

Maico Model RS Group Phonographic Audiometer. *J. Am. Med. Assoc.* **137,** 1535, Aug. 21, 1948.
Mfr: The Maico Company, Inc.
21 N. 3rd St.
Minneapolis 1

Microtone ADC Audiometer. Model 53-A. *J. Am. Med. Assoc.* **146,** 338, May 26, 1951.
Mfr: The Microtone Company
Ford Parkway on the Mississippi
St. Paul 1

Sonotone Screening Audiometer, Model 30. *J. Am. Med. Assoc.* **145,** 33, Jan. 6, 1951.
Mfr: Sonotone Corporation
Elmsford, N.Y.

Western Electric Audiometer, Model 4C. *J. Am. Med. Assoc.* **118,** 1297, April 11, 1942.

Western Electric Audiometer, Model 4CA. *J. Am. Med. Assoc.* **139**, 99, Jan. 8, 1949.

Mfr: Audivox, Inc. Successor to
    Western Electric Hearing
    Aid Division
    259 W. 14th St.
    New York 11

Minimal Requirements for Acceptable Speech Audiometers*

1. SCOPE

Several diagnostic tests of hearing are based on the ability of a listener correctly to repeat or write down words or sentences delivered to him at known acoustic levels. To standardize these tests of hearing it is necessary to specify both the test material, *i.e.*, the words or sentences, their manner of presentation, the acoustic levels to be employed, etc., and also the apparatus to be employed for the presentation. The present specification deals only with the apparatus for delivering such speech tests to the listener, with the general objectives (*a*) that the speech sounds that reach the listener's ear shall be a faithful reproduction, within specified limits of tolerance, of the original spoken or recorded material and (*b*) that the sound pressure levels at which the speech sounds reach the listener's ear shall be known and controllable within specified limits. Such an apparatus is designated a "speech audiometer for diagnostic purposes." With such an instrument and employing appropriate spoken or recorded material it is possible to determine both the "hearing loss for speech" and the "discrimination loss for speech."† The "speech audiometer for diagnostic purposes" which is the subject of this specification is intended for testing one individual at a time and should be distinguished from "screening speech audiometers" designed for rapid approximate testing of large groups of persons simultaneously.

It is anticipated that separate specifications covering suitable test material, and particularly covering recordings of test material, will be prepared at a later date. Certain assumptions concerning these anticipated specifications are evident in this specification.

The normal threshold for speech, sometimes known as the "speech reception threshold," depends not only on the average sensitivity of normal human ears but also on the characteristics of the test material employed, the voice of the speaker and the electroacoustic characteristics of the speech audiometer. One objective of the present specification is to standardize the latter so that when the test material, the characteristics of the recording system, etc., are also specified, a value for the normal threshold for speech, in decibels relative to a standard acoustic reference level, can be determined experimentally. Until such standardization is completed the normal threshold for speech must be determined empirically for each voice and each recording and for each form of speech test.

* Reprinted with permission from *J. Am. Med. Assoc.* (In press).

† These concepts are more fully defined in an article by H. Davis, "The Articulation Area and the Social Adequacy Index for Hearing," *The Laryngoscope*, **58**, (8) 761–778.

2. Definitions

The essential elements of a speech audiometer are (1) a source of speech, either (a) the voice of the operator or (b) a recording, usually a phonograph disc or a magnetic tape, (2) a transducer appropriate to the source; *i.e.*, a microphone, a turntable and phonograph pickup, or a magnetic-tape playback, (3) an amplifier, (4) a meter or other device for monitoring the output of the amplifier to a known or predetermined level, (5) an attenuator, (6) a calibrated earphone or earphones.

A speech audiometer may be a pure tone audiometer (ASA Standard Z24.5-1951) that is provided with an appropriate microphone or playback device and a proper meter or other monitor.

A "recorded-speech audiometer" is a speech audiometer that is provided with a turntable and electrical pickup or a magnetic-tape playback, etc., for use with recorded test material. A "live-voice audiometer" is a speech audiometer that is provided with a microphone for use with the voice of the operator.

The "hearing loss for speech" of an ear is the ratio, expressed in decibels, of the threshold for speech for that ear, determined by an appropriate form of speech test, to the normal threshold for speech determined for that same speech test administered in the same manner.

The "discrimination for speech" or "articulation score" of an ear is the percentage of items in an appropriate form of test, usually monosyllabic words, that is correctly repeated, written down or checked by the listener. This form of test is usually administered at an acoustic level well above the threshold for speech. The normal value of discrimination (or articulation score) for each test must be determined empirically. The "discrimination loss" is the difference, in percentage points, between the normal score for the test and the score obtained for the ear under test.

3. Requirements

General. The general features listed in Section 1.2 shall be provided. A speech audiometer may be a recorded-speech audiometer or a live-voice audiometer or both. No bone conduction receiver is required. No interrupter is required.

Power Supply. The audiometer shall operate by electrical power from one or more of the following sources: battery power supply, direct current at line voltage of 117 volts, alternating current at 60 cps and 117 volts, or such supply as regional requirements demand. The tests specified in Section 3.7 (absolute calibration) shall be made at line voltages of 105 and 125 volts or at the extremes of the usable range of battery voltages recommended by the manufacturer or at proportional voltages above and below those required by regional demands. Tests for compliance with other requirements shall be made at the nominal voltages recommended by the manufacturer.

Battery-operated Instrument. In a battery-operated instrument some means of determining when the loaded limiting battery voltage has been reached must be provided.

Nameplate. The audiometer shall have a nameplate giving the manufacturer's name, the model number, the serial number, the voltage and frequency (or frequencies) of the power supply, and the power consumed by the audiometer.

Headband and Cushions. A spring headband shall be provided to hold the earphone or earphones firmly against the ear. Cushions and/or other coverings for the earphone and the spring tension shall be designed with due consideration of (1) acoustic seal, (2) comfort, (3) ease of rapid and accurate placement and removal, (4) ease of cleaning, and (5) maintenance of the proper size of cavity for which the earphone is calibrated. If only one earphone is provided a dummy earphone with proper cushion or covering to cover and close the opposite ear shall be provided and suitably marked. The headband shall be easily and rapidly adjustable to fit the heads of adults or children.

Earphones. If two or more earphones, substantially identical in appearance and interchangeable in their connections, are furnished with a speech audiometer, each earphone must meet the requirements of over-all acoustic fidelity (3.2) and of distortion (3.6). If a clear color code or else a connector that will not allow connection of an earphone to the wrong circuit is provided, the output of each earphone need meet these specifications only when the earphone is connected to its intended circuit.

If two earphones are provided, a contact shall also be provided on the panel of the instrument whereby the output can be delivered to one or the other earphone. The signal from the earphone nominally "Off" shall be 10 db. below the normal threshold for speech or at least 65 db. below the signal from the receiver nominally "On."

If more than one earphone is provided and the earphones can be disconnected from the main instrument, the output from any earphone remaining connected shall not vary by more than $\frac{1}{2}$ db. when another earphone is disconnected.

Playback and Pickup:

Turntable and Pickup for Phonographic Recordings. In a recorded-speech audiometer a turntable of $33\frac{1}{3}$ rpm shall be provided. A turntable capable of 78.26 and 45 rpm in addition is very desirable. The pickup shall exert a maximum force of not more than 10 grams and shall be supplied with a stylus made of a whole diamond ground so as not to be easily fractured.

Magnetic-tape Playback. If a magnetic-tape playback is provided, it shall be capable of playing tape at speeds of $7\frac{1}{2}$ and 15 inches per second.

Amplifier. An amplifier shall be provided to raise the signal level high enough to produce the necessary sound-pressure output from the earphone. Its performance is adequately specified below in the requirements for over-all acoustic fidelity, necessary output, etc., laid down for the system as a whole.

Provision shall be made for continuous adjustment of the *gain* of the amplifier to accommodate differences of ± 10 db. in the absolute level at which the calibrating tone may be recorded.

Monitor. In a recorded-speech audiometer, a meter or equivalent indicator shall be provided to register the attainment of an appropriate reference level (see Sec. 3.7) with a relative accuracy of ± 1 db. when a calibrating tone of 1000 cps, assumed to be recorded on each disc or tape, is played through the pickup and amplifier. The sensitivity of the meter need only be such as to allow clear indication of the desired reference level. The meter shall be connected immediately ahead of the calibrated attenuator.

In a live-voice audiometer, a VU meter (ASA. Specification No. C165-1942) shall be connected to allow the operator to monitor his voice to an appropriate reference level (see Sec. 3.7) measured at the input to the main attenuator. The amount of amplification provided shall be such that the meter will indicate the required reference level when the operator speaks the phrase: "You will say" in a natural conversational voice at a distance of 6 to 12 inches from the microphone, *according to the calibration employed*. (See Section 3.2.3.) A continuously variable adjustment of the *gain* of the amplifier should be provided, as in a recorded-speech audiometer, to allow adjustment to the voices of different operators.

Attenuator. An attenuator shall be provided with maximum insertion loss of 110 db. with indicated steps of 5 db. *or less. If the indicated steps are 5 db.*, an accessory vernier attenuator with steps of 2 db. or 1 db. and a maximum insertion loss of 10 db. is very desirable.

Each measured difference between the outputs at successive steps of the attenuator shall be not more than 6.5 or less than 3.5 *db. for each indicated interval of 5 db.* The intervals shall be determined by measurement of the voltage at the input to the earphone with the earphone coupled to a National Bureau of Standards 9-A coupler. (See American Standard Z24.5-1951.) The signal shall be a 1000 cps tone.

The measured difference in outputs between any two settings of the attenuator dial shall not differ from the indicated difference by more than ±3.0 db.

Over-all Acoustic Fidelity:

Recorded-speech Audiometer. The response characteristic of a recorded-speech audiometer shall conform to the reproducing standards of the National Association of Radio and Television Broadcasters* within ±5 db. throughout the frequency band 200 to 5000 cps. From 50 to 200 and from 5000 to 10,000 cps the response characteristic of the audiometer may fall below the NARTB standard, but it shall not rise above the standard by more than 5 db. It is implied that the electrical pickup or magnetic-tape playback will be provided with an appropriate equalizing network.

NARTB Reproducing Standard:

The NARTB reproducing standard for lateral recording, relating relative stylus velocity to frequency, is adequately defined by the points in Table 1, based on the NARTB Recording and Reproducing Standards of June, 1950.

Test of Response Characteristic. In determining the over-all acoustic fidelity the output shall be measured as the sound-pressure level developed in a coupler similar to a National Bureau of Standards 9-A coupler. (See Fig. 1 in American Standard Z24.5-1951 or latest revision thereof.)

Live-voice Audiometer. For a live-voice audiometer the system shall be tested by placing the microphone in a free acoustic field at a distance of 6 to 12 inches from the source (exact distance to be that recommended by the manufacturer for the actual use of the microphone) and adjusting the acoustic pressure at the

---

* NARTB Recording and Reproducing Standards, June, 1950, or latest revision thereof. (National Association of Radio and Television Broadcasters, 1771 N Street, N.W., Washington, D.C.)

position occupied by the microphone to the same acoustic pressure (preferably 70 db. referred to 0.0002 microbar) at frequencies of 200, 300, 400, 600, 800, 1000, 1500, 2000, 3000, 4000 and 5000 cps. The orientation of the microphone in the field shall be the same as that recommended by the manufacturer for use relative to the mouth of the operator. The resulting pressures developed in a coupler similar to the National Bureau of Standards 9-A coupler shall not deviate from the pressure developed at 1000 cps by more than ±5.0 db.

TABLE 1. NARTB REPRODUCING STANDARD (JUNE, 1950)*

Frequency	Output in decibels relative to output at 700 cps
100	+13.8
150	+10.5
200	+ 8.0
300	+ 4.8
400	+ 3.0
500	+ 1.7
700	− 0.0
1000	− 1.3
1500	− 2.7
2000	− 4.0
3000	− 6.6
4000	− 8.6
7000	−14.0
10000	−16.0

*NARTB Recording and Reproducing Standards, June, 1950, or latest revision thereof. (National Association of Radio and Television Broadcasters, 1771 N Street, N.W., Washington, D.C.)

Low-frequency Cut-off. In both recorded-speech audiometers and live-voice audiometers it is permissible to introduce into the circuit a high-pass filter with nominal cut-off at 150 cps or lower to suppress undesired low frequencies, including rumble of turntable and hum from the power supply.

Distortion:

Over-all Distortion. For a recorded-speech audiometer no harmonic within 20 db. of the fundamental shall be present in the output when the test frequencies 200, 400, 700, 1000, 2000 or 4000 are played from the NARTB test recording and the attenuator is set to its minimum or so as to produce an acoustic pressure of not less than 120 db. re 0.0002 microbar. The acoustic output shall be measured in a NBS 9-A coupler. For a live-voice audiometer an acoustic signal of sufficient purity (no harmonic within 40 db. of the fundamental) shall be delivered to the microphone at a sound pressure level of 70 db. re 0.0002 microbar. The test frequencies and permissible distortion shall be the same as for a recorded-speech audiometer.

Range of Output and Scale Divisions. The scale marking of the intensity dial (attenuator) shall be adjusted so that 0 hearing loss is indicated when a calibrating tone of 1000 cps brings the monitor meter to its reference level and simultaneously produces an acoustic output of 22.0 ± 4.0 db. re 0.0002 microbar.

The purpose of this requirement is to set the 0 hearing loss for speech at a level 7.5 db. above the "normal" threshold for a pure tone of 1000 cycles as defined in the ASA standard for pure tone audiometers for general diagnostic purposes. This value is subject to future adjustment when additional experiments have been performed to evaluate the normal relation between the threshold for speech (using carefully chosen recorded word tests) and the threshold for a 1000 cycle tone. It is believed that the adjustment will not be more than ±3 db.

The scale of hearing loss shall extend from −10 db. to +100 db. in steps of 5 db. or less.

Noise. The rms weighted electrical background noise from all sources other than surface noise of the recordings shall be at least 50 db. below the level of the signal. The measurement for noise shall be made in the following manner. The amplifier shall be adjusted so that the meter indicates the reference level when the 1000 cycle tone is played (NAB Test recording or equivalent) or a 70 db. acoustic pressure is delivered to the microphone in the case of a live voice speech audiometer. The attenuator shall be set to the 100 db. hearing-loss setting. The acoustic pressure is measured in a NBS 9-A coupler. In testing a phonographic audiometer, the pickup is now placed in "rest" position but the turntable is allowed to revolve. In testing a magnetic-tape playback, the mechanism is activated but no tape is run across the pickup. The total acoustic output in the coupler is measured under these conditions, with no signal. The pressure shall be at least 50 db. below the first measurement.

The direction radiation of noise such as rumble from the turntable or "needle-talk" from the pickup, from chassis, turntable, pickup or playback shall not be loud enough to be audible to a listener with normal hearing who is seated at a distance of 3 feet from the apparatus in the direction which a patient would normally be seated and wearing the earphones, held by the headband provided, as they would be worn under conditions of actual test. During this test the receivers shall be disconnected from the output of the instrument, or equivalent receivers and headband from another instrument may be provided.

Measurement of Weighted Sound Pressure:

The measurement of weighted sound pressures due to noise shall be made with an equipment having the pressure response-frequency characteristics shown in Fig. 2 in American Standard for Audiometers for General Diagnostic Purposes (Z24.5-1951). It mirrors the curve of Minimum Audible Pressure (Sivian and White). The weighted sound pressure due to any frequency distribution of sound energy shall be the sound pressure due to a 1000 cps sound which gives the same reading on the equipment.

Tests for compliance with the requirements of this section shall be made with a power supply voltage TIF (telephone influence factor) of not less than 80 nor more than 120, if d-c power is specified. If a-c power is specified, the voltage TIF shall be not less than 15 nor more than 25. The frequency weighting characteristics* for TIF measurements are as shown in Fig. 3 of the ASA Specification for Audiometers for General Diagnostic Purposes (Z24.5-1951).

Masking. A device to provide a masking noise for the ear not under test is recommended but is not required. If a masking noise is provided it should be sufficient to render completely unintelligible to the normal ear test material delivered at a level 60 db. above the normal threshold for speech. A calibrated volume control should be provided to adjust the masking noise to lower intensities and a scale should indicate the approximate level (in terms of hearing loss) at which such test material is just effectively masked.

Shock Hazard. Audiometers shall be free from electric-shock hazard. A shock hazard shall be considered to exist at an exposed live part if the open-circuit potential is more than 25 volts and the current with a 1500-ohm load is more than 5 milliamperes.†

* A complete description of the manner in which Telephone Influence Factor measurements are made is contained in a paper by J. M. Barstow, P. W. Blye, and H. E. Kent, *Trans. Am. Inst. Elec. Engrs.*, **54**, 1307, 1935.

† This specification is in accordance with the American Standard for Power-operated Radio Receiving Apparatus, C65.1-1942, Section 73 (A).

PART II. SPECIFICATIONS OF THE AMERICAN STANDARDS ASSOCIATION

American Standard Specification for Audiometers for General Diagnostic Purposes*

1. SCOPE AND PURPOSE

1.1 The audiometer covered by this specification is a device designed for general diagnostic use and to determine the hearing acuity of individuals. The audiometer described is an electroacoustic generator with associated air- and bone-conduction receivers, and provides pure tones of selected frequencies and intensities which cover the major portion of the auditory range. A device for interrupting the tone is provided. The results of measurements with this audiometer determine an individual's auditory threshold as a function of frequency.

1.2 This specification has been prepared with the objective that the measurements obtained with any audiometer shall truly represent a comparison of an individual's auditory threshold with the normal threshold.

2. DEFINITIONS

2.1 Normal Threshold of Audibility. The normal threshold of audibility for air conduction at a given frequency is the modal value of the minimum sound pressures, at the entrance to the ear canal, which produce a pitch sensation in a large number of normal ears of individuals between 18 and 30 years of age. The threshold values accepted for the purposes of this specification shall be those determined by the National Health Survey of 1935–36.

2.2 Hearing Loss. The hearing loss of an ear corresponds to the ratio of the threshold of audibility for that ear to the normal threshold of audibility and is expressed in decibels.

3. REQUIREMENTS

3.1 General. Audiometers shall be designed to furnish readings which give an individual's hearing threshold in terms of hearing loss in decibels relative to a reference normal threshold. Provision shall be made for both air- and bone-conduction measurements. The frequencies of the pure tones generated shall be indicated in cycles per second, and the hearing loss shall be indicated in decibels. The only audible sound should be that which is radiated by the air- and bone-conduction receivers; the chassis and audiometer cabinet shall be so constructed that no audible sound is radiated from them. All audiometers shall be designed to operate on one or more of the following electric power supplies: 117 volts, 60 cycle, a-c; 117 volts, d-c; batteries, or such supply as regional requirements demand. They shall have a nameplate giving the manufacturer's name, the serial number, and, if power-line operated, the voltage (or voltages), and frequency (or frequencies) of the power supply, and the power consumed by the audiometer.

3.2 Power Supply. Tests for compliance with the requirements of Section 3.3 shall be made at line voltages of 110 and 125 volts, for audiometers designed

* ASA Z24.5-1951, approved March 21, 1951.

for nominal 117-volt operation, or at the extremes of the usable range of battery voltages recommended by the manufacturer. For audiometers designed for other line voltages, tests shall be made at the extremes of a proportionate range of voltages. Tests for compliance with the requirements of Sections 3.4, 3.5, 3.6, 3.7, and 3.8 shall be made at a line voltage of 117 volts, or at the voltage indicated on the nameplate of the audiometer, or at the battery voltages recommended as operating voltages by the manufacturer. When a range of voltage is indicated on the nameplate, tests shall be made at the mean voltage.

3.3 Frequencies. Audiometers shall produce sounds of at least the following definitely identified frequencies: 125, 250, 500, 1000, 2000, and 4000 cycles per second for both air- and bone-conduction measurements, and also 8000 cycles per second for air-conduction measurements. Each frequency generated by the audiometer shall have a value within ± 5 per cent of the corresponding frequency reading.

3.4 Hearing-loss Intervals and Hearing-loss Range for Air-conduction Measurement. Hearing-loss dial range shall extend from -10 db (below threshold) by intervals of 5 db or less to at least the values given in Table 1.

Each measured difference (interval) between successive hearing-loss readings shall not differ from the nominal interval in decibels by more than 0.3 of the interval at each of the above indicated frequencies. That is, if the nominal interval is 5 db, the measured interval shall be not less than 3.5 db nor more than 6.5 db.

TABLE 1

Frequency reading, cps	Hearing-loss readings, db above threshold
125	65
250	80
500	85
1000	95
2000	95
4000	90
8000	75

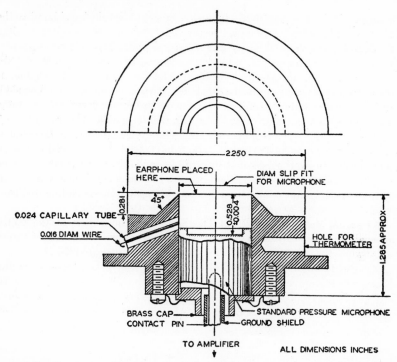

FIG. 1. Coupler for use with air-conduction earphones.* The face of the earphone being calibrated rests on the upper edge with a coupling force equal to the weight of the earphone plus 400 gm. The entire assembly is designed for use with a condenser microphone amplifier.

* The coupler shown in Fig. 1 has been developed by the National Bureau of Standards and is designated as National Bureau of Standards Coupler 9-A. It has been used by audiometer manufacturers and the NBS as a standard coupler for many years. Recently the American Standard Method for the Coupler Calibration of Earphones, Z24.9-1949, has been prepared in which a coupler designated Type-1 is recommended. Adaptation of the Type-1 coupler, or any other coupler, to the different earphones supplied by audiometer manufacturers involves research and consequently would delay the issuance of this Z24.5 standard by one or more years, if any coupler other than the No. 9-A were to be incorporated into this standard. It is planned to rewrite the present standard as soon as the basic research has been completed. The industry will then change gradually from the NBS 9-A to an approved standard coupler. It has been determined that there is but slight measurable difference encountered in the use of these several couplers. (See "Interactions between Microphones, Couplers and Earphones," by K. C. Morrical, J. L. Glaser, and R. W. Benson, *J. Acous. Soc. Am.*, **21**, 190–197, May, 1949.)

The intervals shall be determined by measurement of the electrical input to the earphone, with the earphone coupled to the coupler shown in Fig. 1.

3.5 Sound-pressure Output of the Air-conduction Earphones. Measurements of sound-pressure output of air-conduction earphones shall be made with a coupler having the acoustical characteristics of the coupler shown in Fig. 1. The sound pressure produced by the earphones at each hearing-loss reading shall not differ from the indicated value, as referred to normal threshold, by more than 4 db at the indicated frequencies of 125, 250, 500, 1000, 2000, and by not more than 5 db at frequencies of 4000 and 8000 cycles per second. The sound pressures corresponding to normal threshold have been determined for several types of earphones by the National Bureau of Standards, and are based on the threshold determinations made by the U.S. Public Health Service. The threshold determinations are published in the Preliminary Reports of the National Health Survey Hearing Study Series, Bulletin No. 5, page 10, 1935–36.

3.5.1 *Line Voltage Variation.* The acoustic output level at the 60 db setting shall not depart by more than ± 1 db from its value at the line voltage of 117 volts when the line voltage is varied from 105 volts to 125 volts. In audiometers designed for power sources of other voltages, the output level shall not

TABLE 2. THRESHOLD PRESSURES OF LABORATORY STANDARD EARPHONE*

Frequency, cps	Pressure, db above 1 dyne per cm²
125	−19.5
250	−34.4
500	−49.2
1000	−57.3
2000	−57.0
4000	−58.9
8000	−53.1

* These pressures apply only to the Western Electric Type 705-A Earphone.

depart by more than ± 1 db from its value at normal line voltage when the voltage is varied over an equivalent proportion above and below the normal voltage.

3.5.2 *Loudness Balance.* The sound pressures in this coupler which correspond to normal threshold for any particular type or configuration of earphone are determined by loudness balancing against a laboratory standard earphone.* The loudness balance test should be performed by a jury of not less than six persons with normal hearing.

The threshold pressures† of this earphone are as shown in Table 2.

* The Western Electric 705-A Earphone has been found suitable as a laboratory standard earphone.

† These threshold pressures have been determined by loudness balancing with the earphones used in the National Health Survey Hearing Study.

3.5.3 *Measurement of Sound-pressure Output.* The sound-pressure output of the audiometer shall be measured directly at hearing-loss settings of 60 db. The sound-pressure output may be obtained at all other hearing-loss dial settings by combination of the pressures measured at 60 db with the results of the hearing-loss interval measurements made under Section 3.4. It may be measured acoustically at practical levels, if equipment is available and shall be measured electrically at all other levels.

3.6 Harmonics in the Output of Air-conduction Earphones. The sound pressure of the fundamental signal shall be at least 25 db above the sound pressure of any harmonic. The harmonic shall be measured at the frequencies and hearing-loss readings shown in Table 1, even though some audiometers may be designed with higher maximum intensities. The measurements shall be made with the coupler shown in Fig. 1. The distortion requirements shall apply at all levels up to the values shown in Table 1, but will normally be measured at the values shown in Table 1.

3.7 Noise in Air-conduction Earphones. The rms weighted sound pressure produced by the earphone in the coupler shown in Fig. 1, due to all frequencies except the signal frequency and its harmonics, shall be either less than 1×10^{-3} dynes per cm^2, or at least 60 db below the sound pressure due to the signal frequency and its harmonics at all specifically designated frequencies and hearing-loss dial settings.

3.7.1 *Measurement of Weighted Sound Pressure.* The measurement of weighted sound pressure shall be made with an equipment having the pressure response-frequency characteristics shown in Fig. 2. The weighted sound pressure due to any frequency distribution of sound energy shall be the sound pressure due to a 1000-cycle-per-second sound which gives the same reading on the equipment.

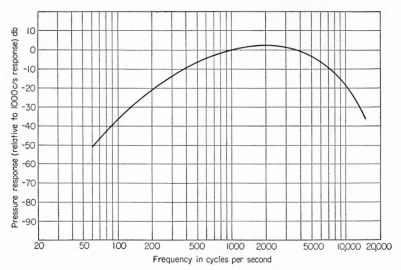

Fig. 2. Pressure response–frequency characteristic of equipment for measurement of noise in air-conduction earphone.*

* This curve is taken from that published in the article entitled "Minimum Audible Sound Fields," by L. J. Sivian and S. D. White, *J. Acous. Soc. Am.*, **4**, 313, 1933, and on page 124 of Hearing, by S. S. Stevens and H. Davis, John Wiley & Sons, Inc., New York.

3.7.2 *Tests for Compliance with Noise Requirements.* Tests for compliance with the requirements of this section shall be made with a power supply voltage TIF (telephone influence factor) of not less than 80, nor more than 120, if d-c power is specified. If a-c power is specified, the voltage TIF shall be not less than 15, nor more than 25. The frequency weighting characteristics* for TIF measurements are as shown in Fig. 3.

All tests for compliance with the noise requirements of this section should be made with the oscillator inoperative but with the remainder of the audiometer circuit in normal operating condition.

3.8 Bone-conduction Receivers. Bone-conduction receivers shall not radiate sound to such an extent that the sound reaching the tympanum through the auditory meatus might influence the validity of the bone-conduction measurement. As judged by an observer with normal hearing, the sound received at the ear via air radiation from the bone conductor shall have a sensation level at least 5 db below the level which the receiver generates by bone conduction when in contact with the head. This measurement is made as follows:

(a) The bone-conduction threshold is determined in the usual manner.

(b) Then, with the receiver in approximately the same position as in the

* A complete description of the manner in which telephone influence factor measurements are made is contained in a paper by J. M. Barstow, P. W. Blye, and H. E. Kent, *Trans. Am. Inst. Elec. Engrs.*, **54**, 1307, 1935.

threshold measurements, the driver element or contact area is covered with the soft flesh at the end of the operator's finger to create a closure comparable to that created when the receiver is on the mastoid. Care should be taken that no direct contact is made between the finger and the skull.

(c) The threshold at which any auditory sensation is perceived should then be noted and should be at least 5 db above the direct bone conduction threshold.

(d) A jury of at least six persons with normal hearing should perform this test and the mean of the results should be taken.

Determination of the air radiation from bone-conduction receivers is not required at frequencies above 2000 cycles per second.

3.9 Shock Hazard. Audiometers shall be free from electric-shock hazard. A shock hazard shall be considered to exist at an exposed live part if the open-circuit potential is more than 25 volts and the current with a 1500-ohm load is more than 5 milliamperes.*

3.10 Audiogram Blanks. The results of hearing-loss measurements made with an audiometer shall be plotted on cross-section paper. The abscissae shall be frequency in cycles per second on a logarithmic scale and the ordinates shall be hearing loss in decibels on a linear scale. One octave on the frequency scale shall be the same distance as 20 decibels on the hearing-loss scale.

3.11 Tone Interrupter. The tone interrupter shall be so designed and constructed that during operation no transients or extraneous frequencies are audible to the normal ear. It is recommended that after operation of the switch the time required for the test tone to rise to a value which is within ± 1 db of the required sound pressure shall be not less than 0.1 second and not more than 0.5 second.

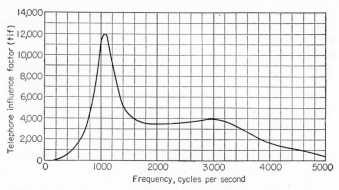

Fig. 3. Frequency weighting network for TIF measurements.

* This specification is in accordance with the American Standard for Power-operated Radio Receiving Apparatus, C65.1-1942, Section 73 (A).

SPEECH MATERIALS FOR AUDITORY TESTS

THE following lists are presented to familiarize the reader with the types of material that are used in the clinical measurement of *Hearing Loss for Speech* and *Discrimination Loss*. They may also serve as sources of test words for those who would like to construct lists for use with the live voice.

Two points of caution must be made. First, if the live voice is used, instead of the recorded version of these tests, the tester must provide himself with suitable means for measuring and controlling the level of speech at the listener's ear. Second, the words in each list are arranged alphabetically, and if tests are constructed from these lists, the reader is cautioned that the word order should be scrambled. Several versions of the same list may be provided by different word orders or scramblings.

TWO-SYLLABLE SPONDEE WORDS

The following lists represent the sources from which two widely used recorded auditory tests have been taken.

Auditory Test No. 9. The first, Auditory Test No. 9 of the Psycho-Acoustic Laboratory, Harvard University, provides a vocabulary of 84 spondee words. Each of two lists, of 42 words each, has been recorded for phonograph use in such a way that the threshold of intelligibility or Hearing Loss for Speech can be measured easily and quickly. Details about the structure of the test and the method of measuring the threshold are given in Hudgins *et al.*

Words Used in Auditory Test No. 9, Psycho-Acoustic Laboratory, Harvard University

LIST I

1. airplane	9. bobwhite	17. drawbridge
2. armchair	10. bonbon	18. earthquake
3. backbone	11. buckwheat	19. eggplant
4. bagpipe	12. coughdrop	20. eyebrow
5. baseball	13. cowboy	21. firefly
6. birthday	14. cupcake	22. hardware
7. blackboard	15. doorstep	23. headlight
8. bloodhound	16. dovetail	24. hedgehog

25. hothouse	31. playground	37. sunset
26. inkwell	32. railroad	38. watchword
27. mousetrap	33. shipwreck	39. whitewash
28. northwest	34. shotgun	40. wigwam
29. oatmeal	35. sidewalk	41. wildcat
30. outlaw	36. stairway	42. woodwork

List II

1. although	15. hotdog	29. playmate
2. beehive	16. housework	30. scarecrow
3. blackout	17. iceberg	31. schoolboy
4. cargo	18. jacknife	32. soybean
5. cookbook	19. lifeboat	33. starlight
6. daybreak	20. midway	34. sundown
7. doormat	21. mishap	35. therefore
8. duckpond	22. mushroom	36. toothbrush
9. eardrum	23. nutmeg	37. vampire
10. farewell	24. outside	38. washboard
11. footstool	25. padlock	39. whizzbang
12. grandson	26. pancake	40. woodchuck
13. greyhound	27. pinball	41. workshop
14. horseshoe	28. platform	42. yardstick

Auditory Tests No. W-1 *and W*-2. More recently a second list has been prepared, consisting of 36 spondee words. These lists have also been recorded both at constant level and at decreasing level (to expedite threshold measurement) as Auditory Tests No. W-1 and W-2, Central Institute For The Deaf, St. Louis, Missouri.[1] Instructions for using these tests are provided by the distributor. A report on the tests is, at the time of this writing, in preparation.

Words Used for Auditory Tests No. W-1 and W-2, Central Institute for the Deaf, St. Louis, Missouri

1. airplane	13. greyhound	25. padlock
2. armchair	14. hardware	26. pancake
3. baseball	15. headlight	27. playground
4. birthday	16. horseshoe	28. railroad
5. cowboy	17. hotdog	29. schoolboy
6. daybreak	18. hothouse	30. sidewalk
7. doormat	19. iceberg	31. stairway
8. drawbridge	20. inkwell	32. sunset
9. duckpond	21. mousetrap	33. toothbrush
10. eardrum	22. mushroom	34. whitewash
11. farewell	23. northwest	35. woodwork
12. grandson	24. oatmeal	36. workshop

[1] These tests are now available on 12-in phonograph records at either 33⅓ or 78 rpm from Technisonic Laboratories, 1201 So. Brentwood Blvd., Brentwood, Missouri.

PB LISTS

Phonetically balanced lists of one-syllable words may be used to measure the articulation score under various experimental conditions and also to measure Discrimination Loss at a high SPL.

Twenty such lists are given in Egan. Each of these may be scrambled several times to provide the user with a large source of PB lists to be used in clinical testing with the live voice. Four of these are given here as samples.

Four Out of the Twenty PB-Lists, Psycho-Acoustic Laboratory, Harvard University

LIST I

1. are	14. dish	27. is	39. ride
2. bad	15. end	28. mange	40. rise
3. bar	16. feast	29. no	41. rub
4. bask	17. fern	30. nook	42. slip
5. box	18. folk	31. not	43. smile
6. cane	19. ford	32. pan	44. strife
7. cleanse	20. fraud	33. pants	45. such
8. clove	21. fuss	34. pest	46. then
9. crash	22. grove	35. pile	47. there
10. creed	23. heap	36. plush	48. toe
11. death	24. hid	37. rag	49. use (yews)
12. deed	25. hive	38. rat	50. wheat
13. dike	26. hunt		

LIST II

1. awe	14. fate	27. need	39. sludge
2. bait	15. five	28. niece	40. snuff
3. bean	16. frog	29. nut	41. start
4. blush	17. gill	30. our	42. suck
5. bought	18. gloss	31. perk	43. tan
6. bounce	19. hire	32. pick	44. tang
7. bud	20. hit	33. pit	45. them
8. charge	21. hock	34. quart	46. trash
9. cloud	22. job	35. rap	47. vamp
10. corpse	23. log	36. rib	48. vast
11. dab	24. moose	37. scythe	49. ways
12. earl	25. mute	38. shoe	50. wish
13. else	26. nab		

List III

1. ache	14. dill	27. neck	39. sped
2. air	15. drop	28. nest	40. stag
3. bald	16. fame	29. oak	41. take
4. barb	17. far	30. path	42. thrash
5. bead	18. fig	31. please	43. toil
6. cape	19. flush	32. pulse	44. trip
7. cast	20. gnaw	33. rate	45. turf
8. check	21. hurl	34. rouse	46. vow
9. class	22. jam	35. shout	47. wedge
10. crave	23. law	36. sit	48. wharf
11. crime	24. leave	37. size	49. who
12. deck	25. lush	38. sob	50. why
13. dig	26. muck		

List IV

1. bath	14. eel	27. new	39. sage
2. beast	15. fin	28. oils	40. scab
3. bee	16. float	29. or	41. shed
4. blonde	17. frown	30. peck	42. shin
5. budge	18. hatch	31. pert	43. sketch
6. bus	19. heed	32. pinch	44. slap
7. bush	20. hiss	33. pod	45. sour
8. cloak	21. hot	34. race	46. starve
9. course	22. how	35. rack	47. strap
10. court	23. kite	36. rave	48. test
11. dodge	24. merge	37. raw	49. tick
12. dupe	25. move	38. rut	50. touch
13. earn	26. neat		

Four new PB lists have been constructed and scrambled to produce a phonographically recorded set of 24 lists, comprising Auditory Test No. W-22, Central Institute For The Deaf, St. Louis, Missouri.[1]

[1] This test is now available on 12-in phonograph records at either 33⅓ or 78 rpm from Technisonic Laboratories, 1201 So. Brentwood Blvd., Brentwood, Missouri.

Lists of Words Used in Auditory Test No. W-22, Central Institute for the Deaf, St. Louis, Missouri

List I

1. ace	14. east	27. mew	39. there (their)
2. ache	15. felt	28. none (nun)	40. thing
3. an	16. give	29. not (knot)	41. toe
4. as	17. high	30. or (oar)	42. true
5. bathe	18. him	31. owl	43. twins
6. bells	19. hunt	32. poor	44. up
7. carve	20. isle (aisle, I'll)	33. ran	45. us
8. chew	21. it	34. see (sea)	46. wet
9. could	22. jam	35. she	47. what
10. dad	23. knees	36. skin	48. wire
11. day	24. law	37. stove	49. yard
12. deaf	25. low	38. them	50. you (ewe)
13. earn (urn)	26. me		

List II

1. ail (ale)	14. else	27. new (knew)	39. star
2. air (heir)	15. flat	28. now	40. tare (tear)
3. and	16. gave	29. oak	41. that
4. bin (been)	17. ham	30. odd	42. then
5. by	18. hit	31. off	43. thin
6. cap	19. hurt	32. one (won)	44. too (two, to)
7. cars	20. ice	33. own	45. tree
8. chest	21. ill	34. pew	46. way (weigh)
9. die (dye)	22. jaw	35. rooms	47. well
10. does	23. key	36. send	48. with
11. dumb	24. knee	37. show	49. young
12. ease	25. live [lɪv]	38. smart	50. yore (your)
13. eat	26. move		

List III

1. add (ad)	14. end	27. nest	39. tan
2. aim	15. farm	28. no (know)	40. ten
3. are	16. glove	29. oil	41. this
4. ate (eight)	17. hand	30. on	42. three
5. bill	18. have	31. out	43. though
6. book	19. he	32. owes	44. tie
7. camp	20. if	33. pie	45. use (yews)
8. chair	21. is	34. raw	46. we
9. cute	22. jar	35. say	47. west
10. do	23. king	36. shove	48. when
11. done (dun)	24. knit	37. smooth	49. wool
12. dull	25. lie (lye)	38. start	50. year
13. ears	26. may		

List IV

1. aid	14. dolls	27. near	39. tin
2. all (awl)	15. dust	28. net	40. than
3. am	16. ear	29. nuts	41. they
4. arm	17. eyes (ayes)	30. of	42. through (thru)
5. art	18. few	31. ought (aught)	43. toy
6. at	19. go	32. our (hour)	44. where
7. bee (be)	20. hang	33. pale (pail)	45. who
8. bread (bred)	21. his	34. save	46. why
9. can	22. in (inn)	35. shoe	47. will
10. chin	23. jump	36. so (sew)	48. wood (would)
11. clothes	24. leave	37. stiff	49. yes
12. cook	25. men	38. tea (tee)	50. yet
13. darn	26. my		

GLOSSARY

This Glossary defines most of the technical terms that are used in the body of the text. Some of the definitions are restricted to the context of the book. In addition, certain technical terms not used earlier are defined, particularly in the field of acoustics, in order to acquaint the reader with *standard definitions*. These are among the items that are followed by an asterisk (*), which indicates quotation, with permission, from *American Standard Acoustical Terminology* (Z24.1-1951). New York: American Standards Association.

Absolute threshold. See **Threshold of audibility.**

Acceleration.* The acceleration of a point is the time rate of change of the velocity of the point.

Acoustics.* Acoustics is the science of sound, including its production, transmission, and effects.

Air Conduction.* Air conduction is the process by which sound is conducted to the inner ear through the air in the outer ear canal as part of the pathway.

Ampere. See **Current.**

Amplifier. An amplifier is a device that enlarges changes in energy. A vacuum-tube amplifier, for example, causes small electrical changes in its grid circuit to appear much larger in its plate circuit.

Amplitude. The amplitude of an oscillating quantity is the value of that quantity. The peak amplitude is the maximum value that the quantity attains, while the instantaneous amplitude is the value of the quantity at any instant.

Amplitude distortion. A system is said to exhibit amplitude distortion when the waveform of the output is not a faithful reproduction of the waveform of the input. Response is nonlinear as a function of amplitude.

Articulation (Per cent articulation) and **Intelligibility (Per cent intelligibility).*** Per cent articulation or per cent intelligibility of a communication system is the percentage of the speech units spoken by a talker or talkers that is understood correctly by a listener or listeners.

Articulation score. See **Articulation.**

Artificial ear.* An artificial ear is a device for the measurement of earphones which presents an acoustic impedance to the earphone equivalent to the impedance presented by the average human ear. It is equipped with a microphone for measurement of the sound pressures developed by the earphone.

Attenuation. Attenuation is a weakening or reduction of energy (*e.g.*, sound or electricity), usually by the dissipation of energy (*e.g.*, by friction or resistance) as heat.

Attenuator (Attenuation network). In electrical circuits an attenuator is a resistive device that is designed to control the ratio of output to input voltages in steps of a decibel or multiples of a decibel.

Audiogram (Threshold audiogram). An audiogram is a graph that shows Hearing Loss (in decibels) for pure tones as a function of frequency.

Audiology. Audiology is that interdisciplinary professional area that has to do with the measurement and treatment of impaired hearing.

Audiometer. An audiometer is an instrument for measuring Hearing Loss. Measurements may be made with speech signals, usually recorded, or with tone signals. (See Appendix A.)

Auditory nervous system. The auditory nervous system is that portion of the central nervous system (CNS) which carries impulses from the cochlear end organs to the auditory cortex.

Auditory system. The auditory system consists of all parts of the ear and of the auditory nervous system that have to do with the process of hearing.

Aural harmonic.* An aural harmonic is a harmonic generated in the auditory mechanism.

Average speech power.* The average speech power for any given time interval is the average value of the instantaneous speech power over that interval.

Basilar membrane. The basilar membrane is the membranous portion of the spiral lamina, which separates the scala media from the scala tympani. It supports the end organs of hearing.

Beats.* Beats are periodic variations that result from the superposition of waves having different frequencies.

Bel.* The bel is a dimensionless unit for expressing the ratio of two values of power, the number of bels being the logarithm to the base 10 of the power ratio.

Binaural. Binaural listening is listening with two ears.

Bone conduction.* Bone conduction is the process by which sound is conducted to the inner ear through the cranial bones.

Capacitance. A capacitor (condenser) has a capacitance of 1 farad if it will store 1 coulomb of electrical charge when a voltage of 1 volt is applied.

Capacitative reactance. Capacitative reactance is a measure of the opposition offered by a given capacitor (condenser) to current flow. The unit of measure is the ohm. The reactance is inversely proportional to the capacitance and to the frequency of the alternating current.

Cochlea. The cochlea is a snail-shell-like cavity in the temporal bone, comprising that part of the labyrinth which contains the essential receptor organs of hearing.

Complex tone.* A complex tone is a sound wave produced by the combination of simple sinusoidal components of different frequencies.

Conditioned response. A conditioned response is made to a stimulus that has come to elicit or evoke the response by being associated with another stimulus that elicited the response in the first place. For example, salivation may be elicited by a sound if the sound has been associated with food previously.

Conductive hearing loss. Conductive hearing loss is produced by lesions of the conducting apparatus, e.g., the external or middle ear.

Condyle. The condyle of the mandible is one of two processes that extend upward into the tissue below the external auditory meatus.

Consonant. Consonants are those speech sounds that involve the obstruction or impeding of the air stream by the articulation of two surfaces. All speech sounds that are not vowels are consonants.

Continuous spectrum.* A continuous spectrum is the spectrum of a wave, the components of which are continuously distributed over a frequency region.

Coupler. See **Artificial ear.**

Cranial bone. The cranial bone is that part of the skull that contains the brain.

Cross-hearing. Cross-hearing takes place when sounds delivered to one ear transmit energy either around or through the head in sufficient quantity to stimulate the opposite ear.

Current. The current in an electric circuit is the rate of electron flow through the circuit. The unit of measure is the ampere. By Ohm's Law, current is defined as the voltage divided by the resistance.

Cycle. A cycle is that portion of a periodic function that occurs in one period.

Decibel.* The decibel is $\frac{1}{10}$ bel. The abbreviation db is commonly used for the term decibel.

Difference limen (Differential threshold) (just noticeable difference).* A difference limen is the increment in a stimulus which is just noticed in a specified fraction of the trials. The relative difference limen is the ratio of the difference limen to the absolute magnitude of the stimulus to which it is related.

Diplacusis binauralis. An observer demonstrates the phenomenon of diplacusis binauralis when two tones of the same frequency, each presented to a different ear, appear to have different pitches.

Discrimination Loss. A Discrimination Loss is the difference between 100 per cent and the percentage of words of a PB list that a listener repeats correctly when the list is presented at an intensity that is so high that a further increase in intensity will not increase the articulation.

Distortion. See **Amplitude** and **Frequency distortion.**

Dyne per square centimeter. See **Microbar.**

Ear. See **External, Middle,** and **Inner ear.**

Eardrum. The eardrum is a conically shaped membrane that is stretched across the end of the external auditory meatus. It marks the boundary between the external and middle ears.

Earphone (Receiver).* An earphone is an electroacoustic transducer intended to be closely coupled acoustically to the ear.

Effective sound pressure (Root-Mean-Square sound pressure).* The effective sound pressure at a point is the root-mean-square value of the instantaneous sound pressures over a time interval at the point under consideration. In the case of periodic sound pressures, the interval must be an integral number of periods or an interval long compared to a period. In the case of nonperiodic sound pressures, the interval should be long enough to make the value obtained essentially independent of small changes in the length of the interval.

Electroacoustic transducer.* An electroacoustic transducer is a transducer for receiving waves from an electric system and delivering waves to an acoustic system, or vice versa.

End organ. The end organ of a receptor system is the mechanism by which stimulus energy is transduced to nervous activity. In hearing, the end organ within the cochlea usually refers to the organ of Corti.

Energy. Energy is a measure of the capacity of a body to do work or of work that is done. The unit of measure is the erg, 1 erg being expended when a mass of 1 gm is accelerated 1 cm per second per second.

Equal-loudness contour. See **Loudness contour.**

Erg. See **Energy.**

Eustachian tube. The Eustachian, or auditory, tube is a canal, lined by mucous membrane, with bony and cartilaginous support, connecting the pharynx with the middle ear.

External auditory meatus (Ear canal). The external auditory meatus is a canal that extends from the pinna inward to the eardrum.

External ear. The external ear consists of the pinna and the external auditory meatus.

Fatigue. Auditory fatigue is the difference (in decibels) between the threshold of audibility after acoustic stimulation and the threshold before such stimulation. The amount of fatigue must be stated for a given time or as a function of time.

Filter. See **High-pass filter** and **Low-pass filter.**

Formant. A formant is a peak in the acoustic spectrum of a sound. Most vowels, for example, may be characterized by the first two or three formants.

Free field.* A free field is a field (wave or potential) in a homogeneous isotropic medium free from boundaries. In practice it is a field in which the effects of the boundaries are negligible over the region of interest.

Free progressive wave (Free wave).* A free progressive wave is a wave in a medium free from boundary effects. A free wave in a steady state can only be approximated in practice.

Frequency of a periodic quantity.* The frequency of a periodic quantity, in which time is the independent variable, is the number of periods occurring in unit time. Unless otherwise specified, the unit is the cycle per second.

Frequency distortion. A system is said to exhibit frequency distortion when it performs better at some frequencies than at others. Response is nonlinear as a function of frequency.

Frequency-vs.-response characteristic. See **Response.**

Fundamental frequency.* The fundamental frequency of a periodic quantity is the frequency of a sinusoidal quantity which has the same period as the periodic quantity.

Harmonic. A harmonic is a component of a complex tone whose frequency is an integral multiple of the fundamental frequency of the complex tone.

Hearing Loss (Deafness). The Hearing Loss for a sound is the difference (in decibels) between the threshold for that sound and the corresponding normal threshold.

Hearing Loss for Speech.* Hearing Loss for Speech is the difference in decibels between the speech levels at which the average normal ear and the defective ear, respectively, reach the same intelligibility, often arbitrarily set at 50 per cent.

High-pass filter.* A high-pass filter is a wave filter having a single transmission band, extending from some critical or cutoff frequency, not zero, up to infinite frequency.

Impedance.* An impedance is the complex ratio of a forcelike quantity (force, pressure, voltage, temperature, or electric field strength) to a related velocitylike quantity (velocity, volume velocity, current, heat flow, or magnetic field strength).

Inductance. An inductor (coil) has an inductance of 1 henry if it self-induces a back EMF of 1 volt when a current change of 1 amp passes through it.

Inductive reactance. Inductive reactance is a measure of the opposition to current flow offered by an inductor (coil). The unit of measure is the ohm. Inductive reactance is directly proportional to the inductance and to the frequency of alternating current.

Inner ear. The inner ear consists of the membranous and osseous labyrinths.

Instantaneous sound pressure.* The instantaneous sound pressure at a point is the total instantaneous pressure at that point minus the static pressure at that point. The commonly used unit is the microbar.

Instantaneous speech power.* The instantaneous speech power is the rate at which sound energy is being radiated by a speech source at any given instant.

Intelligibility. See **Articulation.**

Intensity Level (Specific sound-energy flux level) (Sound-energy flux density level).* The Intensity Level, in decibels, of a sound is 10 times the logarithm to the base 10 of the ratio of the intensity of this sound to the reference intensity. The reference intensity shall be stated explicitly.

Just noticeable difference. See **Difference limen.**

Labyrinth. The labyrinth is the system of intercommunicating canals and cavities that makes up the inner ear.

Level above threshold (Sensation Level).* The level above threshold of a sound is the pressure level of the sound in decibels above its threshold of audibility for the individual observer.

Line spectrum.* A line spectrum is the spectrum of a wave, the components of which are confined to a number of discrete frequencies.

Localization (Auditory localization). When a listener is asked to localize a sound, he is expected to report the direction of the sound source, or its distance, or both. In physiology, *localization* is also used to refer to a place in the nervous or other systems where a certain process is mediated.

Loudness.* Loudness is the intensive attribute of an auditory sensation, in terms of which sounds may be ordered on a scale extending from soft to loud.

Loudness contours.* Loudness contours are curves which show the related values of Sound Pressure Level and frequency required to produce a given loudness sensation for the typical listener.

Loudness Level.* The Loudness Level, in phons, of a sound is numerically equal to the sound pressure level in decibels, relative to 0.0002 microbar, of a simple tone of frequency 1000 cps which is judged by the listeners to be equivalent in loudness.

Loud-speaker (Speaker).* A loud-speaker is an electroacoustic transducer usually intended to radiate acoustic power effectively at a distance in air.

Low-pass filter.* A low-pass filter is a wave filter having a single transmission band extending from zero frequency up to some critical or cutoff frequency, not infinite.

Magnetic recorder.* A magnetic recorder is equipment incorporating an electromagnetic transducer and means for moving a ferromagnetic recording medium relative to the transducer for recording electric signals as magnetic variations in the medium.

Mandible. The mandible is the jawbone.

Masking.* Masking is the amount by which the threshold of audibility of a sound is raised by the presence of another (masking) sound. The unit customarily used is the decibel.

Masking audiogram.* A masking audiogram is a graphical presentation of the masking due to a stated noise. This is plotted, in decibels, as a function of the frequency of the masked tone.

Mastoid. The mastoid process extends downward from the temporal bone behind the external auditory meatus.

Maximum sound pressure.* The maximum sound pressure for any given cycle of a periodic wave is the maximum absolute value of the instantaneous sound pressure occurring during that cycle. The commonly used unit is the microbar.

Mechanical phonograph recorder (Mechanical recorder).* A mechanical phonograph recorder is an equipment for transforming electric or acoustic signals into mechanical motion of approximately like form and inscribing such motion in an appropriate medium by cutting or embossing.

Method of adjustment (Method of average error). The method of adjustment is one of three classic psychophysical procedures for measuring either the differential or the absolute threshold. The observer controls the independent stimulus dimension and sets it according to experimental instructions, e.g., "just audible," "just noticeably different," "just intelligible," etc.

Method of constant stimuli. The method of constant stimuli is one of three classic psychophysical procedures for measuring the differential or absolute threshold. Stimuli are presented in discrete categories of the independent-stimulus dimension. The observer responds with a "yes" or "no," "same" or "different" after each stimulus presentation.

Method of limits (Method of serial exploration). The method of limits is one of three classic psychophysical procedures for measuring the differential or absolute threshold. In the method of limits the experimenter gradually increases or decreases either a stimulus dimension or a difference between two stimuli and notes the change in the observer's response (e.g., from audibility to inaudibility, or vice versa).

Microbar, Dyne per square centimeter.* A microbar is a unit of pressure commonly used in acoustics. One microbar is equal to 1 dyne/cm^2.

Microphone.* A microphone is an electroacoustic transducer which responds to sound waves and delivers essentially equivalent electric waves.

Middle ear. The middle ear consists of the cavity containing the ossicles, the Eustachian tube, and the mastoid cells.

Modulation. The modulation of any periodic function is a periodic change in one or several of the dimensions of the function. Amplitude or frequency modulation involves periodic changes of the amplitude or frequency, respectively, of a periodic function.

Monaural. Monaural listening is listening with one ear.

Natural frequency. See **Resonant frequency.**

Noise.* Noise is any undesired sound. By extension, noise is any unwanted disturbance within a useful frequency band, such as undesired electric waves in any transmission channel or device.

Normal threshold of audibility. See Appendix A.

Octave. An octave is the interval between two tones when they are separated either by a frequency ratio of 2:1 or by a musical interval of 12 semitones.

Ohm. See **Impedance, Reactance,** and **Resistance.**

Oscillation (Vibration).* Oscillation is the vibration, usually with time, of the magnitude of a quantity with respect to a specified reference when the magnitude is alternately greater and smaller than the reference.

Oscillator. An oscillator is a device used to generate oscillations. A pure-tone oscillator is used to generate sinusoidal oscillations.

Ossicle. The auditory ossicles are the three small suspended bones in the middle ear. The chain of ossicles is connected to the eardrum peripherally and to the oval-window membrane centrally.

Otology. Otology is that branch of medicine that is concerned with the ear.

Oval window. The oval window is an opening in the bone between the middle ear and the scala vestibuli of the inner ear. The stapes (third ossicle) is attached to a membrane that is stretched across this window.

Particle velocity.* In a sound wave the particle velocity is the velocity of a given infinitesimal part of the medium, with reference to the medium as a whole, due to the sound wave. The commonly used unit is the centimeter per second.

Peak sound pressure.* The peak sound pressure for any specified time interval is the maximum absolute value of the instantaneous sound pressure in that interval. The commonly used unit is the microbar.

Peak speech power.* The peak speech power is the maximum value of the instantaneous speech power within the time interval considered.

Perceptive (nerve-type) hearing loss. The perceptive hearing loss involves pathologic conditions of the end organs or nervous system central to the oval window.

Period (Primitive period).* The period of a periodic quantity is the smallest value of the increment of the independent variable for which the function repeats itself.

Phase of a periodic quantity.* The phase of a periodic quantity, for a particular value of the independent variable, is the fractional part of a period through which the independent variable has advanced, measured from an arbitrary origin.

Phon.* The phon is the unit of loudness level.

Phonetically balanced list. A PB list is a list of monosyllabic words that contains a distribution of speech sounds that approximates the distribution of the same sounds as they occur in conversational American English.

Phonetics. Phonetics is the study of the description and analysis of the sounds of speech.

Phonograph (Phonographic reproducer). A mechanical phonographic reproducer is a device designed to transform mechanical signals, such as those made by a mechanical recorder, into electric or acoustic signals.

Pinna (Auricle). The pinna is that portion of the external ear that projects outward from the side of the head.

Pitch.* Pitch is that attribute of auditory sensation in terms of which sounds may be ordered on a scale extending from low to high, such as a musical scale.

Power. Power is the rate at which energy is expended or work is done. The unit of measure is the watt. Electrical power is the product of voltage times current.

Pressure. Pressure is a measure of force divided by the area to which the force is applied. Usually measured in dynes per square centimeter.

Pressure spectrum level.* The pressure spectrum level of a sound at a specified frequency is the effective Sound Pressure Level for the sound energy contained within a band 1 cps wide, centered at the specified frequency. Ordinarily this has significance only for sound having a continuous distribution of energy within the frequency range under consideration. The reference pressure should be explicitly stated.

Psychoacoustics. Psychoacoustics is that branch of psychophysics that has to do with acoustic stimuli.

Psychophysics. Psychophysics is the study of the relations between physical stimuli and the responses to which they give rise.

Pure tone. See **Simple tone**.

Reactance. See **Capacitative reactance** and **Inductive reactance**.

Receiver. See **Earphone**.

Recruitment. Recruitment is a phenomenon associated with certain types of hearing loss in which the loudness of tones appears to increase more rapidly than normal when the growth of loudness is related to logarithmic increments of the stimulus intensity above the threshold.

Resistance. A resistor has a resistance of 1 ohm when an applied voltage of 1 volt produces a current of 1 amp. Resistance is the nonreactive component of electrical impedance. By Ohm's Law, resistance equals the voltage divided by the current.

Resonance. Resonance is the property of a mechanical or electrical system of oscillating at a particular frequency with minimum dissipation of energy.

Resonant frequency.* A resonant frequency is a frequency at which resonance exists.

Response.* The response of a device or system is a quantitative expression of the output as a function of the input under conditions which must be explicitly stated. The response characteristic, often presented graphically, gives the response as a function of some independent variable such as frequency or direction.

Round window. The round window is an opening in the bone between the middle ear and the scala tympani of the inner ear. The round-window membrane is stretched across it.

Screening. Audiometric screening is a method or group of methods designed to separate individuals whose thresholds lie above the normal from those whose thresholds lie at or below the normal threshold. Both speech and pure tones are used as test signals.

Sensation. Within the context of this book, a sensation is said to have occurred when an observer responds in an appropriate way after a stimulus has been presented.

Sensation Level. See **Level above threshold.**

Simple tone (Pure tone).* A simple tone is a sound wave, the instantaneous sound pressure of which is a simple sinusoidal function of the time.

Sinusoid. A sinusoid is any waveform that has the same shape as a sine wave, a graph relating the sine of an angle to the size of the angle.

Sone.* The sone is a unit of loudness. By definition, a simple tone of frequency 1000 cps, 40 db above a listener's threshold, produces a loudness of 1 sone. The loudness of any sound that is judged by the listener to be n times that of the 1-sone tone is n sones.

Sound.* Sound is an alteration in pressure, stress, particle displacement, particle velocity, etc., which is propagated in an elastic material, or the superposition of such propagated alterations.

Sound energy.* The sound energy of a given part of a medium is the total energy in this part of the medium minus the energy which would exist in the same part of the medium with no sound waves present.

Sound field.* A sound field is a region containing sound waves.

Sound intensity. (Specific sound-energy flux) (Sound-energy flux density).* The sound intensity in a specified direction at a point is the average rate of sound energy transmitted in the specified direction through a unit area normal to this direction at the point considered. The commonly used unit is the erg per second per square centimeter, but sound intensity may also be expressed in watts per square centimeter.

Sound-level meter.* A sound-level meter is an instrument including a microphone, an amplifier, an output meter, and frequency weighting networks for the measurement of noise and sound levels in a specified manner; the measurements are intended to approximate the loudness level which would be obtained by the more elaborate ear-balance method.

Sound pressure. See **Effective, Instantaneous, Maximum,** and **Peak sound pressure.**

Sound Pressure Level.* The Sound Pressure Level, in decibels, of a sound is 20 times the logarithm to the base 10 of the ratio of the pressure of this sound to the reference pressure. The reference pressure shall be explicitly stated.

Spectrum.* The spectrum of a wave is the distribution in frequency of the magnitudes (and sometimes phases) of the components of the wave. Spectrum also is used to signify a continuous range of frequencies, usually wide in extent, within which waves have some specified common characteristic, *e.g.*, audio-frequency spectrum, radio-frequency spectrum, etc.

Speech. Speech is one process by which human beings communicate with other human beings. (We have restricted the use of the term to those instances in which sounds are produced by a talker and are received by a listener.) The term may refer to physiologic, psychologic, or physical aspects of the process.

Speech power. See **Average, Instantaneous,** and **Peak speech power.**

Spondee. A spondaic foot contains two syllables with equal stress on both. Spondaic words are used in tests for the threshold of intelligibility.

Threshold of audibility (Threshold of detectability).* The threshold of audibility for a specified signal is the minimum effective sound pressure of the signal that is capable of evoking an auditory sensation in a specified fraction of the trials. The characteristics of the signal, the manner in which it is presented to the listener, and the point at which the sound pressure is measured must be specified.

Threshold of feeling (or **discomfort, tickle,** or **pain**).* The threshold of feeling (or discomfort, tickle, or pain) for a specified signal is the minimum effective sound pressure of that signal which, in a specified fraction of the trials, will stimulate the ear to a point at which there is the sensation of feeling (or discomfort, tickle, or pain).

Threshold of intelligibility. The threshold of intelligibility for speech is the level at which the speech must be presented in order that the listener may repeat correctly 50 per cent of the items.

Timbre (Musical quality).* Timbre is that attribute of auditory sensation in terms of which a listener can judge that two sounds similarly presented and having the same loudness and pitch are dissimilar.

Time-error. Auditory time-error is a phenomenon that is demonstrated when a shift or constant error in the judgment of a psychological dimension of a sound occurs as a function of the time of separation between the sound and a standard reference sound with which it is compared.

Tinnitus. When an observer reports that he hears sounds in the absence of any external acoustic stimulation, he is said to have tinnitus.

Tone.* A tone is a sound wave capable of exciting an auditory sensation having pitch.

Transformer. A transformer is a device by which electrical current in one coil produces current flow in a second coil when the electromagnetic fields of both coils overlap.

Vacuum tube. A vacuum tube is any device in which the flow of electric current is controlled by having free electrons emitted by a cathode and attracted by an anode. One application is the amplifier.

Velocity.* The velocity of a point is the time rate of change of a position vector of that point with respect to an inertial frame.

Volt. See **Voltage.**

Voltage. Voltage is the difference in electromotive force between two points. The unit of measurement is the volt. By Ohm's Law, voltage is defined as current times resistance.

VU meter (Volume-level indicator). A VU meter (volume-unit meter) is a voltmeter that is specifically designed for monitoring speech and music.

Vowel. A vowel, one of two types of speech sounds, is a continuous complex sound initiated by the vocal cords and modified by the nasal, oral, and pharyngeal cavities.

Watt. See **Power.**

Wave.* A wave is a disturbance which is propagated in a medium in such a manner that at any point in the medium the displacement is a function of the time, while at any instant the displacement at a point is a function of the position of the point. Any physical quantity which has the same relationship to some independent variable (usually time) that a propagated disturbance has, at a particular instant, with respect to space, may be called a wave.

Waveform. The waveform of a sound is a graph showing the instantaneous amplitude, pressure, or intensity as a function of time.

BIBLIOGRAPHY

Angell, J. R., and W. Fite. (1901) The monaural localization of sound. *Psychol. Rev.*, **8**, 225–246.

Banister, H. (1934) Audition: I. Auditory phenomena and their stimulus correlates. Chap. 16 in C. Murchison (Ed.), *A Handbook of General Experimental Psychology*. Worcester: Clark University Press.

Bárány, E. (1938) A contribution to the physiology of bone conduction. *Acta oto-laryng., Stockh.*, Suppl. 26.

Beasley, W. C. (1938) *National Health Survey, Hearing Study Series. Bulletin No. 5*. Washington: U.S. Public Health Service.

Békésy, G. v. (1932) Zur Theorie des Hörens bei der Schallaufnahme durch Knochenleitung. *Ann. Physik.*, **13**, 111–136.

Békésy, G. v. (1936a) Über die Herstellung und Messung langsamer sinusförmiger Luftdruckschwankungen. *Ann. Physik.*, **25**, 413–432.

Békésy, G. v. (1936b) Über die Hörschwelle und Fühlgrenze langsamer sinusförmiger Luftdruckschwankungen. *Ann. Physik.*, **26**, 554–566.

Békésy, G. v. (1941) Über die Schallausbreitung bei Knochenleitung. *Z.Hals-Nas.-u. Ohrenheilk.*, **47**, 430–442.

Békésy, G. v. (1947) A new audiometer. *Acta oto-laryng., Stockh.*, **35**, 411–422.

Békésy, G. v. (1948) Vibration of the head in a sound field and its role in hearing by bone conduction. *J. Acoust. Soc. Amer.*, **20**, 749–760.

Békésy, G. v. (1949) The structure of the middle ear and the hearing of one's own voice by bone conduction. *J. Acoust. Soc. Amer.*, **21**, 217–232.

Békésy, G. v., and W. A. Rosenblith. (1951) The mechanical properties of the ear. Chap. 27 in S. S. Stevens (Ed.), *Handbook of Experimental Pscyhology*. New York: Wiley.

Beranek, L. L. (1949) *Acoustic Measurements*. New York: Wiley.

Bloomer, H. (1942) A simple method for testing the hearing of small children. *J. Speech Disorders*, **7**, 311–312.

Bonvallet, G. L. (1950) Levels and spectra of transportation vehicle noise. *J. Acoust. Soc. Amer.*, **22**, 201–205.

Bordley, J. E., and W. G. Hardy. (1949) A study in objective audiometry with the use of a psychogalvanic response. *Ann. Otol., etc., St. Louis*, **58**, 751–759.

Bordley, J. E., W. G. Hardy, and C. P. Richter. (1948) Audiometry with the use of galvanic skin resistance response: a preliminary report. *Johns Hopk. Hosp. Bull.*, **82**, 569.

Boring, E. G. (1942) *Sensation and Perception in the History of Experimental Psychology*. New York: Appleton-Century-Crofts.

Breakey, M. R. (1948) *Inter-comparisons of Articulation Tests on Hard-of-hearing and Normal Hearing Subjects*. St. Louis, Mo.: Washington University, M.S. (Educ.) thesis.

Brogden, W. J., and G. A. Miller. (1947) Physiological noise generated under earphone cushions. *J. Acoust. Soc. Amer.*, **19**, 620–623.

Bronstein, A. J. (1936) Sensibilization of the auditory organ by acoustic stimuli. *Bull. Biol. Méd. exp., U.R.S.S.*, **1**, 274–275, 276–277, 347–349.

de Bruine-Altes, J. C. (1946) *The Symptom of Regression in Different Kinds of Deafness* (thesis). Groningen: J. B. Wolters.

Bunch, C. C. (1943) *Clinical Audiometry*. St. Louis: Mosby.

Burr, E. G., and H. Mortimer. (1939) Improvements in audiometry at Montreal General Hospital. *Canad. Med. Ass. J.*, **40**, 22–27.

Carhart, R. (1946a) Monitored live-voice as a test of auditory acuity. *J. Acoust. Soc. Amer.*, **17**, 339–349.

Carhart, R. (1946b) Speech reception in relation to pattern of pure tone loss. *J. Speech Disorders*, **11**, 97–108.

Carhart, R. (1950) Clinical application of bone conduction audiometry. *Arch. Otolaryng., Chicago*, **51**, 1–10.

Carhart, R., and C. Hayes. (1949) Clinical reliability of bone conduction audiometry. *Laryngoscope, St. Louis*, **59**, 1084–1101.

Caussé, R., and P. Chavasse (1941) Récherches sur le seuil de l'audition binauriculaire comparé au seuil monauriculaire en fonction de la fréquence. *C. R. Soc. Biol. Paris*, **135**, 1272–1275.

Caussé, R., and P. Chavasse (1942a) Différence entre le seuil de l'audition binauriculaire et le seuil monauriculaire en fonction de la fréquence. *C. R. Soc. Biol. Paris*, **136**, 301.

Caussé, R., and P. Chavasse (1942b) Différence entre l'écoute binauriculaire et monauriculaire pour la perception des intensités supraliminaires. *C. R. Soc. Biol. Paris*, **136**, 405.

Caussé, R., and P. Chavasse (1947) Études sur la fatigue auditive. *Année psychol.*, 1942–1943, **43–44**, 265–298.

Churcher, B. G., A. J. King, and H. Davies. (1934) The minimum perceptible change of intensity of a pure tone. *Phil. Magazine*, **18**, 927–939.

Coombs, C. H. (1938) Adaptation of the galvanic response to auditory stimuli. *J. Exp. Psychol.*, **22**, 244–268.

Davis, H. (1947) *Hearing and Deafness*. New York: Rinehart (formerly Murray Hill).

Davis, H. (1948) The articulation area and the social adequacy index for hearing. *Laryngoscope, St. Louis*, **58**, 761–778.

Davis, H., *et al.* (1946) The selection of hearing aids. *Laryngoscope, St. Louis*, **56**, 85–115 (Part I), 135–163 (Part II).

Davis, H., *et al.* (1947) *Hearing Aids; An Experimental Study of Design Objectives*. Cambridge, Mass.: Harvard University Press.

Davis, H., *et al.* (1950) Temporary deafness following exposure to loud tones and noise. *Acta oto-laryng., Stockh.*, Suppl. 88.

Denes, P., and R. E. Naunton. (1950) The clinical detection of auditory recruitment. *J. Laryng.*, **64**, 375–398.

Dishoeck, H. A. E. van, and J. L. van Gool. (1948) The detailed audiogram. *Arch. Otolaryng., Chicago*, **47**, 149–154.

Dix, M. R., and C. S. Hallpike. (1947) The peep-show: a new technique for pure-tone audiometry in young children. *Brit. Med. J.*, **2**, 719–731.

Dix, M. R., C. S. Hallpike, and J. D. Hood. (1948) Observations upon the loudness recruitment phenomenon with especial reference to the differential diagnosis of disorders of the internal ear and eighth nerve. *Proc. Roy. Soc. Med.*, **41**, 516–526.

Doerfler, L. G. (1948) Neurophysiological clues to auditory acuity. *J. Speech & Hearing Disorders*, **13**, 227–232.

Doerfler, L. G. and K. Stewart. (1946) Malingering and psychogenic deafness. *J. Speech Disorders*, **11**, 181–186.

Egan, J. P. (1948) Articulation testing methods. *Laryngoscope, St. Louis*, **58**, 955–991.

Egan, J. P., and H. W. Hake. (1950) On the masking pattern of a simple auditory stimulus. *J. Acoust. Soc. Amer.*, **22**, 622–630.

Ewing, I. R., and A. W. G. Ewing, (1944) The ascertainment of deafness in infancy and early childhood. *J. Laryng.*, **59**, 309–333.

Falconer, G. A., and H. Davis. (1947) The intelligibility of connected discourse as a test for the "threshold for speech." *Laryngoscope, St. Louis*, **57**, 581–595.

Finch, G., and E. Culler. (1934) Effects of protracted exposure to a loud tone. *Science*, **80**, 41–42.

Fletcher, H. (1929) *Speech and Hearing*. New York: Van Nostrand.

Fletcher, H. (1950) A method of calculating hearing loss for speech from an audiogram. *J. Acoust. Soc. Amer.*, **22**, 1–5.

Fletcher, H., and W. A. Munson. (1933) Loudness, its definition, measurement and calculation. *J. Acoust. Soc. Amer.*, **5**, 82–108.

Fletcher, H., and J. C. Steinberg. (1929) Articulation testing methods. *Bell System Tech. J.*, **8**, 806–854.

Fowler, E. P. (1928) Marked deafened areas in normal ears. *Arch. Otolaryng., Chicago*, **8**, 151–155.

Fowler, E. P. (1947) Tests for hearing. In E. P. Fowler, Jr. (Ed.), *Loose-leaf Medicine of the Ear*. New York: Nelson.

Fowler, E. P., Jr. (1949) Standard audiogram recording. *Acta oto-laryng., Stockh.*, Suppl. 78, 173–182.

French, N. R., and J. C. Steinberg. (1947) Factors governing the intelligibility of speech sounds. *J. Acoust. Soc. Amer.*, **19**, 90–119.

Froeschels, E. (1946) Testing the hearing of young children. *Arch. Otolaryng., Chicago*, **43**, 93–98.

Froeschels, E., and H. Beebe. (1946) Testing the hearing of newborn infants. *Arch. Otolaryng., Chicago*, **44**, 710–714.

Gardner, M. B. (1947a) Short duration auditory fatigue as a method of classifying hearing impairment. *J. Acoust. Soc. Amer.*, **19**, 178–190.

Gardner, M. B. (1947b) A pulse-tone clinical audiometer. *J. Acoust. Soc. Amer.*, **19**, 592–599.

Garner, W. R. (1947) Auditory thresholds of short tones as a function of repetition rates. *J. Acoust. Soc. Amer.*, **19**, 600–608.

Garner, W. R., and G. A. Miller. (1947) The masked threshold of pure tones as a function of duration. *J. Exp. Psychol.*, **37**, 293–303.

Garrett, H. E. (1951) *Great Experiments in Psychology* (3d ed.) New York: Century.

Goldstein, M. A. (1933) *Problems of the Deaf.* St. Louis: Laryngoscope Press.

Guilford, J. P. (1936) *Psychometric Methods.* New York: McGraw-Hill.

Haggard, E. A., and R. Gerbrands. (1947) An apparatus for the measurement of continuous changes in palmar skin resistance. *J. Exp. Psychol.,* **37,** 92–98.

Hallpike, C. S., and J. D. Hood. (1951) Some recent work on auditory adaptation and its relationship to the loudness recruitment phenomenon. *J. Acoust. Soc. Amer.,* **23,** 270–274.

Hardy, W. G. (1948) Special techniques for the diagnosis and treatment of psychogenic deafness. *Ann. Otol. etc., St. Louis,* **57,** 65–95.

Hardy, W. G., and J. E. Bordley. (1951) Special techniques in testing the hearing of children. *J. Speech & Hearing Disorders,* **16,** 123–131.

Harris, J. D. (1945) Group audiometry. *J. Acoust. Soc. Amer.,* **17,** 73–76.

Harris, J. D. (1946) Free voice and pure-tone audiometry for routine testing of auditory acuity. *Arch. Otolaryng., Chicago,* **44,** 452–467.

Harris, J. D. (1948a) Discrimination of pitch: suggestions toward method and procedure. *Amer. J. Psychol.,* **61,** 309–322.

Harris, J. D. (1948b) *Some Suggestions for Speech Reception Testing.* New London, Conn.: Naval Medical Research Laboratory, Report No. 2, Project NM-003-021.

Harris, J. D. (1950) *Studies in Short-duration Auditory Fatigue. II. The Effect of the Duration of the Stimulating Tone; III. The Effect of the Interval between Stimuli.* New London, Conn.: Naval Medical Research Laboratory, Report No. 168, **9,** 291–300.

Harris, J. D., and C. K. Myers. (1950) *Loudness Perception for Pure Tones and for Speech.* New London, Conn.: Naval Medical Research Laboratory, Report No. 156, **9,** 97–127.

Harris, J. D., A. I. Rawnsley, and P. A. Kelsey. (1950) *Studies in Short-duration Auditory Fatigue. I. Frequency Differences as a Function of Intensity.* New London, Conn.: Naval Medical Research Laboratory, Report No. 167, **9,** 278–290.

Hawkins, J. E., Jr., and S. S. Stevens. (1950) The masking of pure tones and of speech by white noise. *J. Acoust. Soc. Amer.,* **22,** 6–13.

Hilgard, E. M., and D. G. Marquis. (1940) *Conditioning and Learning.* New York: Appleton-Century-Crofts.

Hirsh, I. J. (1947) Clinical application of two Harvard auditory tests. *J. Speech Disorders,* **12,** 151–158.

Hirsh, I. J. (1948a) Binaural summation and interaural inhibition as a function of the level of masking noise. *Amer. J. Psychol.,* **61,** 205–213.

Hirsh, I. J. (1948b) The influence of interaural phase on interaural summation and inhibition. *J. Acoust. Soc. Amer.,* **20,** 536–544.

Hirsh, I. J. (1948c) Binaural summation—a century of investigation. *Psychol. Bull.,* **45,** 193–206.

Hirsh, I. J. (1950a) The relation between localization and intelligibility. *J. Acoust. Soc. Amer.,* **22,** 196–200.

Hirsh, I. J. (1950b) Binaural hearing aids: A review of some experiments. *J. Speech & Hearing Disorders*, **15**, 114–123.

Hirsh, I. J., and I. Pollack. (1948) The role of interaural phase in loudness. *J. Acoust. Soc. Amer.*, **20**, 761–766.

Hirsh, I. J., and W. D. Ward. (1952) Recovery of the auditory threshold after strong acoustic stimulation. *J. Acoust. Soc. Amer.*, **24**, 131–141.

Hirsh, I. J., and F. A. Webster. (1949) Some determinants of interaural phase effects. *J. Acoust. Soc. Amer.*, **21**, 496–501.

Hood, J. D. (1950) Studies in auditory fatigue and adaptation. *Acta oto-laryng., Stockh.*, Suppl. 92.

Hovland, C. I. (1937a) The generalization of conditioned responses: I. The sensory generalization of the conditioned responses with varying frequencies of tone. *J. Gen. Psychol.*, **17**, 235–248.

Hovland, C. I. (1937b) The generalization of conditioned responses. IV. The effects of varying the amounts of reinforcement upon the degree of generalization of conditioned responses. *J. Exp. Psychol.*, **21**, 261–276.

Hovland, C. I., and A. H. Riesen. (1940) Magnitude of galvanic and vasomotor response as a function of stimulus intensity. *J. Gen. Psychol.*, **23**, 103–121.

Hudgins, C. V. (1950) A progress report of an acoustic training experiment for profoundly deaf children. *J. Acoust. Soc. Amer.*, **22**, 675. (Abstract.)

Hudgins, C. V., et al. (1947) The development of recorded auditory tests for measuring hearing loss for speech. *Laryngoscope, St. Louis*, **57**, 57–89.

Huizing, H. C. (1942) Die Bestimmung der Regression bei der Gehörprüfung und der physikalische, physiologische und psychologische Zusammenhang bei der Gehörprothese. *Acta oto-laryng., Stockh.*, **30**, 487–499.

Huizing, H. C. (1948) The symptom of recruitment and intelligibility of speech. *Acta oto-laryng., Stockh.*, **36**, 346–355.

Huizing, H. C. (1949) The relation between auditory fatigue and recruitment. *Acta oto-laryng., Stockh.*, Suppl. 78, 169–172.

Johnson, A. M. (1913) Audition and habit formation in the dog. *Behavior Monogr.*, **2**, No. 3.

Johnston, P. W. (1948) The Massachusetts hearing test. *J. Acoust. Soc. Amer.*, **20**, 697–703.

Keaster, J. (1947) A quantitative method of testing the hearing of young children. *J. Speech Disorders*, **12**, 159–160.

Kelley, N. H., and S. N. Reger. (1937) The effect of binaural occlusion of the external auditory meati on the sensitivity of the normal ear for bone conducted sound. *J. Exp. Psychol.*, **21**, 211–217.

Keys, J. W. (1947) Binaural versus monaural hearing. *J. Acoust. Soc. Amer.*, **19**, 629–631.

Kinsler, L. E., and A. R. Frey. (1950) *Fundamentals of Acoustics*. New York: Wiley.

Knapp, P. H., and B. H. Gold. (1950) The galvanic skin response and diagnosis of hearing disorders. *Psychosom. Med.*, **12**, 6–22.

Knudsen, V. O. (1923) The sensibility of the ear to small differences in intensity and frequency. *Physic. Rev.*, **21**, 84–103.

Knudsen, V. O., and C. M. Harris. (1950) *Acoustical Designing in Architecture.* New York: Wiley.

Kobrak, H. G. (1948) The present status of objective hearing tests. *Ann. Otol. etc., St. Louis,* **57,** 1018–1026.

Kryter, K. D. (1946) Effects of ear protective devices on the intelligibility of speech in noise. *J. Acoust. Soc. Amer.,* **18,** 413–417.

Kryter, K. D. (1950) The effects of noise on man. *J. Speech & Hearing Disorders,* Suppl. 1.

Langenbeck, B. (1950a) Die Geräuschaudiometrie als diagnostische Methode. *Z. Laryngol. Rhinol. Otol.,* **29,** 103–121.

Langenbeck, B. (1950b) Die Geräuschaudiometrie als diagnostische Methode. II. Schwellennahe und schwellenferne Geräuschaudiogramme. *Z. Laryngol. Rhinol. Otol.,* **29,** 470–487.

Langenbeck, B. (1950c) Geräuschaudiometrische Diagnostik. Die Absolutauswertung. *Arch. Ohr. u. Z. Hals Heilkunde.,* **158,** 458–468.

Lemon, H. B., and M. Ference, Jr. (1946) *Analytical Experimental Physics* (rev. ed.). Chicago: University of Chicago Press.

Licklider, J. C. R. (1944) *The Effects of Amplitude Distortion upon the Intelligibility of Speech.* Cambridge, Mass.: Psycho-Acoustic Laboratory, OSRD Report No. 4217.

Licklider, J. C. R. (1946) The effects of amplitude distortion upon the intelligibility of speech. *J. Acoust. Soc. Amer.,* **18,** 429–434.

Licklider, J. C. R. (1948) The influence of interaural phase relations upon the masking of speech by white noise. *J. Acoust. Soc. Amer.,* **20,** 150–159.

Licklider, J. C. R. (1951) Basic correlates of the auditory stimulus. Chap. 25 in S. S. Stevens (Ed.), *Handbook of Experimental Psychology.* New York: Wiley.

Licklider, J. C. R., and G. A. Miller. The perception of speech. Chap. 26 in S. S. Stevens (Ed.), *Handbook of Experimental Psychology.* New York: Wiley.

Lowy, K. (1942) Cancellation of the electrical cochlear response with air- and bone-conducted sound. *J. Acoust. Soc. Amer.,* **14,** 156–158.

Lüscher, E., and J. Zwislocki (1947) The decay of sensation and the remainder of adaptation after short pure-tone impulses on the ear. *Acta oto-laryng., Stockh.,* **35,** 428–445.

Lüscher, E., and J. Zwislocki. (1948) Eine einfache Methode zur monauralen Bestimmung des Lautstärkeausgleiches. *Arch. Ohr.-, Nas.-, u. KehlkHeilk,* **155,** 323.

Lüscher, E., and J. Zwislocki. (1949a) A simple method for indirect monaural determination of the recruitment phenomenon (Difference Limen in intensity in different types of deafness). *Acta oto-laryng., Stockh.,* Suppl. 78, 156–168.

Lüscher, E., and J. Zwislocki. (1949b) Adaptation of the ear to sound stimuli. *J. Acoust. Soc. Amer.,* **21,** 135–139.

de Maré, G. (1937) Ein neues Phänomen in Ohr: Nachwirkende Verdeckung. (A new auditory phenomenon: after-effect masking.) *Skand. Arch. Physiol.,* **77,** 57–58.

de Maré, G. (1939) Audiometrische Untersuchungen über das Verhalten des normalen und schwerhörigen Ohres bei funktioneller Belastung, nebst Bemerkungen zur Theorie des Gehörs. *Acta oto-laryng., Stockh.,* Suppl. 31.

Martin, N. A. (1946) Psychogenic deafness. *Ann. Otol., etc., St. Louis*, **55**, 81–87.

Michels, M. W., and C. T. Randt. Galvanic skin response in the differential diagnosis of deafness. *Arch. Otolaryng., Chicago*, 1947, **45**, 302–311.

Miller, G. A. (1947a) The masking of speech. *Psychol. Bull.*, **44**, 105–129.

Miller, G. A. (1947b) Sensitivity to changes in the intensity of white noise and its relation to masking and loudness. *J. Acoust. Soc. Amer.*, **19**, 609–619.

Miller, G. A. (1951) *Language and Communication*. New York: McGraw-Hill.

Miller, G. A., and W. R. Garner. (1944) Effect of random presentation on the psychometric function: implications for a quantal theory of discrimination. *Amer. J. Psychol.*, **57**, 451–467.

Miller, G. A., G. Heise, and W. Lichten. (1951) The intelligibility of speech as a function of the context of the test materials. *J. Exp. Psychol.*, **41**, 329–335.

Miller, G. A., F. M. Wiener, and S. S. Stevens. (1946) *Transmission and Reception of Sounds under Combat Conditions.* Summary technical report of Division 17, National Defense Research Committee.

Montgomery, H. C. (1932) Do our ears grow old? *Bell. Lab. Rec.*, **10**, 311–313.

Morgan, C. T., and E. Stellar. (1950) *Physiological Psychology* (2d ed.) New York: McGraw-Hill.

Munson, W. A., and M. B. Gardner. (1950) Loudness patterns—a new approach. *J. Acoust. Soc. Amer.*, **22**, 177–190.

Munson, W. A., and F. M. Wiener. (1950) Sound measurements for psychophysical tests. *J. Acoust. Soc. Amer.*, **22**, 382–386.

Myers, C. K., and J. D. Harris. (1949) *The Inherent Stability of the Auditory Threshold.* New London, Conn.: Naval Medical Research Laboratory, Report No. 3.

Newhart, H., and S. N. Reger. (1945) Syllabus of audiometric procedures in the administration of a program for the conservation of hearing in school children. *Trans. Amer. Acad. Ophthal. Oto-laryng.*, Suppl. 49, p. 28.

Newman, E. B. (1933) The validity of the just noticeable difference as a unit of psychological magnitude. *Trans. Kans. Acad. Sci.*, **36**, 172–175.

Newman, E. B. (1948) Hearing. Chap. 14 in E. G. Boring, H. S. Langfeld, and H. P. Weld (Eds.), *Foundations of Psychology.* New York: Wiley.

Olson, H. F., and F. Massa. (1939) *Applied Acoustics* (2d ed.). Philadelphia: Blakiston.

Peyser, A. (1940) Zur Methodik einer otologischen Prophylaxis der industriellen Lärmschwerhörigkeit. *Acta oto-laryng., Stockh.*, **28**, 443–462.

Pohlman, A. G., and F. W. Kranz. (1924) Binaural minimum audition in a subject with ranges of deficient acuity. *Proc. Soc. Exp. Biol., N.Y.*, **21**, 335.

Pollack, I. (1948a) Monaural and binaural threshold sensitivity for tones and for white noise. *J. Acoust. Soc. Amer.*, **20**, 52–57.

Pollack, I. (1948b) The atonal interval. *J. Acoust. Soc. Amer.*, **20**, 146–149.

Pollack, I. (1949) Specification of sound pressure levels. *Amer. J. Psychol.*, **62**, 412–417.

Postman, L. J. (1946) The time-error in auditory perception. *Amer. J. Psychol.*, **59**, 193–219.

Postman, L. J., and J. P. Egan. (1949) *Experimental Psychology: An Introduction.* New York: Harper.

Potter, R. K., and G. E. Peterson. (1948) The representation of vowels and their movements. *J. Acoust. Soc. Amer.*, **20**, 528–535.

Potter, R. K., G. A. Kopp, and H. C. Green. (1947) *Visible Speech*. New York: Van Nostrand.

Reger, S. N. (1936) Differences in loudness response of the normal and hard-of-hearing ear at intensity levels slightly above the threshold. *Ann. Otol., etc., St. Louis*, **45**, 1029–1039.

Reger, S. N., and H. A. Newby. (1947) A group pure-tone hearing test. *J. Speech Disorders*, **12**, 61–66.

Richter, C. P., and F. P. Whelan. (1949) Description of a skin-galvanometer that gives a graphic record of activity in the sympathetic nervous system. *J. Neurosurg:*, **6**, 279–284.

Riesz, R. R. (1928) Differential intensity sensitivity of the ear for pure tones. *Physic. Rev.*, **31**, 867–875.

Rosenblith, W. A. (1942) Industrial noises and industrial deafness. *J. Acoust. Soc. Amer.*, **13**, 220–225.

Rosenblith, W. A., and G. A. Miller. (1949) The threshold for continuous and interrupted tones. *J. Acoust. Soc. Amer.*, **21**, 467 (Abstract).

Rudmose, H. W. (1950) Free-field thresholds *vs.* pressure thresholds at low frequencies. *J. Acoust. Soc. Amer.*, **22**, 674 (Abstract).

Rudmose, H. W., *et al.* (1948) Voice measurements with an audio spectrometer. *J. Acoust. Soc. Amer.*, **20**, 503–512.

Rüedi, L., and W. Furrer. (1946) Physics and physiology of acoustic trauma. *J. Acoust. Soc. Amer.*, **18**, 409–412.

Rüedi, L., and W. Furrer. (1947) *Das akustische Trauma*. Basel: Karger.

Sacia, C. F., and C. J. Beck. (1926) The power of fundamental speech sounds. *Bell System. Tech. J.*, **5**, 393–403.

Seashore, C. E. (1938) *Psychology of Music*. New York: McGraw-Hill.

Shaw, W. A. (1945) *Measurements of Insulation and Sensitivity of Service Headsets*. Cambridge, Mass.: Psycho-Acoustic Laboratory, OSRD Report No. 6113.

Shaw, W. A., E. B. Newman, and I. J. Hirsh. (1947) The difference between monaural and binaural thresholds. *J. Exp. Psychol.*, **37**, 229–242.

Shower, E. G., and R. Biddulph. (1931) Differential pitch sensitivity of the ear. *J. Acoust. Soc. Amer.*, **3**, 275–287.

Silverman, S. R., C. E. Harrison, and H. S. Lane. (1946) *Tolerance for Pure Tones and for Speech in Normal and Hard-of-hearing Ears*. St. Louis: Central Institute for the Deaf, OSRD Report 6303.

Sivian, L. J., and S. D. White. (1933) On minimum audible sound fields. *J. Acoust. Soc. Amer.*, **4**, 288–321.

Skinner, B. F. (1938) *The Behavior of Organisms*. New York: Appleton-Century-Crofts.

Skinner, B. F. (1950) Personal communication.

Smith, M. H., and J. C. R. Licklider. (1949) Statistical bias in comparisons of monaural and binaural thresholds: Binaural summation or supplementation. *Psychol. Bull.*, **46**, 278–284.

Steinberg, J. C., and M. B. Gardner. (1937) The dependence of hearing impairment on sound intensity. *J. Acoust. Soc. Amer.*, **9**, 11–23.

Steinberg, J. C., and M. B. Gardner. (1940) On the auditory significance of the term hearing loss. *J. Acoust. Soc. Amer.*, **11**, 270–277.

Steinberg, J. C., and W. A. Munson. (1936) Deviations in the loudness judgments of 100 people. *J. Acoust. Soc. Amer.*, **8**, 71–80.

Steinberg, J. C., H. C. Montgomery, and M. B. Gardner. (1940) Results of the World's Fair hearing tests. *J. Acoust. Soc. Amer.*, **12**, 290–301.

Stevens, S. S. (1934) The attributes of tones. *Proc. Nat. Acad. Sci., Wash.*, **20**, 457–459.

Stevens, S. S. (1948) Sensation and psychological measurement. Chap. 11 in E. G. Boring, H. S. Langfeld, and H. P. Weld (Eds.), *Foundations of Psychology*. New York: Wiley.

Stevens, S. S. (1951) Mathematics, measurement and psychophysics. Chap. 1 in S. S. Stevens (Ed.), *Handbook of Experimental Psychology*. New York: Wiley.

Stevens, S. S., and H. Davis. (1938) *Hearing: Its Psychology and Physiology*. New York: Wiley.

Stevens, S. S., and E. B. Newman. (1936) The localization of actual sources of sound. *Amer. J. Psychol.*, **48**, 297–306.

Stevens, S. S., J. Miller, and I. Truscott. (1946) The masking of speech by sine waves, square waves, and regular and modulated pulses. *J. Acoust. Soc. Amer.*, **18**, 418–424.

Stevens, S. S., C. T. Morgan, and J. Volkmann. (1941) Theory of the neural quantum in the discrimination of loudness and pitch. *Amer. J. Psychol.*, **54**, 315–335.

Thorndike, E. L. (1898). Animal intelligence. *Psychol. Rev.* Monogr. Suppls. II, No. 4 (whole No. 8).

Unger, M. (1939) Objective measurement of hearing. *Arch. Otolaryng., Chicago*, **29**, 621–623.

Utley, J. (1949) Suggestive procedures for determining auditory acuity in very young acoustically handicapped children. *Eye, Ear, Nose & Throat Monthly*, **228**, 590–595.

de Vries, H. (1948) The minimum audible energy. *Acta oto-laryng., Stockh.*, **36**, 230–235.

Waetzmann, E., and L. Keibs. (1936) Hörschwellenbestimmungen mit dem Thermophon und Messungen am Trommelfell. *Ann. Physik., Lpz.*, **26**, 141–144.

Wallach, H. (1939) On sound localization. *J. Acoust. Soc. Amer.*, **10**, 270–274.

Wallach, H., E. B. Newman, and M. R. Rosenzweig. (1949) The precedence effect in sound localization. *Amer. J. Psychol.*, **62**, 315–336.

Watson. L. A., and T. Tolan. (1949) *Hearing Tests and Hearing Instruments*. Baltimore: Williams & Wilkins.

Wegel, R. L. (1932) Physical data and physiology of excitation of the auditory nerve. *Ann. Otol., etc., St. Louis*, **41**, 740–779.

Wegel, R. L., and C. E. Lane. (1924) The auditory masking of one pure tone by another and its probable relation to the dynamics of the inner ear. *Physic. Rev.*, **23**, 266–285.

Wheeler, D. E. (1949) Detection of noise susceptible ears. *Laryngoscope, St. Louis*, **59**, 1328–1338.

Wiener, F. M., and D. A. Ross. (1946) The pressure distribution in the auditory canal in a progressive sound field. *J. Acoust. Soc. Amer.*, **18**, 401–408.

Wiener, F. M., *et al.* (1944) *Response Characteristics of Interphone Equipment*—IV. Cambridge, Mass: Electro-Acoustic Laboratory, Harvard University, OSRD Report No. 3105.

Wilson, W. H. (1943) Prevention of traumatic deafness: A preliminary report. *Arch. Otolaryng., Chicago*, **37**, 757–767.

Wilson, W. H. (1944) Prevention of traumatic deafness: further studies. *Arch. Otolaryng., Chicago*, **40**, 52–59.

Witting, E. G., and W. Hughson. (1940) Inherent accuracy of a series of repeated clinical audiograms. *Laryngoscope, St. Louis*, **50**, 259–269.

Wolfle, H. M. (1932) Conditioning as a function of the interval between the conditioned and the original stimulus. *J. Gen. Psychol.*, **7**, 80–103.

Wood, A. (1941) *Acoustics*. New York: Interscience Publishers.

Woodworth, R. S. (1938) *Experimental Psychology*. New York: Holt.

Yerkes, R. M., and S. Morgulis. (1909) The method of Pavlov in animal psychology. *Psychol. Bull.*, **6**, 257–273.

NAME INDEX

Page numbers in **boldface** type refer to entries in the Bibliography

SUBJECT INDEX

Page numbers in **boldface** type refer to definitions in the Glossary

A

Acoustic trauma (*see* Fatigue, auditory)
Acoustics, 18, **334**
Acuity, 89*n*., 188–189
Adaptation (*see* Fatigue, auditory)
Air conduction, 243, **334**
American Medical Association (AMA), 293–294
  Council on Physical Medicine and Rehabilitation, 72, 108, 284, 304–320
American Standards Association (ASA), 72, 108, 321–327
Ammeter, 42, 61
Ampere, 37, **334**
Amplifier, 53–54, 69–70, **334**
  hearing-aid, 80
Amplitude distortion, 64, 167, **334**
Articulation score, 132–133, **334**
  factors that determine, 133–142
Articulation vs. gain function, 133–135, 143, 146
Artificial ear, 91–92, **334**
Attenuator, 61, 70–71, **334**
Attributes, psychological, 203–207
  measurement of, 206–207
Audibility, threshold of, 343
  (*See also* Threshold, absolute)
Audiogram, 109–110, 283–287, **334**
  air-conduction, 283–286
  bone-conduction, 286–287
Audiometer, pure-tone, 71–74, 168, **335**
  Békésy, 115–116, 222, 286
  specification for, 304–313, 321–327
  use of, 110–114
  screening, specification for, 311–314

Audiometer, speech, 81–83
  specification for, 314–320
Audiometry, clinical, 89, 108–117, 276–301
  aims of, 277–281
  pulse-tone, 100, 114–115, 280–281
  speech, 143–153, 288–293
  live-voice, 82, 142, 289–291
  materials for (*see* Word lists)
Auditory training, evaluation of, 299–300
Aural harmonics, 167
Autonomic nervous system, 259, 269, 274

B

Beats, 167, 196, **335**
Bel, 58–59, **335**
Bell Telephone Laboratories, 114, 131, 229
Binaural hearing, 231–240, **335**
  and hearing aids, 240–241
  (*See also* Localization)
Bone conduction, 242–248, 253–254, **335**
  absolute vs. relative, 249–251
  by air, 246–248
  compression, 245–246
  inertia, 244–245
Bone-conduction tests (*see* Test, Rinne, Schwabach, Weber)
Bone-conduction vibrator, 249, 287

C

Calibration, earphone, 91–93
Capacitance, 46–48, 61, **335**
Capacitative reactance, 47–48, **335**

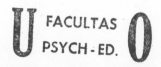